Handbook of Neonatal Infections
A Practical Guide

Commissioning Editor: Maria Khan
Project Editor: Rachel Robson
Project Supervisor: Mark Sanderson

Typeset by J&L Composition Ltd, Filey, North Yorkshire
Printed in China
NPCC/01

Handbook of Neonatal Infections
A Practical Guide

Professor David Isaacs

Department of Immunology and Infectious Diseases,
The New Children's Hospital,
Royal Alexandra Hospital for Children,
Parramatta, NSW, Australia

and

Professor E. Richard Moxon

Department of Paediatrics,
John Radcliffe Hospital,
Oxford, UK

W. B. SAUNDERS

London • Edinburgh • New York • Philadelphia • Sydney • Toronto

WB SAUNDERS A Division of Harcourt Brace and Company Limited
© Harcourt Brace and Company 1999. All rights reserved.

 is a registered trademark of Harcourt Brace and Company Limited

First published 1999

ISBN 0-7020-2477-5

British Library Cataloguing in Publication Data
A catalogue record for this book is available from the British Library

Library of Congress Cataloging in Publication Data
A catalog record for this book is available from the Library of Congress

Medical knowledge is constantly changing. As new information becomes
available, changes in treatment, procedures, equipment and the use of
drugs becomes necessary. The authors and Publishers have, as far as it is
possible, taken care to ensure that the information given in the text is
accurate and up to date. However, readers are strongly advised to
confirm that the information, especially with regard to drug usage,
complies with latest legislation and standards of practice.

The
Publisher's
policy is to use
**paper manufactured
from sustainable forests**

Contents

Preface

Remington and Klein's *Infectious Diseases of the Fetus and Newborn Infant* is one of the finest reference works in paediatrics. It is comprehensive and learned, a veritable fount of wisdom. A publisher once asked us, 'What is wrong with the book?' 'Nothing', we replied. 'If you were writing a book on neonatal infections, what would you do differently?' she asked. That is a different question and explains why we ever wrote a book on neonatal infections in the first place.

Remington and Klein does not fit in the pocket. It is not easy bedtime reading, and of course it never set out to be. It is a reference work. As practising paediatricians, as well as paediatric infectious disease specialists, we set out to write a highly practical book on neonatal infections. Our aim was to try to help practising and training neonatologists with the day-to-day decisions on care of babies with possible, probable or proven infections.

When is it best to start antibiotics? When should they be stopped? Which antibiotic should be used? How can infections be prevented? How should outbreaks be managed? How to cope with multi-resistant organisms? In 1991, we published a book *Neonatal Infections* (Oxford, Butterworth–Heinemann) which was an attempt at writing a practical, readable book on neonatal infections to complement, not to rival, Remington and Klein. We hope that a *Handbook of Neonatal Infections* will act as a handbook for ready reference but also a book to read about principles of preventing and managing neonatal infections.

We would like to acknowledge our discussions with colleagues and friends in Oxford (Andrew Wilkinson, Peter Hope, David Lindsell, Simon Dobson, Robert Booy, Paul Heath) and in Sydney (Heather Jeffery, Lyn Gilbert, David Henderson-Smart, Nick Evans, Phil Beeby, Peter Barr, Guan

Koh, Julian Wojtulewicz, Rob Halliday) which have helped form our ideas on neonatal infections. We would like to thank Jonathan Austyn and Katharine Wood of the University of Oxford for their excellent lectures which formed the basis for much of the chapter on immunity. The drawings were done by the Department of Medical Illustration, John Radcliffe Hospital, Oxford and by Kate Hilliger of the Medical Education Department, New Children's Hospital, Sydney. Pixie Maloney in Medical Photography, Sydney was a continual help. The secretarial work was done with enormous skill by Francine Sanhard, with help from Jennifer Cook.

Chapters were kindly reviewed by a large number of colleagues. In addition to those already mentioned, we would like to acknowledge with gratitude the contributions of Carole Baker and Morven Edwards in Houston, Texas, Amanda Ogilvy-Stuart in Oxford, Margaret Burgess, David Burgner, Jonathan Craig, Andrew Daley, Joanne Ging, Deborah Lewis, Maura McDonnell, David McIntosh, Jenny Royle and Melanie Wong in Sydney, David Brewster in Darwin, David Tudehope and James King in Brisbane, Tors Clothier in Alice Springs, Andrew Kemp in Melbourne, Ross Messer in Cairns, C.T. Lim, Jacquie Ho and Zabidi in Malaysia, Adedayo Kimiki in Papua New Guinea, and nursing staff in Oxford, Sydney and Mulago Hospital, Kampala, Uganda. Many of the above have helped collect surveillance data on neonatal infections, as have our colleagues in the Australasian Study Group for Neonatal Infections.

Finally, we would like to thank the medical students, junior doctors, nurses and paramedical staff whose dedication, energy and skill have helped to keep newborn babies alive and well, and whose questions have stimulated the contents of this book.

David Isaacs
E. Richard Moxon

Abbreviations

AAP	American Academy of Pediatrics
ADCC	antibody-dependent cellular cytotoxicity
ADH	antidiuretic hormone
AIDS	acquired immune deficiency syndrome
AZT	azidothymidine (zidovudine)
BCG	bacille Calmette-Guérin
CDC	Communicable Disease Centers
CIE	countercurrent immunoelectrophoresis
CMV	cytomegalovirus
CNS	central nervous system
CPAP	constant positive airway pressure
CRP	C-reactive protein
CSF	cerebrospinal fluid
CT	computed tomography
CTL	cytotoxic T lymphocyte
CVS	congenital varicella syndrome
DIC	disseminated intravascular coagulation/ coagulopathy
DNA	deoxyribonucleic acid
DTP	diphtheria, tetanus, pertussis
DTPA	diethylenetriamine penta-acetate
EBV	Epstein–Barr virus
EEG	electroencephalogram
ECG	electrocardiogram
ELISA	enzyme-linked immunosorbent assay
EPEC	enteropathogenic *Escherichia coli*
ESBL	extended-spectrum β-lactamase-producing Gram-negative
ESR	erythrocyte sedimentation rate
ETA	endotracheal (tube) aspirate

ETEC	enterotoxigenic *Escherichia coli*
FTA	fluorescent treponemal antibody
G-CSF	granulocyte colony-stimulating factor
G6PD	glucose-6-phosphate dehydrogenase
GBS	group B streptococcus
GFR	glomerular filtration rate
GI	gastrointestinal
GM-CSF	granulocyte–macrophage colony-stimulating factor
GMP	guanosine monophosphate
HBcAg	hepatitis B core antigen
HBeAg	hepatitis B e antigen
HBIg	hepatitis B immunoglobulin
HBsAg	hepatitis B surface antigen
HIV	human immunodeficiency virus
HLA	human leucocyte antigen
HSV	herpes simplex virus
HSVE	herpes simplex virus encephalitis
ICP	intracranial pressure
IDU	idoxuridine
IF	immunofluorescence
IFN	interferon
IgA	immunoglobulin A
IgG	immunoglobulin G
IgM	immunoglobulin M
IL	interleukin
i.m.	intramuscular
IMV	intermittent mandatory ventilation
IPPV	intermittent positive-pressure ventilation
i.v.	intravenous
IVDU	intravenous drug user
IVIG	intravenous immunoglobulin
IVH	intraventricular haemorrhage
IVP	intravenous pyelography
LSCS	lower segment caesarean section
LP	lumbar puncture

LPA	latex particle agglutination
MBC	minimum bactericidal concentration
MCU	micturating cysto-urethrography
MIC	minimum inhibitory concentration
MRSA	methicillin-resistant *Staphylococcus aureus*
NBT	nitro-blue tetrazolium
NEC	necrotizing enterocolitis
NK	natural killer
NPA	nasopharyngeal aspirate
OPV	oral polio vaccine
PaO_2	arterial partial pressure of oxygen
PCP	*Pneumocystis carinii* pneumonia
PCR	polymerase chain reaction
PRP	polyribosyl ribitol phosphate
PUJ	pelvi-ureteric junction
RBC	red blood cell
RDS	respiratory distress syndrome
RNA	ribonucleic acid
RSV	respiratory syncytial virus
SCBU	special care baby unit
SPA	suprapubic aspirate
TB	tuberculosis
THAM	tris-hydroxymethyl aminomethane
TMP-SMX	trimethoprim–sulphamethoxazole
TORCH	*Toxoplasma gondii*, rubella, cytomegalovirus, herpes simplex virus
TPHA	*Treponema pallidum* haemagglutinating antibody
TTN	transient tachypnoea of the newborn
UAC	umbilical arterial catheter
UTI	urinary tract infection
VA	ventriculoatrial
VDRL	Venereal Disease Research Laboratory
VLBW	very low birthweight
VP	ventriculoperitoneal
VUJ	vesico-ureteric junction

VUR	vesico-ureteric reflux
VZV	varicella-zoster virus
WBC	white blood cell
ZIG	zoster immune globulin

1 | Pathogenesis and epidemiology

PATHOGENESIS

The incidence of infection is higher in the neonatal period than at any other time in life, even if preterm babies are excluded. Some of the factors that determine this increased susceptibility to infection are summarized in Table 1.1. In addition to the immaturity of the immune system, which is discussed in detail in Chapter 2, there are several reasons why preterm babies are more susceptible to infection than term babies (Table 1.2). Many studies have shown that the incidence of infection increases with falling birthweight or gestation and that low birthweight is the single most important independent variable in predisposing to sepsis.

EARLY-ONSET SEPSIS

The fetus and newborn infant are exposed to infection in unique ways. The amniotic fluid is bacteriostatic or bactericidal for many organisms, with the exception of group B streptococci. Thus, despite the fact that the maternal genital tract and rectum are frequently colonized with potential pathogens, amnionitis is rare and most babies are not born infected.

Immaturity of the immune system
  Poor humoral response to organisms (IgG and IgA)
  Relatively poor neutrophil response
  Relatively poor complement activity
  Possibly impaired macrophage function
  Relatively poor T cell function
Exposure to microorganisms from the maternal genital tract
  Ascending infection via amniotic fluid
  Transplacental haematogenous spread
Exposure to viruses from mother without antibody
  Antenatal, e.g. rubella, CMV, HIV
  Viraemic spread, e.g. chickenpox
  Perinatal, e.g. herpes simplex virus, hepatitis B
Peripartum factors
  Trauma to skin, vessels, etc. during parturition
  Scalp electrodes and other invasive obstetric procedures
Portals of colonization and subsequent invasion
  Umbilicus
  Mucosal surfaces
  Eye
  Skin
Exposure to organisms postnatally: exposure in neonatal unit or lying-in wards to organisms from other babies
  Overcrowding
  Understaffing

Table 1.1 Reasons for increased susceptibility to infection in the neonatal period (term infants)

Nevertheless, amnionitis can occur. Sometimes this produces maternal symptoms or signs of frank chorioamnionitis with fever, a tender uterus and purulent, foul-smelling amniotic fluid. More commonly, however, amnionitis is asymptomatic and the amniotic fluid is not frankly purulent or even cloudy. There is good evidence that infection of the amniotic fluid can actually initiate preterm labour, possibly through the formation of bacterial products with prostaglandin-like activity.

The amniotic fluid is in continual contact with the fetal lungs *in utero* and, although the latter are collapsed, ascending infection causing pneumonia and secondary septicaemia is

Immunological
    Reduced transplacental transfer of maternal IgG
    Relative immaturity of all immune mechanisms
Exposure to microorganisms from maternal genital tract
    Preterm labour may be precipitated by infection (chorioamnionitis)
Invasive procedures
    Endotracheal tubes
    Intravascular catheters
    Chest drains
    Cerebrospinal fluid shunts
Increased postnatal exposure
    Organisms from other babies on neonatal unit
    Overcrowding and understaffing
Poor surface defences
    Skin thin, easily traumatized
Conditions predisposing to sepsis
    Prolonged artificial ventilation
    Intravenous feeding
    Necrotizing enterocolitis
Antibiotic pressures
    Resistant organisms
    Fungal infection

Table 1.2 Reasons for greater susceptibility to infection of preterm infants

probably the most important route of early-onset sepsis. Certainly, most babies with sepsis in the first 48 hours postnatally present with pneumonia as well as septicaemia.

Babies with group B streptococcal pneumonia are frequently septicaemic at delivery. This might suggest transplacental haematogenous spread from a maternal septicaemia, but there is little evidence to support this mechanism in most instances of early-onset sepsis. It is more likely that the bacteraemia occurs secondary to multiplication of organisms within the fetal lung.

Benirschke [1] proposed ascending infection as the major cause of early-onset sepsis. To examine this hypothesis he looked at infections occurring in twin pregnancies. Given that twins *in utero* can lie either horizontally or vertically,

Benirschke suggested that, if the twins were horizontal (the commonest position), twin one would be affected by ascending infection before twin two, whereas, if they were vertical, simultaneous infection was likely (see Figure 1.1). In the former case, twin one alone or both twins would be infected; in the latter case, both twins were likely to be infected. Of the 23 infected twin pregnancies that he studied, both twins were infected in 7 cases, twin one alone in 16, but in no case was twin two alone infected.

Although most early-onset sepsis is probably caused by ascending infection, there are exceptions. In infection with *Listeria monocytogenes*, transplacental haematogenous spread is probably the most important mechanism. A history of maternal flu-like illness with fever, often two or more weeks before delivery, is usual. Signs of neonatal infection are often present at birth, and the placenta often shows granulomata and inflammatory changes suggestive of placental infection. However, some babies with early-onset *Listeria* infection also have pneumonia, implying that both transplacental and ascending infection may occur simultaneously.

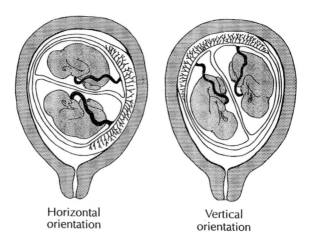

Horizontal
orientation

Vertical
orientation

Figure 1.1 Different intrauterine orientations

There is a clear distinction between the pathogenetic mechanisms causing early- and late-onset sepsis. We have conventionally used a cut-off point of age 48 hours to distinguish early from late sepsis. The rationale for using 48 hours is shown in Figure 1.2, which shows the organisms causing sepsis in 241 episodes affecting 234 babies in Australasian neonatal units over 2 years.

Some authorities have used 7 days as the cut-off between early and late sepsis: clearly, this will mean that 'early-onset' sepsis includes a number of babies with coagulase-negative staphylococcal infection. A cut-off of 5 days is reasonable, but the clearest distinction comes at 2 days. However, this does not mean that infection occurring in the first 48 hours after birth will not include occasional cases of nosocomial infection. Indeed, coagulase-negative staphylococcal and *Staphylococcus aureus* septicaemia may occur within 48 hours of birth.

Occasionally, early-onset sepsis occurs in babies delivered by caesarean section through intact membranes. Although rare, these infections suggest either that transplacental spread has

Organism	Cases	Meningitis	Deaths
Group B streptococcus	107	21	10
Escherichia coli	26	3	6
Listeria monocytogenes	6	1	1
Streptococcus pneumoniae	5	1	1
Staphylococcus aureus	4	1	0
Streptococcus viridans	3	0	0
Enterococci	3	0	0
Other Gram-negative	3	0	0
Haemophilus influenzae	2	0	1
Anaerobes	2	0	0
Total	161	27 (16.8%)	19 (11.8%)
Data from refs [16] and [20]			

Table 1.3 Organisms causing septicaemia or meningitis in the first 48 hours after birth, Australia, 1992–94

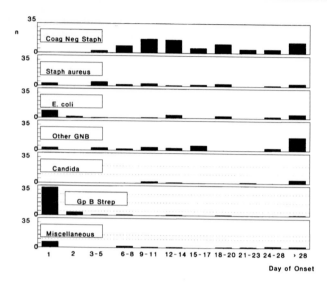

Figure 1.2 Timing of neonatal septicaemia or meningitis. Time of first positive culture in 234 babies with 241 episodes of systemic sepsis, Australasia, 1992–93 (Reproduced with permission from ref. [16].) [GNB = Gram negative bacilli]

occurred, or that bacteria can cross intact membranes to set up an amnionitis, or that colonization has occurred at operation and led to rapid spread of infection.

Skin trauma during delivery may provide a portal of entry for microorganisms. Instrumentation of the baby before delivery, for example with scalp electrodes, vacuum extraction or forceps, is particularly likely to damage the skin, and skin sepsis, osteomyelitis and disseminated sepsis may occur.

The well-documented maternal risk factors for early-onset sepsis are spontaneous preterm onset of labour (with or without membrane rupture), prolonged rupture of the membranes, and maternal fever [2]. Approximately 75% of all cases of early-onset sepsis are associated with one or more such risk factors; the remaining 25% of cases occur in term babies without recognized predisposing factors. Perinatal asphyxia has also been described as a risk factor for sepsis, but it is not clear whether this causes sepsis or is a sign of pre-existing sepsis. Gluck and colleagues [3] noted that 20% of babies with sepsis had severe respiratory depression at birth requiring artificial intubation. Risk factors for early-onset sepsis are considered further in Chapter 6.

Empirical antibiotic treatment of early-onset sepsis needs to cover primarily streptococcal and Gram-negative infections. At present, early-onset staphylococcal sepsis is rare enough that no authorities, to our knowledge, yet advocate the inclusion of a penicillinase-resistant penicillin in empirical therapy for early onset sepsis. Penicillin or ampicillin and an aminoglycoside provide excellent cover for almost all pathogens encountered.

LATE-ONSET SEPSIS

Early- and late-onset infections have a different pathogenesis. In early-onset infections (whether ascending or transplacental), sepsis occurs rapidly and babies are often systemically infected at delivery. In late-onset infections, in contrast, the organism first colonizes the baby and only later invades to cause sepsis. The most important sites colonized are the upper respiratory tract, conjuctivae, other mucosal surfaces, umbilicus and skin. Because the time interval between colonization and invasion will vary, it is clear that the distinction between early- and late-onset sepsis is an artificial one, based on the timing of onset of signs and symptoms of infection.

The organisms causing late-onset sepsis in Australasian neonatal units over a 1-year period, 1992–93, are shown in Table 1.4. As discussed by Gladstone *et al.* [4], there has been a change in the organisms predominantly causing late-onset sepsis in neonatal units in industrialized countries. Whereas *S. aureus*, β-haemolytic streptococci and, later, Gram-negative organisms used to predominate, there has been an increasing trend to infections with 'commensal species' such as coagu-lase-negative staphylococci and fungi. This reflects the greater survival of extremely low birthweight babies, who are at risk of sepsis with commensals because of their degree of immunological immaturity, the invasiveness and duration of the

Organism	n	Deaths due to sepsis	Deaths possibly due to sepsis	Meningitis
Coagulase-negative staphylococci	124	0	2	0
Staphylococcus aureus	25	3	0	3
Escherichia coli	20	2	1	4
Klebsiella species	9	2	1	1
Pseudomonas species	8	4	0	0
Candida species	7	1	1	2
Enterobacter species	5	3	0	0
Group B streptococcus	5	0	0	1
Anaerobes	5	2	0	1
Enterococci	4	0	0	0
Acinetobacter species	3	0	0	1
Serratia species	2	0	0	0
Others	3	0	0	0
Total	220	17 (7.7%)	5	13 (5.9%)

Table 1.4 Organisms causing 220 episodes of late-onset septicaemia or meningitis in 194 babies over 48 hours old in Australasian neonatal units, 1992–93

procedures needed to keep them alive, and the use of antibiotics and parenteral nutrition which favour selection of commensals.

The selection of empirical antibiotics for treating suspected late-onset sepsis will partly depend on local circumstances, such as the prevalence of resistant organisms. However, anti-staphylococcal antibiotics and Gram-negative cover are priorities: a penicillinase-resistant penicillin such as fluclo-xacillin or vancomycin is usual, combined with an aminoglyco-side or a third-generation cephalosporin. The merits of these combinations will be considered in detail in Chapter 6.

FACTORS PREDISPOSING TO SEPSIS

The organisms causing late-onset sepsis on a neonatal unit are evidently very different from those causing sepsis in term babies at home. The organisms causing sepsis in a neonatal intensive care unit are very similar to those in an adult intensive care unit: Gram-negative enteric bacilli and staphylococci pre-dominate. Neonates may become colonized with these organ-isms, as well as enterococci, group B streptococci and other organisms, at the time of delivery (sometimes called 'auto-infection'), but may also become colonized from other babies (hospital-acquired or nosocomial infection, from the Greek: *nosocomos* = hospital).

Neonatal units and, indeed, postnatal wards are often over-crowded and understaffed. Crowded wards [5,6] and increases in workload [7] have been shown to lead to increased spread of colonizing organisms and to an increase in the incidence of nosocomial infections.

Babies receiving intensive care are subjected to other inva-sive procedures. Intravascular cannulas, particularly if they remain in place for some time, are a potent source of infection. As might be expected, skin organisms such as *Staphylococcus epidermidis* and *S. aureus* are a common source of infection of these cannulas. *S. epidermidis,* an organism of relatively low virulence, adapts well to colonization of foreign bodies such as indwelling cannulas. It has the capacity to erode into, and gain sustenance from, the plastic cannulas and to secrete a protective 'slime' layer resulting in the formation of micro-colonies on the cannula.

Intravenous feeding is another risk factor for developing sepsis. Not only can the cannulas used for such feeding become infected, but the intravenous fluids themselves can provide a culture medium for microorganisms. If quality control is lax, i.v. fluids can readily become contaminated with organisms such as *S. epidermidis* and Enterobacteriaceae. Fat emulsions are also excellent growth media for fungi such as *Malassezia furfur*, and i.v. feeding is associated with an increased risk of systemic candidiasis.

One of the most important risk factors for late sepsis is prolonged endotracheal intubation for ventilatory support [6,8]. Humidified air provides an excellent growth medium for hydrophilic organisms such as Gram-negative bacilli, and the mucociliary clearance mechanisms are bypassed by the endotracheal tube. Routine suctioning of the endotracheal tube has been shown frequently to cause a transient bacteraemia [9] and, especially in the presence of vascular endothelial damage or an indwelling cannula, this may lead to sustained bacteraemia.

Necrotizing enterocolitis or lesser degrees of necrosis of the gut mucosa can provide a ready portal of entry for gut organisms such as Gram-negative bacilli and anaerobes. This subject is dealt with in detail in Chapter 13.

Because sepsis can be rapidly fatal and the signs of sepsis are non-specific, antibiotics are used liberally in neonatal units. This 'antibiotic pressure' may select for antibiotic-resistant organisms. Resistant organisms are not necessarily more virulent than other organisms: there is some evidence that amino-glycoside-resistant Gram-negative bacilli may be less virulent than sensitive ones [8,10]. Nevertheless, some methicillin-resistant *Staphylococcus aureus* (MRSA) seem to exhibit enhanced virulence and can cause serious outbreaks of systemic infection. The indiscriminate use of antibiotics also selects for colonization by, and infection with, fungi: the duration of prior antibiotic therapy for a baby is one of the most important risk factors for the development of systemic candidiasis.

PORTALS OF ENTRY

The umbilical cord is an important potential portal of entry of bacteria. In the 1950s, *Staphylococcus aureus* sepsis was widespread in the USA and UK. It was almost certainly no coincidence that these outbreaks resolved at the time that umbilical cord care (antisepsis), i.e. cleaning the umbilical stump with powerful antiseptics, became universal [11]. Whenever this lesson has been forgotten and umbilical cord care relaxed, outbreaks of impetigo and systemic staphylococcal sepsis tend to occur and remind us of the predilection of *S. aureus* for the umbilical stump, and of its ability to spread to the skin and thence to cause disseminated sepsis [12].

The skin of the newborn, and particularly that of preterm infants, is thin and susceptible to trauma, both during delivery and subsequently. Skin sepsis is common in the neonatal period, usually with *S. aureus*; skin abscesses in babies receiving intensive care may also be caused by Gram-negative bacilli, *Staphylococcus epidermidis* and fungi. Organisms may be inoculated directly into areas of traumatized skin or may be blood-borne and seed embolically. Neonatal conjunctivitis is common, possibly because immunoglobulin A (IgA) production in tears is poor. Conjunctivitis may be caused by organisms acquired in hospital, such as *S. aureus* and *Pseudomonas aeruginosa*, or during passage through an infected vaginal canal, such as *Chlamydia trachomatis* or *Neisseria gonorrhoeae*.

Urinary tract infections are rare, and when they do occur are often associated with structural abnormalities causing urinary stasis.

Ischaemic lesions of the gastrointestinal tract secondary to necrotizing enterocolitis, Hirschsprung's disease or other diseases causing bowel obstruction and/or vascular damage can lead to septicaemia due to the passage of organisms from the bowel flora (enteric bacilli, anaerobes) through the necrotic bowel wall.

VIRUS INFECTIONS

Virus infections are often more severe in the neonatal period than at any other time in life, including infections occurring in severely immunocompromised patients. Infections caused by enteroviruses, herpes simplex virus and varicella-zoster virus can be devastating and rapidly fatal. In all these examples, previous maternal infection protects the baby, by transplacental passage of maternal antibody; in contrast, peripartum primary maternal infection is associated with more severe disease, as there is a large inoculum of virus and little or no passively acquired antibody to protect the baby.

VIRULENCE

Thus far, we have concentrated on host factors in the pathogenesis of neonatal infection and have paid little attention to the organisms and their virulence. It is clear that the different patterns of sepsis seen with different organisms are, in part, attributable to the different propensity with which they colonize epithelial surfaces and invade the bloodstream and meninges to cause severe sepsis.

Some organisms cause meningitis in a high proportion of cases (e.g. group B streptococci and *Listeria*); others do so much more rarely (e.g. *Staphylococcus epidermidis*). Meningitis results from high-level bacteraemia and the causative organisms must multiply efficiently in the vascular spaces or seed the blood from extravascular sites in order to cause a sufficient bacteraemia to lead to meningitis. They must also cross the 'blood–brain barrier' and multiply in the meninges.

There may also be variation in virulence within strains. For example, group B streptococci can be subdivided into subtypes I, II and III. These are found with approximately equal frequency in the maternal vaginal tract and also cause early-onset sepsis, suggesting that, for early sepsis, environmental factors are as important as any particular interstrain variation in virulence. Late-onset group B streptococcal septicaemia and meningitis, however, is largely caused by subtype III organisms, implying that these are more pathogenic than the other subtypes.

Clones of group B streptococcus of high virulence have been identified in the United States and may explain the relatively high incidence of neonatal group B streptococcal infection in the USA, despite levels of maternal colonization comparable to those in other countries. Because newborns, particularly preterm infants, are immunologically immature, they may become infected with organisms of low virulence that normally cause only opportunist infections. A number of organisms that rarely cause serious disease in older children may cause neonatal septicaemia and even meningitis; examples are α-haemolytic streptococci, anaerobes and fungi.

INOCULUM EFFECT

Severity of disease is determined in part by the size of the inoculum of potentially pathogenic organisms. The inoculum size may help to explain the observation that 'vertical' infections caused by bacteria or viruses are generally far more severe than postnatally acquired infections with the same organisms. For example, early-onset group B streptococcal infection has a worse prognosis than the late-onset infection.

EPIDEMIOLOGY

INCIDENCE

The incidence of neonatal sepsis varies with a number of different factors, some of which are considered below. In the United States, the incidence of neonatal infection has varied from 1 to 8.1 per 1000 live births [13], although in one region the rate has remained fairly constant over many years at 2–4 cases per 1000 live births [4,14].

ORGANISMS

The organisms causing early-onset sepsis reflect the vaginal flora of pregnant women. The prevalent organisms may vary rapidly over time, and may be altered by external factors. In the UK, all pregnant women are screened for syphilis and gonorrhoea and treated if positive. As a consequence, neonatal infection with these organisms is very rare, but this is not the case in many other parts of the world. There may be marked geographical variations: maternal carriage of group B streptococci has approximately the same prevalence in the UK and USA, but neonatal group B streptococcal infection is 3 to 10 times more common in the USA than in the UK. There is evidence that particularly virulent clones of group B streptococci may circulate in the USA and be responsible for the increased rate of neonatal sepsis. There are also annual fluctuations in the incidence of neonatal group B streptococcal infection in the same institution that are not easily explicable.

The organisms causing early-onset sepsis in the UK [15] are remarkably similar to those in Australia (Table 1.3, Figure 1.2) and in the United States [4]. Group B streptococcus predominates, followed by *Escherichia coli* and then miscellaneous Gram-positive and Gram-negative organisms.

The organisms causing infection in the first 24–48 hours after birth are distinctly different from those causing sepsis after 48 hours of age (Figure 1.2). Late-onset infections, as already emphasized, can result from invasion of organisms colonizing the maternal genital tract or from the environment and it has been noted that the organisms colonizing babies and causing sepsis on a neonatal unit may change with time, for no apparent reason. In Oxford, although no deliberate attempts were made to eliminate any particular organisms, nor alter antibiotic policy significantly over the 5 years 1984–89, there were none the less marked fluctuations in the organisms causing sepsis from year to year (see Figure 1.3). In 1984–85, *Pseudomonas aeroginosa* predominated, to be succeeded by enterococci and *Klebsiella oxytoca* in 1985–87. No babies colonized with *Pseudomonas* were detected from 1986 to 1988. Over the years 1986–89 *Staphylococcus epidermidis* became the major pathogen causing septicaemia; less than one-half of these cases were associated with infected intravascular cannulas.

Despite these variations, the annual total number of cases of late-onset sepsis remained constant, as if babies were

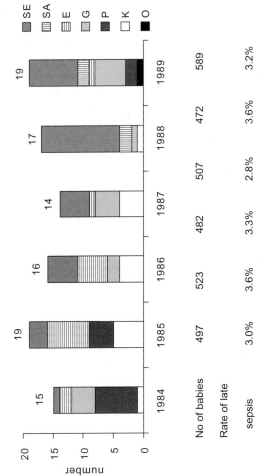

Figure 1.3 Organisms causing late-onset septicaemia or meningitis, John Radcliffe Hospital, Oxford, 1984-89. SE, *Staphylococcus epidermidis*; SA, *Staphylococcus aureus*; E, enterococci; G, Gram-negative bacilli; P, *Pseudomonas*; K, *Klebsiella*; O, other

predestined by their degree of immunocompromise to develop sepsis with whichever organisms colonized them.

A corollary is that it may be preferable to be colonized with a relatively benign organism, such as *S. epidermidis*, rather than more virulent Gram-negative organisms. Indeed, in the USA in the 1960s, deliberate attempts were made to colonize babies with benign strains of *S. aureus*, in order to compete with more virulent strains of *S. aureus* causing nursery outbreaks. Such 'neonatal germ warfare' may be needed again in future, for example if multiresistant organisms become a particular problem.

GEOGRAPHICAL

The major geographical variations in organisms causing sepsis largely reflect differences between industrialized and non-industrialized countries. The organisms causing sepsis, of both early and late onset, in Australia, North America and the UK are very similar [15,16].

Group B streptococcus (GBS) has been an uncommon cause of early-onset sepsis in non-industrialized countries. However, Malaysia, which is becoming increasingly industrialized, now has the same rate of early-onset GBS sepsis as the UK [17], whereas historically in Malaysia most early-onset infections have been with Gram-negative enteric bacilli [18].

Listeria causes a significant proportion of all early-onset infections in France, Germany and Switzerland, although these infections may occur mainly in epidemics; however, it is a relatively uncommon cause of sepsis in the UK, North America and Australia [19]. This may be because maternal listeriosis is associated with diet, e.g. the consumption of soft cheeses.

The organisms causing late-onset infections in babies on neonatal units largely reflect the prevailing intensive care flora, although there has been a major change in recent years in industrialized countries from Gram-negative enteric bacilli to coagulase-negative staphylococci causing the majority of episodes of late sepsis. In contrast, in non-industrialized countries with little or no access to intensive care, Gram-negative enteric bacilli have persisted as the major late-onset pathogens. Some pathogens causing frequent infections in developing countries, such as *E. coli* and *Klebsiella* species, are also found in industrialized countries. Others, such as *Salmonella* species, are almost exclusive to non-industrialized countries.

Neonatal tetanus is one of the major killers of babies worldwide: in non-industrialized countries this is commonly caused by the application of mud, ghee or other contaminated materials to the umbilical stump, compounded by the low level of tetanus immunization of mothers.

There are also regional differences within countries and sometimes between hospitals which are geographically close. Such differences may be due to identifiable environmental factors such as hygiene or antibiotic pressures, but often the cause remains obscure.

RACE AND SOCIO-ECONOMIC STATUS

It is not easy to tease out the relative importance of race and socio-economic status. The rate of early-onset group B streptococcal sepsis in Australian Aborigines is 5.2 per 1000 live births, over three times the rate in non-Aborigines [20]. However, the rate of many other infections is also high in Aborigines and this is due to poverty, it is believed, rather than to racial characteristics.

Similar considerations apply to other racial groups. For example, black American infants dying within 48 hours of birth had a significantly higher rate of pneumonia than white infants (28% versus 11%) in one study [21] and than either Puerto Rican or white infants in another study (38%, 22%, 20% respectively) [22]. The latter study also showed an inverse relationship between the incidence of pneumonia and household income.

AGE AND BIRTHWEIGHT

Gestational age is one of the most important factors in determining the incidence of sepsis. There is an inverse correlation between gestational age or birthweight and the incidence of group B streptococcal sepsis [2], suggesting that this is an important determinant in early-onset sepsis. In several studies, late-onset sepsis has been shown to display a similar relationship (see Table 1.5). The risk of both early- and late-onset sepsis increases markedly in very preterm babies, particularly those weighing less than 1000 g at birth.

In a sample of Australasian neonatal units, wide variations in rates of late-onset sepsis were found when numbers of episodes of sepsis were compared as a proportion of numbers of admissions or as a proportion of baby-days [23]. However, when babies were stratified by birthweight, the differences between the units disappeared: the rate of late-onset sepsis for any given birthweight was identical between each of six units (Table 1.5). No difference in rates of late-onset sepsis between term babies and those weighing between 2000 and 2499 g was found (Table 1.5), but there was a >20-fold increase in babies <1000 g at birth. Systemic candidiasis is rare, except in babies of very low birthweight (<1500 g).

The effects of postnatal age are less clear-cut, but in general the incidence of infection decreases with increasing postnatal age. This is because early-onset and late-onset infections relate to the special conditions of exposure already outlined, and because of increasing immunological maturity with age. Nevertheless, the risk of sepsis remains high for very preterm infants, particularly those requiring long-term respiratory support and intravenous feeding.

SEX

Early-onset sepsis affects both sexes equally, implying that overwhelming exposure is a more important determinant than host factors in the pathogenesis of early-onset sepsis. In late-onset sepsis, when host factors might be expected to be more important, boys are more susceptible in almost all studies, and may have more than twice the incidence.

Hospital	No. of babies with late sepsis/No. of babies admitted to neonatal unit					
	<999 g (%)	1000–1499 g (%)	1500–1999 g (%)	2000–2499 g (%)	≥2500 g (%)	Total (%)*
Adelaide	12/37 (32.4)	8/68 (11.8)	3/113 (2.7)	1/150 (0.7)	2/267 (0.7)	26/635 (4.1)
Brisbane	12/80 (15.0)	11/124 (8.9)	0/188	2/255 (0.8)	3/531 (0.6)	28/1178 (2.4)
Christchurch	7/25 (28.0)	7/48 (14.6)	3/90 (3.3)	1/87 (1.1)	6/287 (2.1)	24/537 (4.5)
Melbourne	7/47 (14.9)	6/76 (7.9)	3/134 (2.2)	1/151 (0.7)	5/487 (1.0)	22/895 (2.5)
Perth	20/81 (24.7)	16/143 (11.2)	4/213 (1.9)	1/291 (0.3)	1/768 (0.1)	42/1496 (2.8)
Sydney	12/40 (30.0)	11/104 (10.6)	2/129 (1.6)	0/141	0/559	25/973 (2.6)
Total	70/310 (22.6)	59/563 (10.5)	15/867 (1.7)	6/1075 (0.6)	17/2899 (0.6)	165/5714 (2.9)

Data from ref. [23].
*χ^2 = 7.06, 5 d.f. P>0.1.

Table 1.5 Proportion of babies developing late-onset sepsis by birthweight in tertiary neonatal units attached to maternity hospitals in Australia and New Zealand, 1992–93

MULTIPLE PREGNANCIES

Preterm twins are at greater risk (nearly five times) of group B streptococcal infection than preterm singletons [24], and the first-born twin is at greater risk of early-onset infection than the second [1].

MORTALITY AND MORBIDITY

Many factors influence mortality and morbidity from bacterial infections. One of the most important is whether infection is due to early-onset (ascending or transplacental) or late-onset (hospital-acquired) infection. Although there has been a general improvement in the mortality rate from early-onset sepsis, this nevertheless remains as high as 25–50% in many centres. In Oxford over the 5 years from 1984 to 1989, the mortality rate from early-onset sepsis was 28%. In contrast, the mortality rate from late-onset bacterial sepsis was considerably lower: in Oxford, only 3 of 77 episodes (4%) were responsible for babies' deaths over the same period. In Australian studies, the mortality rate from early-onset sepsis was 15% in 1993 and 10% in 1994, whereas that from late-onset sepsis was 9% and 8% respectively [16, 23].

Mortality from early-onset sepsis increases with falling birthweight in Australia, with a mortality rate of 2% for babies over 2500 g at birth, compared with 37.5% for those under 1000 g [23]. In contrast, the mortality rate from late-onset sepsis did not vary significantly with birthweight or gestational age; this somewhat surprising finding may be due to selection bias in that the neonatal units selected for this study were almost all tertiary referral centres. Such selection bias would also explain the relatively high mortality rate from late-onset sepsis; in other studies it is around 5% [13].

In a study from the USA, Naeye estimated that amniotic fluid infection was responsible for 17% of perinatal deaths, of which about two-thirds were neonatal deaths [25]. A far more conservative definition of perinatal infection led Edouard and Alberman to attribute only 1.3–1.8% of perinatal deaths in the UK from 1966 to 1978 to infection [26].

There may be considerable morbidity not just from bacterial meningitis but from pneumonia, which may contribute to chronic lung disease, and from other infections. Furthermore, viral and parasitic infections may be severe, particularly congenital infections acquired early in gestation and those acquired around delivery.

SUMMARY

- The incidence of infection is higher in the neonatal period than at any other time in life.
- Early-onset sepsis is usually due to ascending infection from organisms colonizing the maternal genital tract or rectum and causes pneumonia; transplacental haematogenous spread is less common.
- Late-onset sepsis is caused by organisms acquired perinatally or by those acquired nosocomially, often through invasive procedures.
- The incidence of sepsis is inversely proportional to birthweight or gestational age at birth.
- Low birthweight is the most important factor predisposing to sepsis.
- Over 20% of babies with birthweight under 1000 g, but less than 1% with birthweight over 2000 g on neonatal units, develop late-onset sepsis.
- The mortality rate of late-onset sepsis is inversely related to birthweight.
- The mortality rate from early-onset sepsis (10–30%) is higher than that from late-onset sepsis (5–10%).

References

1 Benirschke K. Routes and types of infection in the fetus and newborn. *Am J Dis Child* 1960; **99**: 714–21.
2 Boyer KM, Gadzala CA, Burd LI *et al.* Selective intrapartum chemoprophylaxis of group B streptococcal early-onset disease. I. Epidemiologic rationale. *J Infect Dis* 1983; **148**: 795–801.

3 Gluck L, Wood HF & Fousek MD. Septicemia of the newborn. *Pediatr Clin North Am* 1966; **13**: 1131–48.

4 Gladstone IM, Ehrenkranz RA, Edberg SC & Battimore RS. A ten-year review of neonatal sepsis and comparison with the previous fifty-year experience. *Pediatr Infect Dis J* 1990; **9**: 819–25.

5 Goldmann DA, Leclair J & Macone A. Bacterial colonization of neonates admitted to an intensive care unit. *J Pediatr* 1978; **69**: 193–7.

6 Goldmann DA, Durbin WA & Freeman J. Nosocomial infections in a neonatal intensive care unit. *J Infect Dis* 1981; **144**: 449–59.

7 Isaacs D, Catterson J, Hope PL *et al.* Factors influencing colonisation with gentamicin resistant Gram negative organisms in the neonatal unit. *Arch Dis Child* 1988; **63**: 533–5.

8 Isaacs D, Wilkinson AR & Moxon ER. Surveillance of colonisation and late-onset septicaemia in neonates. *J Hosp Infect* 1987; **10**: 114–19.

9 Storm W. Transient bacteremia following endotracheal suctioning in ventilated newborns. *Pediatrics* 1980; **65**: 487–90.

10 White RD, Townsend TR, Stephens MA & Moxon ER. Are surveillance of resistant enteric bacilli and antimicrobial usage among neonates in a newborn intensive care unit useful? *Pediatrics* 1981; **68**: 1–4.

11 Johnson JD, Malachowski NC, Vosti KL & Sunshine P. A sequential study of various modes of skin and umbilical care and the incidence of staphylococcal colonization and infection in the neonate. *Pediatrics* 1976; **58**: 354–61.

12 Verber IG & Pagan FS. What cord care – if any? *Arch Dis Child* 1993; **68**: 594–6.

13 Klein JO & Marcy SM. Bacterial sepsis and meningitis. In: Remington JS & Klein JO (eds) *Infectious Diseases of the Fetus and Newborn Infant*, 4th edn. Philadelphia: WB Saunders, 1995: 835–90.

14 Freedman RM, Ingram DL, Gross I *et al.* A half century of neonatal sepsis at Yale. *Am J Dis Child* 1981; **135**: 140–4.

15 Isaacs D & Moxon ER. *Neonatal Infections*. Oxford: Butterworth-Heinemann, 1991.

16 Isaacs D, Barfield C, Grimwood K *et al.* Systemic bacterial and fungal infections in infants in Australian neonatal units. *Med J Aust* 1995; **162**: 198–201.

17 Beng LH & Ho J. Neonatal group B streptococcal infection in a Malaysian general hospital. *Malay J Child Health* 1995; **7**: 32–7.

18 Lim NL, Chor CY, Wong YH, Boo NY & Kasin MS. Bacteraemic infection in a neonatal intensive care unit. A 9 month survery. *Med J Malaysia* 1995; **50**: 52–8.

19 Gellin BG & Broome CV. Listeriosis. *JAMA* 1989; **261**: 1313–20.
20 Australasian Study Group for Neonatal Infections (ASGNI). Early-onset group B streptococcal infections in Aboriginal and non-Aboriginal infants. *Med J Aust* 1995; **163**: 302–6.
21 Fujikura T & Froehlich LA. Intrauterine pneumonia in relation to birth, weight and race. *Am J Obstet Gynecol* 1967; **97**: 81–4.
22 Naeye RL, Dellinger WS & Blanc WA. Fetal and maternal features of antenatal bacterial infections. *J Pediatr* 1971; **79**: 733–9.
23 Isaacs D, Barfield C, Clothier T *et al*. Late onset infections of infants in neonatal units. *J Paediatr Child Health* 1996; **32**: 158–61.
24 Pass MA, Khare S & Dillon HC Jr. Twin pregnancies: incidence of group B streptococcal colonization and disease. *J Pediatr* 1980; **97**: 635–7.
25 Naeye RL. Causes of perinatal morbidity in the US Collaborative Perinatal Project. *JAMA* 1977; **238**: 228–9.
26 Edouard L & Alberman E. National trends in the certified causes of perinatal mortality, 1966 to 1978. *Br J Obstet Gynaecol* 1980; **87**: 833–8.

2 | Immunity

INTRODUCTION

Infection is more common in the neonatal period than at any other time in life. This is partly attributable to exposure to large numbers of organisms, but is also due to a relative failure of the neonatal host defences to clear microorganisms from blood and tissues. The 'immune deficiency' of newborn infants is relative rather than absolute: babies rarely become infected with opportunistic organisms such as *Pneumocystis carinii* unless their immunity is further compromised. Systemic fungal infections occur almost exclusively in low birthweight babies who are further compromised by parenteral nutrition through central venous cannulas and by receiving broad-spectrum antibiotics for long periods (see Chapter 15). Most neonatal infections are caused by organisms that are also capable of causing infection in older children and adults, but neonatal infection is usually more severe and more likely to disseminate and be fatal.

The basis of the defective immunity in the newborn period can be illustrated by considering the mechanisms involved in protection against infection. Invading microorganisms may be thought of as predominantly extracellular or intracellular (Table 2.1). This convenient oversimplification allows us to examine adult host defence mechanisms and the ways in which the newborn is relatively poor in overcoming infection.

Extracellular organisms are mainly bacteria, both Gram-positive bacteria such as group B streptococci and staphylococci, and Gram-negative organisms such as *Escherichia coli*. These organisms are predominantly cleared by phagocytosis by polymorphonuclear leukocytes (neutrophils or granulocytes). Phagocytosis is enhanced if the surface of the organism is altered by being coated with antibody and complement (opsonization).

Once infection is established within cells, intracellular organisms such as *Listeria*, *Salmonella*, *Mycobacterium tuberculosis*, viruses and parasites are protected from antibodies, complement and neutrophil phagocytosis. In these circumstances other host defence mechanisms, which rely on recognition of infected cells as well as of infecting organisms, are required. Cells of the macrophage/monocyte lineage are the most important phagocytic cells in combating intracellular infection. Natural killer cells recognize and destroy infected cells non-specifically, whereas recognition of infected cells by thymus-derived (T) lymphocytes is an antigen-specific, immune mechanism. Macrophages/monocytes interact with T lymphocytes, which themselves produce soluble proteins

Mechanism	Extracellular organisms	Intracellular organisms
Non-immune	Neutrophils Complement	Natural killer cells Macrophage/monocyte
Immune	B lymphocytes Antibody	T lymphocytes Cytotoxicity Delayed-type hypersensitivity Memory

Table 2.1 Different host defence mechanisms predominantly employed in response to extracellular and intracellular microorganisms

(lymphokines) that enhance the activity of macrophages/monocytes and natural killer cells. Thus there is interaction between cells, resulting in amplification of the immune response to intracellular organisms.

In this chapter, we deal first with immune (antigen-specific) and non-immune host cellular defences against invading microorganisms and the extent to which such cellular defences are immature or defective in the neonatal period. We then illustrate the neonatal response to infection with different groups of organisms.

ANTIGEN-SPECIFIC IMMUNE RESPONSES

ANTIBODY PRODUCTION

Antibody molecules share certain structural features (see Figure 2.1). Their main role is to coat the surface of microorganisms and alter the surface structure (opsonize them), rendering the

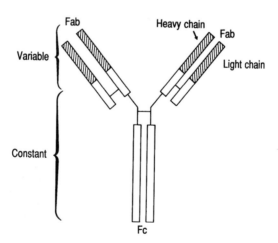

Figure 2.1 Antibody molecule. There are two antigen-binding sites (Fab) with variable regions (shaded) allowing different specificities of antigen recognition. The Fc region is constant, allowing recognition by cell receptors

organisms more susceptible to phagocytosis. This process is particularly important in recovery from infections caused by extracellular organisms. Although antibody may be important in preventing infection and reinfection with intracellular organisms, it is less important in recovery from acute infection due to these organisms.

Antibodies are produced by plasma cells derived from B lymphocytes or B cells, lymphocytes which have immunoglobulins on their surface. The 'B' stands for the bursa of Fabricius, the organ in birds in which such cells develop. The equivalent human fetal organ is the liver, and B cells bearing surface immunoglobulin appear in the fetal liver from about 8 weeks' gestation.

B cells differentiate into plasma cells with the assistance of cells called helper T lymphocytes or T helper (Th) cells, which express the CD4 antigen (formerly called OKT4) on their surface.

B cells will respond to unaltered or 'native' antigens and do not require antigens to be 'processed' by other cells (see below) in order to recognize them. B cells secrete five different classes of immunoglobulin (G, A, M, D or E), according to which heavy chain (see Figure 2.1) is incorporated into the immunoglobulin (Ig) molecule.

Immunoglobulin G (IgG)

The human newborn initially produces relatively little IgG compared with older children and adults, and IgG levels remain low until 4–6 months postnatally (Figure 2.2). This is frequently forgotten when trying to diagnose viral infections: it is not useful to look for a rise in IgG titre in the neonatal period.

Fetal and neonatal IgG are acquired transplacentally from the mother. Placental transfer occurs in two ways, passively and actively. Passive transfer of IgG increases progressively from about 17 weeks' gestation and most IgG transfer occurs in the last trimester. By 30 weeks' gestation, the fetal serum IgG level is about half that at full term. The active, enzymatic transfer is primarily a regulatory mechanism allowing compensation for abnormally high or low levels of maternal IgG [1]. Levels

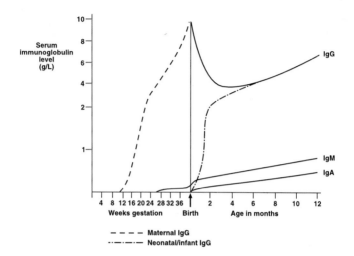

Figure 2.2 Changes in serum immunoglobulin levels in the fetus and infant over time

of IgG in the full-term newborn are equal to or even slightly greater than adult levels. The proportions of IgG subclasses in the newborn are the same as in the mother (IgG1, 70%; IgG2, 20%; IgG3, 7%; IgG4, 3%). IgG2, produced primarily in response to polysaccharides, has the shortest half-life, and newborns and infants mount a poor antibody response to polysaccharide antigens, such as the outer capsule of capsulated organisms like group B streptococcus, *E. coli* K1 and *Streptococcus pneumoniae*.

Immunoglobulin A (IgA)

The newborn is also poor at producing IgA, the antibody present on mucosal surfaces which is important in protection against respiratory and gastrointestinal pathogens. Furthermore, IgA does not cross the placenta. There are two forms of IgA: serum IgA and secretory IgA. Serum IgA is virtually absent at birth and adult levels are not achieved until about 10 years of age. Secretory IgA, however, appears soon after birth and reaches adult levels by 3–6 months of age [2]. Produced in exocrine gland secretions, it is a dimeric molecule composed of two IgA molecules joined by a J (joining) chain and a secretory component (see Figure 2.3). Plasma cells in the gland produce IgA and J chain, whereas epithelial cells contribute the secretory component. Secretory IgA is not found in tears until 10–20 days after birth, which may partly explain the propensity of neonates to conjunctivitis. Secretory cells do not appear in the intestinal mucosa until about 4 weeks postnatally, but colostrum and breast milk do contain secretory IgA, so that the incidence of respiratory and gastrointestinal infections is lower in breastfed infants. The protective effect of IgA is an important reason for early introduction of enteral feeds with breast milk for preterm babies.

Immunoglobulin M (IgM)

IgM is a single molecule at the cell surface, but when secreted it can form a pentameric structure in the serum, in conjunction with the same joining J chain as appears in secretory IgA (see Figure 2.4). Because each IgM molecule has two antigen-

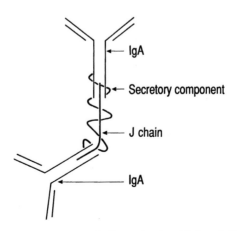

Figure 2.3 Secretory IgA molecule. Two molecules of IgA are held together by a joining (J) chain and secretory component to form a dimer

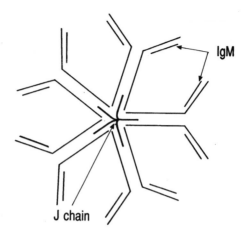

Figure 2.4 IgM molecule. Pentameric structure of IgM in serum with five antibody molecules joined by J chain

binding sites (Fab), each pentamer has 10 binding sites. IgM binds to antigen, forming a lattice structure. It is more effective than IgG in binding to endotoxin from Gram-negative organisms, and is the only immunoglobulin other than IgG to bind and activate complement. IgM has a major role in recovery from Gram-negative sepsis and it has been found that IgM-enriched intravenous immunoglobulin is more effective than normal immunoglobulin in treating neonatal sepsis [3].

The fetus can produce IgM from about 30 weeks' gestation. As this immunoglobulin does not cross the placenta, the detection of IgM specific to a given organism, e.g. rubella, in cord blood indicates congenital infection. Babies born before 30 weeks' gestation are at increased risk of infection because transplacental passage of maternal IgG is relatively poor and IgM production occurs at only a low level.

Immunoglobulin D (IgD)

The role of IgD is uncertain and it is found in only low levels in serum. There is evidence that IgD can cross the placenta and can activate the classical pathway of complement.

Immunoglobulin E (IgE)

IgE does not cross the placenta and very little is produced in the neonatal period. Some workers have found that cord blood IgE levels correlate with the subsequent development of symptomatic atopy, but absolute levels are too low to be of useful predictive value [4]. It has been suggested that IgE specific to respiratory syncytial virus (RSV) may appear in the nasopharynx of infected babies and its persistence may contribute to recurrent wheezing [5].

ANTIGEN PRESENTATION

T lymphocytes do not recognize antigens unless they are first 'processed' and presented on the surface of antigen-presenting cells. The latter are phagocytic cells which ingest the microorganism and process it by degrading its proteins to small peptides which are transported to, and presented on, the cell surface. Almost any cell can be an antigen-presenting cell but the most important are probably macrophages and monocytes. Macrophages possess receptors to the Fc portion of the antibody molecule which allow them to associate with organisms coated with antibody (see Figure 2.5). Macrophage complement

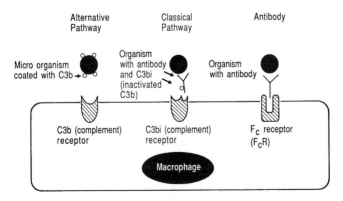

Figure 2.5 Mechanisms by which macrophages recognize microorganisms using surface receptors. (Courtesy of Dr Jonathan Austyn, Nuffield Department of Surgery, Oxford)

receptors bind to two different C3 breakdown products, C3b and its further degradation product, inactivated C3b (C3bi). The macrophage therefore can recognize organisms through three distinct immune mechanisms (Figure 2.5), and although macrophages can ingest organisms without previous exposure to the organism they can also use immune recognition. Activated macrophages can kill organisms using the same respiratory burst as neutrophils (see below).

When macrophage and monocyte function is studied in newborn infants it is found that interleukin 1 (IL-1) production is normal but that chemotaxis, phagocytosis and antigen processing are all variably diminished. Furthermore neonatal macrophages are less readily activated by lymphokines, such as interferon-γ (IFNγ). As lymphokines are relatively poorly produced by neonatal T lymphocytes there is a cumulative defect in response to intracellular organisms.

T LYMPHOCYTES (CELLULAR IMMUNITY)

T lymphocytes (thymus-derived lymphocytes) are responsible for cellular or cell-mediated immunity. They recognize, through specific T cell receptors, antigens that have been processed (degraded to peptides) and presented on the surface of antigen-presenting cells. The antigen-presenting cell presents degraded antigen in association with its own major histocompatibility complex (MHC) or human leukocyte antigen (HLA) molecule on the cell surface (see Figure 2.6). T cells recognize processed antigen through a receptor which has constant and variable regions, analogous to immunoglobulin. Once the T cell has recognized processed antigen it starts to proliferate. It may then either mature into a 'memory cell' which becomes quiescent but can recognize the same antigen if re-exposed, or into an 'effector cell' responsible either for destroying infected cells (cytotoxic T cell) or for helping B cells to produce antibody (T helper cell). Cytotoxic T cells are important in recovery from infection with intracellular pathogens, particularly viruses. T cells are also responsible for delayed-type hypersensitivity, important in recovery from tuberculosis.

T cells produce soluble proteins or lymphokines, such as the interleukins and immune interferon (interferon-γ). The lymphokines can act on B cells, natural killer cells (see below), macrophages and activated T cells themselves to recruit these cells to the site of infection and amplify the immune response.

T cell function is only marginally poorer in preterm and full-term neonates than in adults. Immunization with BCG (bacille Calmette-Guérin) is as protective at birth as in older children, suggesting near-normal delayed-type hypersensitivity. Graft rejection is active at birth.

Neonatal T cells can proliferate and produce lymphokines in response to appropriate stimuli, although some workers have found lower levels of lymphokine production (e.g. interferon-γ) in newborns than in adults. Some babies as young as 3 weeks old have been shown to mount a cytotoxic T-lymphocyte response to infection with respiratory syncytial virus [6]. Newborns and infants will not mount an antibody response to polysaccharide antigens such as the capsules of *Haemophilus*

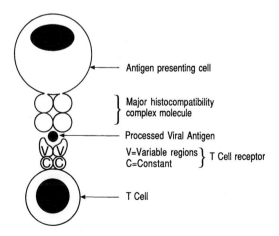

Figure 2.6 A T cell uses a T cell receptor to recognize 'processed viral antigen' (degraded to a peptide) presented on the surface of an antigen-presenting cell in association with a molecule of its major histocompatibility complex

influenzae type b or pneumococcus, but if the capsular poly-saccharide is linked to a T cell-dependent antigen such as diphtheria toxoid, babies as young as 2 months may make an antibody response to both the diphtheria toxoid and the capsular polysaccharide (see Chapter 21).

Most T cells have receptors with two α chains and two β chains. αβ T cells depend on the thymus for development and can only recognize processed antigens presented by class I or II MHC molecules (Figure 2.5). In contrast, γδ T cells, which have receptors with γ and δ chains, develop even when there is complete thymic aplasia and do not require class I or II MHC. γ T cells are thought to be important in neonatal immunity, acting as a first-line defence against a variety of intracellular (e.g. *Mycobacterium*) and extracellular (e.g. *Staphylococcus*) pathogens [7].

ANTIBODY-DEPENDENT CELLULAR CYTOTOXICITY (ADCC)

ADCC, the importance of which in most infections is unknown, depends on cytotoxic (killer) cells recognizing organisms coated with antibody, presumably via Fc receptors, and effecting cell lysis. Various cell types including killer cells, macrophages and granulocytes are capable of ADCC. The process is augmented by interferon.

NON-IMMUNE RESPONSES

NEUTROPHILS

Polymorphonuclear leukocytes, or neutrophils, are important in phagocytosing extracellular organisms such as *Staphylococcus aureus*. To kill these organisms, neutrophils need to be able to detect them and move towards them (chemotaxis), adhere to them (adhesion), ingest them (phagocytosis) and kill them by intracellular generation of toxic oxygen metabolites such as superoxide ions (respiratory burst). Studies of neutrophil func-tion in the neonatal period have shown moderately reduced chemotaxis and reduced expression of receptors, particularly in preterm babies [8].

The main problem appears to be that there is a diminished bone marrow reserve of immature neutrophils. If infection leads to peripheral destruction of neutrophils, the neutrophil reserve rapidly becomes depleted, resulting in neutropenia. Neutropenia is relatively common in neonatal bacterial infections and is associated with a worse prognosis.

COMPLEMENT

The complement system consists of a series of proteins which interact in a sequence or cascade to generate other proteins responsible for important defences to microorganisms (chemotaxis, opsonization and cell lysis). The complement system also regenerates its component proteins so that complement activation continues in the presence of infecting organisms. The central event in the complement cascade is the conversion of C3 to the activated molecule C3b. This can be achieved either by the classical pathway or the alternative pathway (see Figure 2.7). The classical pathway requires the presence of antibody and

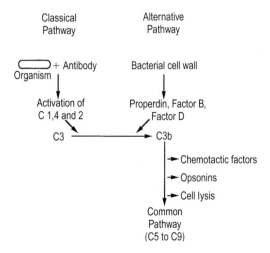

Figure 2.7 Simplified representation of the complement cascade

is best activated by immune complexes. The alternative pathway can be activated by bacterial cell wall products, such as endotoxin or polysaccharide, in the absence of antibody. However, antibody may augment alternative pathway-mediated killing. Both pathways catalyse the conversion of C3 to C3b by an enzyme, C3 convertase. This then leads to a series of reactions, the common pathway. This pathway generates chemotactic factors which attract inflammatory cells, anaphylatoxins which increase vascular permeability and hence access of inflammatory cells, opsonins which coat microorganisms, and the terminal membrane attack complex which punches holes in cell walls and lyses them. An important feature is that the complement cascade occurs on the cell surface of the infecting organism.

The complement cascade amplifies the response: a single IgG molecule can generate 10 000 membrane attack complexes.

Complement levels in the term newborn are approximately one-half those of normal adults, and preterm babies have even lower levels [9].

NATURAL KILLER CELLS

Morphologically, natural killer (NK) cells resemble large granular lymphocytes, but they probably derive from a lineage distinct from B and T cells. They kill virus-infected cells, some microorganisms and tumour cells spontaneously, and do not require antigen processing or MHC recognition. NK activity is stimulated by interferon and is generally somewhat lower in neonates than in adults. NK cells are particularly important in recovery from infections with herpesviruses [10]. In neonates there are fewer NK cells and they respond less well to interferons [11].

INTERFERON (IFN) PRODUCTION

There are five known types of interferon: IFNα, IFNβ and IFNγ are the main types, while IFN-W and IFN-T, produced by trophoblastic cells in early pregnancy, have only recently been described [12].

IFNα can be produced by almost any nucleated cell in the body while IFBβ is produced by fibroblasts and epithelial cells in response to various stimuli, particularly virus infections. The interferons act on neighbouring cells, stimulating them to produce various antiviral proteins that render the cell resistant to viral infection.

The production of IFNα and IFNβ is not a specific immune mechanism: they can be produced in response to a wide range of viruses and can protect against a number of different viruses.

IFNα is produced locally in most respiratory virus infections before antibody can be detected and is probably one of the most important mechanisms of recovery from such infections. Production of IFNα and IFNβ appears to be quantitatively normal in the neonatal period, even by preterm neonates.

IFNγ, or immune interferon, in contrast to IFNα, is produced by T cells on re-exposure to an antigen to which they have already been sensitized and is thus an immune mechanism. Although IFNγ has antiviral properties, its major role is as a modulator of the immune response. Macrophages and monocytes are activated by IFNγ, thus improving their ability to process and present antigen, whereas NK cells and the cells responsible for ADCC are activated to increase lysis of virus-infected cells. In the newborn period less IFNγ is produced, and macrophages, NK cells and ADCC cells are less sensitive to its action.

The various interactions between immune and non-immune responses to infection are summarized in Figure 2.8.

FIBRONECTIN

Fibronectin is a glycoprotein present in soluble form in the plasma, but also in cells or tissues. It enhances adhesion and chemotaxis of neutrophils and monocytes, and also enhances binding of bacteria like group B streptococcus and staphylococci to these phagocytes. When fibronectin binds to specific receptors present on phagocytic cells, this stimulates the production of cytokines such as tumour necrosis factor.

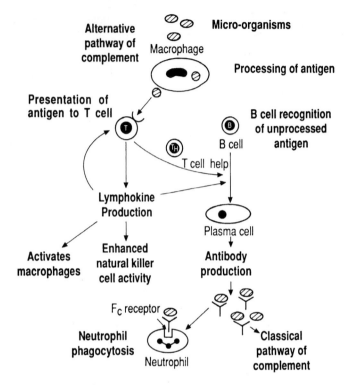

Figure 2.8 Immune (specific) and non-immune mechanisms interacting in response to infection

Plasma fibronectin is produced by the liver; fibroblasts and endothelial cells are among the cell types that produce cellular or tissue fibronectin.

In neonates, and particularly preterm neonates, plasma fibronectin levels are lower than in older children [13]. Prospective studies have not shown that low plasma fibronectin levels predispose to sepsis, but rather that sepsis causes levels to fall in preterm babies [14].

IMMUNOLOGICAL RESPONSE TO INFECTION

PYOGENIC BACTERIA

Pyogenic bacteria are extracellular organisms. They generally colonize a mucocutaneous surface before invasion. In the neonate, production of secretory IgA and fibronectin, which would normally decrease bacterial adherence, is relatively poor.

Once the organism is locally established, the most important defence mechanism is phagocytosis and killing by neutrophils, enhanced by opsonization by specific antibody and complement (see Figure 2.9). The relative importance of these factors may vary depending on the organism, e.g. defects in the terminal components of the complement pathway are peculiarly associated with *Neisseria* infections. In general, however, invasive disease with pyogenic organisms such as group B streptococci is more likely in the absence of type-specific antibody. The ready depletion of the pool of neutrophil precursors means that neutropenia, an unusual occurrence in older children, readily occurs in neonatal infections with pyogenic organisms.

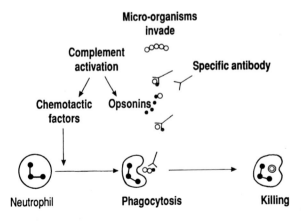

Figure 2.9 Host defences against infection with pyogenic bacteria

VIRUSES

A critical factor determining the severity of most neonatal virus infections is the timing of infection. The fetus is poorly protected against viruses so that intrauterine infection readily occurs. Infections in the first trimester, the time of maximum organogenesis, are most likely to be teratogenic. Infections acquired just before or at delivery are often severe because there is a large amount of virus and little or no maternal antibody. Enterovirus and varicella-zoster virus infections due to postnatal acquisition of the same virus, even in the absence of maternal antibody, are generally relatively mild. On the other hand, postnatal herpes simplex virus infection in the absence of maternally acquired antibody may be devastating. This suggests that the newborn may be able to mount an immune response to slow-growing or less virulent viruses, but not to rapidly multiplying, virulent viruses like herpes simplex.

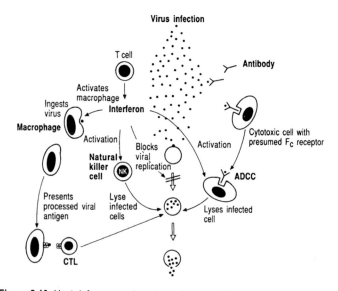

Figure 2.10 Host defences against virus infection. ADCC, antibody-dependent cellular cytoxicity; CTL, cytotoxic T lymphocyte; NK, natural killer cell

Apart from antibody, important early mechanisms in limiting viral replication are probably interferons, NK cells and ADCC, which act in the presence of maternal IgG (Figure 2.10). IgM directed against viruses can be produced by neonates, but is less efficient at neutralizing virus than IgG and will not sensitize virus-infected cells to lysis by effector cells. Neonatal IgG production is poor, so the newborn without specific maternal IgG is disadvantaged in combating virus infections. ADCC cannot operate in the absence of IgG, NK cell activity is generally lower in newborns, and IFNγ (but not IFNα) production is diminished. The role of cytotoxic T lymphocytes (CTLs) in clearing infection has not been well established in newborns.

INTRACELLULAR PATHOGENS

The immunological response to intracellular pathogens other than viruses is predominantly mediated by cellular immunity. *Listeria*, *Salmonella* and *Mycobacterium tuberculosis* are facultative intracellular pathogens, whereas *Chlamydia trachomatis*

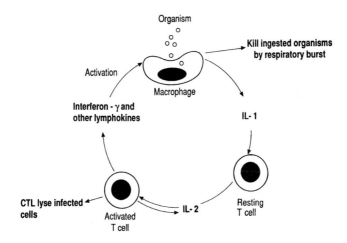

Figure 2.11 Host defences against intracellular pathogens. IL-1, IL-2, interleukins 1 and 2; CTL, cytotoxic T lymphocytes

and *Toxoplasma gondii* are obligate intracellular pathogens. In animals, macrophage depletion increases susceptibility to *Listeria*, whereas T cell depletion increases susceptibility to all intracellular pathogens, and immunity to intracellular pathogens can be restored by passive transfer of sensitized T cells.

Monocytes and macrophages produce interleukins, messenger proteins which activate T cells, whereas T cells produce lymphokines, including IFNγ, which activates macrophages, and interleukin 2 (IL-2), which activates T cells. Thus there is amplification of the cellular response to infections (see Figure 2.11). The cytokine-dependent interaction between T lymphocytes and macrophages is poor in neonates [15] and largely explains the increased susceptibility to intracellular pathogens.

SUMMARY

- The susceptibility of newborns to infection is largely due to immaturity of the immune system.
- Susceptibility to infection increases with prematurity.
- Transplacental IgG passage occurs mainly in the third trimester of pregnancy, and a fetus at 30 weeks' gestation has a serum IgG level about 50% of the adult level.
- Mucosal IgA is absent at birth. Full-term but not preterm newborns rapidly produce secretory IgA, though serum IgA concentration remains low.
- Neonatal T cell function is relatively unimpaired; fungal infections are a major problem only in extremely low birthweight babies.
- Neonatal neutrophils function reasonably well, but the neutrophil storage pool is easily reduced; neutropenia is not uncommon in sepsis and is a poor prognostic sign.
- Complement activity in the full-term newborn is about half that of normal adults, while levels are even lower in preterm babies.

References

1 Gitlin D, Kumate J, Urrusti J & Morales C. The selectivity of the human placenta in the transfer of plasma proteins from mother to fetus. *J Clin Invest* 1964; **43**: 1938–51.

2 Gleeson M, Cripps AW, Clancy RL *et al.* Ontogeny of the secretory immune system in man. *Aust NZ J Med* 1982; **12**: 256–8.

3 Haque KN, Remo C & Bahakim H. Comparison of two types of intravenous immunoglobulins in the treatment of neonatal sepsis. *Clin Exp Immunol* 1995; **101**: 328–33.

4 Young MC & Geha RS. Ontogeny and control of human IgE synthesis. *Clin Immunol Allerg* 1985; **5**: 339–49.

5 Welliver RC, Wong DT, Sun M *et al.* The development of respiratory syncytial virus-specific IgE and the release of histamine in nasopharyngeal secretions after infection. *N Engl J Med* 1981; **305**: 841–6.

6 Isaacs D, Bangham CRM & McMichael AJ. Cell-mediated cytotoxic response to respiratory syncytial virus in infants with bronchiolitis. *Lancet* 1987; **ii**: 769–71.

7 Morita CT, Parker CM, Brenner MB *et al.* TCR usage and functional capabilities of human αδ T cells at birth. *J Immunol* 1994; **153**: 3979–80.

8 Kemp AS & Campbell DE. The neonatal immune system. *Semin Neonatal* 1996; **1**: 67–75.

9 Miller ME. *Host Defenses in the Human Neonate*. New York: Grune & Stratton, 1978.

10 Biron CA, Byron KS & Sullivan JL. Severe herpesvirus infections in an adolescent without natural killer cells. *N Engl J Med* 1989; **320**: 1731–5.

11 Kohl S. The neonatal human's immune response to herpes simplex infection: a critical view. *Pediatr Infect Dis J* 1989; **8**: 67–74.

12 Stuart-Harris R & Penny R. *Clinical Applications of the Interferons*. London: Chapman & Hall, 1997.

13 Dyke MP & Forsyth KD. Plasma fibronectin levels in extremely preterm infants in the first 8 weeks of life. *J Paediatr Child Health* 1994; **30**: 36–9.

14 Dyke MP & Forsyth KD. Decreased plasma fibronectin concentrations in preterm infants with septicaemia. *Arch Dis Child* 1993; **68**: 557–60.

15 Wilson CB. Immunologic basis for increased susceptibility of the neonate to infection. *J Pediatr* 1986; **108**: 1–12.

3 | Clinical manifestations

INTRODUCTION

It is well known that the signs of neonatal bacterial sepsis are often non-specific and may be clinically indistinguishable from those occurring in non-infectious conditions, as well as being very similar to the signs of severe fungal and severe viral infection. Rapid deterioration is usual if the appropriate treatment is not given to a baby with bacterial sepsis, so that antibiotics must be prescribed early if sepsis is suspected. A clinical diagnosis of sepsis should carry greater weight than any rapid diagnostic laboratory test for sepsis, such as blood count or serum C-reactive protein (CRP), since no test has 100% sensitivity. If the doctor or nurse suspects sepsis, then empirical therapy should be started. There is no substitute for clinical skills in the management of sepsis.

SEPTICAEMIA

The signs of septicaemia vary somewhat according to whether the sepsis is acquired by vertical infection (early onset) or following colonization and later invasion (late onset). In general, early-onset sepsis is far more likely to be associated with respiratory distress and babies are more likely to be shocked, whereas the onset of symptoms is often, but by no means always, more insidious in late-onset sepsis.

FEVER

Only about one-half of the babies with proven sepsis are febrile; about 15% have hypothermia or temperature instability, while the remaining babies, about one-third, are normothermic. Thus, although fever should suggest infection, the absence of fever certainly does not exclude it. Fever is an important defence mechanism against infection and failure to mount a febrile response may contribute to the poor outlook in neonatal infections.

TACHYCARDIA

In one study of babies less than 72 hours old, almost half of the babies with sustained tachycardia >160 beats per minute were septic with positive blood cultures, giving a specificity of nearly 50%. Furthermore, tachycardia was a sensitive index of sepsis, being present in 12 of 13 babies with proven sepsis [1]. No similar evaluation has been made of tachycardia in late-onset sepsis.

The specificity of tachycardia with respect to diagnosing sepsis is unstudied, but hypovolaemia from any cause, cardiac problems, drugs and many conditions other than sepsis will cause tachycardia. Nevertheless, it can be a useful sign.

RESPIRATORY DISTRESS

In early-onset sepsis, the clinical picture may be identical to that of hyaline membrane disease (idiopathic respiratory distress syndrome), with tachypnoea, intercostal recession, cyanosis, grunting and flaring of the alar nasae. Furthermore, the chest radiograph may show a generalized fine granularity, focal pneumonic changes or even be completely normal.

In late-onset sepsis, with or without pneumonia, respiratory distress is less common. Tachypnoea may occur in bacterial meningitis due to central stimulation of the respiratory centres with or without acidosis.

LATE TACHYPNOEA

If a baby is initially well, without respiratory distress, it is unusual for the baby to develop later tachypnoea at a few days of age. If a baby develops tachypnoea for the first time at 3–7 days of age, and pneumonitis is present, herpes simplex virus (HSV) infection should be excluded urgently by immuno-fluorescence of a nasopharyngeal aspirate (HSV typically presents at 5–10 days of age). Other causes of late tachypnoea include respiratory syncytial virus, Chlamydia and cardiac causes such as anomalous pulmonary venous drainage. Cytomegalovirus pneumonitis usually presents after 4 weeks of age.

APNOEA

Apnoea is common in septic babies, but apnoea of prematurity occurs in a large proportion of preterm babies. The two types of apnoea ('septic' and apnoea of prematurity) cannot be readily distinguished by the duration, frequency or severity of the episodes, nor by the response to theophylline derivatives, because apnoea may temporarily respond to aminophylline in babies with sepsis.

JAUNDICE

Jaundice occurs in up to one-third of babies with sepsis. For unknown reasons, jaundice is particularly associated with Gram-negative infections, particularly of the urinary tract, but may also occur in group B streptococcal and other Gram-positive infections. The hyperbilirubinaemia is characteristically conjugated, although it may sometimes be predominantly unconjugated [2]. The mechanism is unknown.

HEPATOMEGALY

Hepatomegaly of moderate degree occurs in about one-third of cases of sepsis, often in association with jaundice.

SPLENOMEGALY

This is rarely described in reported series of septic babies, but this may be because of difficulty in eliciting the sign. If present, it suggests bacterial sepsis or intrauterine infection.

SKIN LESIONS

Petechial rash is a feature of congenital infections, but also occurs in immune thrombocytopenia and can result from disseminated intravascular coagulopathy (DIC) in severe sepsis. Very occasionally, meningococcal infection can present in the neonatal period with purpura. A raised papular rash is often present in early-onset listeriosis. A fine macular rash is fairly common in enteroviral infections and also occurs in congenital syphilis. Vesicular lesions, as well as purpura or erythema, may occur in herpes simplex virus infection. Ecthyma gangraenosum, necrotic skin lesions, may occur in *Pseudomonas* sepsis or sepsis due to fungi (Figure 3.1), while sclerema can occur in babies with advanced sepsis from any cause.

Omphalitis may range from a slightly red skin around the umbilicus to a purulent discharge with spreading necrosis of surrounding tissues (necrotizing fasciitis) which can be caused by *Staphylococcus aureus*, but also by Gram-negative bacteria and anaerobes [3].

LETHARGY, IRRITABILITY, ANOREXIA

Non-specific symptoms of lethargy or irritability and, in term infants, poor feeding are present in more than one-half of all babies with sepsis. The baby who 'handles well' may, nevertheless, be infected.

VOMITING, ABDOMINAL DISTENSION

Failure to tolerate enteral feeds, causing abdominal distension or vomiting due to ileus, is a common and important early sign

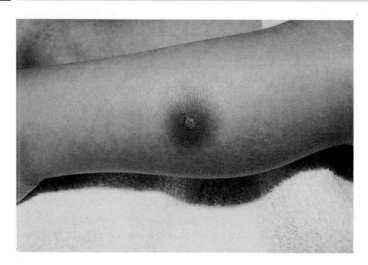

Figure 3.1 Ecthyma gangraenosum, associated with *Pseudomonas* or fungal sepsis

of sepsis. Babies with staphylococcal septicaemia may be diagnosed as having necrotizing enterocolitis (NEC) because of prominent abdominal signs. For this reason, it is important that the empirical antibiotic treatment of NEC should include staphylococcal cover.

MENINGITIS

The signs of meningitis do not differ markedly from those of systemic sepsis without meningeal involvement. Babies often look mottled, are pale and poorly perfused. Neck rigidity is rare in neonatal meningitis and a full or bulging fontanelle is seen in less than one-third of these babies [4]. Convulsions occur in <50%. Irritability is common, as is lethargy. Fever occurs in only about 60%. The cry may be high-pitched, suggesting cerebral irritation.

The clinical diagnosis of meningitis, particularly in preterm babies, is difficult and, unless there are good reasons for not performing a lumbar puncture, a sample of cerebro-spinal fluid (CSF) should be examined and cultured in all cases of suspected neonatal sepsis (see Chapter 5).

URINARY TRACT INFECTION

The signs of urinary tract infection (UTI) are no more specific than those of septicaemia or meningitis. Although there is a well-recognized association between UTI and jaundice [5], jaundice is actually present in <20% of babies with UTI [6]. Other signs of UTI, such as gastrointestinal manifestations (vomiting, abdominal distension, diarrhoea), irritability, lethargy and fever, are variably present and do not distinguish babies with UTI, which is frequently associated with bacter-aemia in the newborn period, from those with sepsis without UTI.

OSTEOMYELITIS OR SEPTIC ARTHRITIS

The clinical features of osteomyelitis and septic arthritis are described in detail in Chapter 10. Either or both conditions may present insidiously with the baby afebrile and feeding well, but with progressive enlargement of a bone or joint, or alternatively with pseudoparesis of a limb, mimicking Erb's palsy (osteomyelitis of the humerus or clavicle) or foot drop. Alter-natively, the onset may be abrupt, with signs indistinguishable from systemic sepsis until multiple areas of bony involvement become apparent.

VIRAL INFECTIONS

Systemic viral infections may present with a clinical picture similar to that of bacterial sepsis, whereas respiratory viruses tend to cause milder, but often equally non-specific, signs (see Chapter 16).

ENTEROVIRUS INFECTIONS

About half of all vertically (maternally) acquired enterovirus infections are associated with a history of peripartum maternal illness. This may be fever, gastroenteritis, upper respiratory tract infection or severe abdominal pain mimicking appendicitis. Babies classically present at 3–5 days, although occasionally at birth and as late as 7 days, with fever, irritability or lethargy, rash, abdominal distension, vomiting and poor feeding. Most develop hepatomegaly with a severe bleeding diathesis. Tachycardia or heart failure due to myocarditis is most likely with coxsackievirus infections, but can also occur with echovirus infections. Meningitis with or without typical signs may occur. The timing of the onset of illness, the severe bleeding and the maternal history all help to suggest a diagnosis of enteroviral infection.

Hospital-acquired enteroviral infections may cause diarrhoea, respiratory signs (apnoea, tachypnoea, recession, increased oxygen requirements), rash, signs of meningitis or myocarditis, or may be completely asymptomatic.

HERPES SIMPLEX VIRUS INFECTION

Herpes simplex virus (HSV) infection may be localized to the skin (usually causing vesicular lesions), eye (keratitis, conjunctivitis, cataracts, chorioretinitis), oral cavity (ulcers) or central nervous system (CNS). Alternatively, it may be disseminated, involving the liver, the above organs plus the lungs, gastrointestinal tract and other organs. Disseminated infection presents with a sepsis-like picture; a bleeding diathesis is common. CNS involvement often results in intractable convulsions. Fever, jaundice, apnoeic episodes, lethargy or irritability, poor feeding, abdominal distension or vomiting, and respiratory distress may all occur. The time of onset of signs is variable. Occasionally babies are born with skin or eye lesions, but usually these present in the first week. Isolated CNS infection, presenting with lethargy, irritability, poor feeding and convulsions, tends to be later, usually between 7 and 30 days.

RESPIRATORY VIRUSES

Infections with several respiratory viruses, notably respiratory syncytial virus (RSV), influenza virus, parainfluenza viruses and rhinoviruses, can present a similar non-specific clinical picture. Apnoeic episodes, respiratory distress with or without added pulmonary shadowing and increased oxygen requirements, lethargy and irritability are all common. Rhinitis is uncommon in neonatal respiratory viral infection.

FUNGAL INFECTIONS

Fungal infections (see also Chapter 15) mainly affect preterm infants with birthweight <1500 g, particularly those babies who have received prolonged courses of antibiotics or total parenteral nutrition. The clinical picture closely mimics bacterial sepsis. The only clinical distinguishing features may be oropharyngeal candidiasis (often not present despite systemic fungal infections), fungal skin abscesses or endophthalmitis, which sometimes accompanies fungaemia. It is important to consider fungal infections early, as fungi often grow slowly, if at all, in blood cultures. Very low birthweight (VLBW) babies with fungaemia are often thrombocytopenic. Empirical antifungal therapy for VLBW babies with suspected fungal sepsis is often necessary [7] and should perhaps be considered more often for VLBW thombocytopenic babies not responding rapidly to antibiotics.

CONCLUSION

In certain tribes in Papua New Guinea, there is a cultural response to illness of any kind, which is to groan, clutch the abdomen and complain of abdominal pain, regardless of the site of pathology. The newborn infant presents a similar problem in that the signs of sepsis, whether attributable to different bacteria, viruses or fungi, are non-specific. Not only is it difficult to predict clinically what sort of organism is causing sepsis, but non-infectious conditions, such as patent ductus arteriosus, may cause an almost identical clinical picture. It is clear that the paediatrician will treat many babies with antibiotics and must rely heavily on the laboratory to confirm or refute a suspicion of sepsis and to identify the causative organisms.

SUMMARY

- The clinical signs of sepsis are often non-specific.
- A clinical diagnosis of sepsis overrules any rapid diagnostic laboratory test, and empirical antibiotics should be started on suspicion of sepsis.
- About 30% of babies with sepsis are normothermic, roughly 50% are febrile and about 15% are hypothermic.
- Tachypnoea occurring at a few days of age in a baby without previous respiratory distress may be due to HSV pneumonitis.
- Fungal infections, often in babies <1500 g in birthweight, may present with non-specific clinical signs and thrombocytopenia, and empirical therapy should be considered.

References

1 Graves GR & Rhodes PG. Tachycardia as a sign of early onset neonatal sepsis. *Pediatr Infect Dis J* 1984; **3**: 404–6.

2 Hamilton JR & Sass-Kortsak A. Jaundice associated with severe bacterial infection in young infants. *J Pediatr* 1963; **63**: 121–8.

3 Mason WH, Andrews R, Ross LA & Wright HT. Omphalitis in the newborn infant. *Pediatr Infect Dis J* 1989; **8**: 521–5.

4 Klein JO & Marcy SM. Bacterial sepsis and meningitis. In: Remington JS & Klein JO (eds) *Infectious Diseases of the Fetus and Newborn Infant*, 4th edn. Philadelphia: WB Saunders, 1995: 835–90.

5 Seeler RA & Hahn K. Jaundice in urinary tract infection in infancy. *Am J Dis Child* 1969; **118**: 553–8.

6 Klein JO & Long SS. Bacterial infections of the urinary tract. In: Remington JS & Klein JO (eds) *Infectious Diseases of the Fetus and Newborn Infant*, 4th edn. Philadelphia: WB Saunders, 1995: 925–34.

7 McDonnell M & Isaacs D. Neonatal systemic candidiasis. *J Paediatr Child Health* 1995; **31**: 490–2.

4 | Rapid laboratory diagnosis

INTRODUCTION

Babies with sepsis can deteriorate rapidly, and empirical antibiotics are started whenever sepsis is suspected. On average, about nine babies are treated with antibiotics and found not to have sepsis for every one who is septic. Many attempts have been made to use laboratory tests to identify those babies with sepsis, and hence to reduce the number of non-septic babies receiving antibiotics.

Evaluating these tests, or combinations of them, involves determining their validity in clinical situations using the following formulae:

	Abnormal test(s)	Normal test(s)
Septic	a	b
Non-septic	c	d

The sensitivity of the test(s) is given by: $a/(a + b) \times 100$
The specificity of the test(s) is given by: $d/(c + d) \times 100$
The positive predictive value (PPV) is given by: $a/(a + c) \times 100$
The negative predictive value (NPV) is given by: $d/(b + d) \times 100$

Any rapid laboratory test for sepsis cannot afford to miss a single case, i.e. the sensitivity should be 100%. As this is impossible to achieve, a clinical diagnosis of sepsis is sufficient, whatever the laboratory results, to start empirical antibiotic therapy.

Table 4.1 lists a number of laboratory tests that have been used to aid the rapid diagnosis of sepsis.

HAEMATOLOGICAL INVESTIGATIONS

TOTAL WHITE CELL COUNT

The total peripheral blood white cell count is of limited use in evaluating a baby for suspected sepsis: about one-third of all babies with sepsis have normal white cell counts, and about one-half of all those babies evaluated for sepsis who have abnormal white cell counts are not, in fact, infected. White cell counts may be $>50 \times 10^9$/L (50 000/mL) in healthy newborns in the first 24 hours of life. A white count should always be performed in suspected sepsis. A low total white cell count is an ominous finding in such a baby and, although neutropenia is

Haematological	Total white cell count
	Neutrophil count
	Immature neutrophil count (band forms)
	Immature to total white cell (I:T) ratio
	Neutrophil morphology
	Platelet count
	ESR, micro-ESR
	Haematological profile
	Nitro-blue tetrazolium test (NBT)
Immunological	Serum acute-phase reactants, e.g. C-reactive protein (CRP)
	Cytokines, e.g. IL-6
Microbiological	CSF microscopy
(see Chapter 5)	Buffy coat microscopy
	Urine microscopy
	Bacterial antigen detection
	Polymerase chain reaction
	Viral antigen detection

Table 4.1 Laboratory tests used to aid rapid diagnosis of sepsis

more often (over 80%) caused by non-infectious factors such as birth asphyxia, it indicates a worse prognosis if the baby is, indeed, infected [1].

NEUTROPHIL COUNT

Because the total white cell count is an unreliable indicator of sepsis, the total neutrophil count has been used as an alternative measure. It is important to relate this to the age of the baby, as the normal range of neutrophil counts varies with age, being far higher in the first 24 hours after birth (Figure 4.1) [2]. At presentation, up to one-third of babies with proven sepsis have normal neutrophil counts, the rest being either high or low. Neutropenia in association with infection is particularly suggestive of severe sepsis and, as this finding suggests depletion of the granulocyte pool in the bone marrow, is a poor prognostic sign.

Immature neutrophils

Immature neutrophils are seen in the peripheral blood of even healthy preterm babies. Most are non-segmented neutrophils, also known as band or stab forms. In sepsis, an increased number of immature neutrophils enters the circulation from the bone marrow, causing a so-called 'shift to the left' in the blood film. Because the bone marrow granulocyte pool is quickly exhausted in neonatal sepsis, there is rarely an increase in the total immature neutrophil count in septic babies and this value alone is an unreliable indicator. As the total white count also tends to drop, the ratio of immature to total white cells is more reliable (see below).

Neutrophil ratios

Various methods of describing the ratio of immature to mature neutrophils have been examined to quantify the 'left shift'. These include the ratio of band to segmented forms, the ratio of immature to segmented neutrophils and the ratio of all immature or just band forms to the total neutrophil count. In studies of many different variables that might indicate sepsis, the

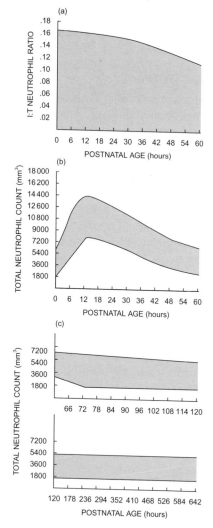

Figure 4.1 (a) The immature to total neutrophil ratio in normal newborn infants. The upper limit from age 60 hours to 28 days is 0.12. (b) The normal total neutrophil count during the first 60 hours. (c) The normal total neutrophil count from age 60 hours to 28 days is 1750–5400 per mm³. Shaded areas indicate normal values. (Reproduced with permission from ref. [2])

immature to total white cell count (I:T) ratio has proved the single most sensitive indicator of sepsis, particularly early-onset sepsis [2,3] (Figure 4.1). The I:T ratio has a sensitivity of about 90% and a specificity of about 80% for early sepsis, lower for late sepsis, so a number of cases will still be missed if this is used as the only indicator of sepsis (Table 4.2).

Rozycki *et al.* [13] found that 13 (21%) of 61 babies with early sepsis had a normal white cell profile (total neutrophil count, total immune neutrophil count and I:T ratio) early in their illness, so that if sepsis was strongly suspected but the white cell profile was normal it was important to repeat the profile within a few hours.

Neutrophil morphology

Although there may be morphological changes, such as vacuoles, toxic granules and Dohle bodies, in the white cells in bacterial infections, these changes are non-specific and may be seen in white cells from normal babies. Occasionally organisms may be seen inside the white cells of septicaemic babies, an ominous finding.

PLATELET COUNT

Thrombocytopenia may be caused by bacterial endotoxin acting directly on platelets or damaging endothelium and causing mild thrombosis, or by cytokines. It is present in about 50% of cases of sepsis. Established disseminated intravascular coagulation (DIC) is rare in neonatal sepsis. Platelet counts fall late in disease and thrombocytopenia may also be caused by birth

	Sensitivity (%)	Specificity (%)	PPV (%)	NPV (%)	Refs
For early sepsis	90–100	50–78	26–52	99–100	3,4
For late sepsis	29–58	78–82	11–26	50–55	5,6
For all	25–100	50–82	11–52	99–100	2–12

Table 4.2 Immature to total white cell count (I:T) ratio in neonatal sepsis

asphyxia, among other conditions. Thus, although thrombocytopenia may indicate sepsis, it is a finding of relatively low sensitivity and specificity. We have found the progressive development of thrombocytopenia to be a useful indicator of continuing sepsis when managing babies with *Staphylococcus epidermidis* septicaemia. Most babies with fungaemia have thrombocytopenia [14], so fungal infection should be considered if very low birthweight babies develop thrombocytopenia.

ERYTHROCYTE SEDIMENTATION RATE (ESR)

The ESR test usually requires too much blood, but can be modified to use very small samples [3]. The ESR tends to rise too late in most infections (not until 24–48 hours after onset) to be of great diagnostic value. It has, however, been used as part of a sepsis screen in a study by Philip [15].

HAEMATOLOGICAL PROFILE

Rodwell *et al.* [1,10] used a scoring system based on various white cell parameters (totals and ratios) and platelet count to assess babies with suspected sepsis. They found that if three or more parameters were abnormal, this identified 96% of septic babies with a specificity of 86%. The use of scoring systems using multiple parameters increases the sensitivity at the cost of reduced specificity, and for early sepsis gives little added benefit above the I:T ratio (Table 4.3).

NITRO-BLUE TETRAZOLIUM (NBT) TEST

Phagocytosing, but not resting, neutrophils will generate free oxygen radicals that will reduce the dye NBT to a purple colour due to formazan. This colour change can be detected using

	Sensitivity (%)	Specificity (%)	PPV (%)	NPV (%)	Refs
Immediate test	63–68	45-55	43–46	70	1–3,10
12–24 hours later	93–100	50–73	56-73	100	1–3,10

Table 4.3 Haematological scoring systems in neonatal sepsis

spectrophotometric techniques. The NBT test may be abnormal in normal preterm neonates and is less sensitive and harder to standardize than many of the other tests described.

IMMUNOLOGICAL INVESTIGATIONS

SERUM ACUTE-PHASE REACTANTS

Acute-phase reactants are serum proteins produced primarily in the liver but also, in the case of orosomucoid, in the intestine in response to various stimuli. These stimuli include bacterial infection, but also other forms of stress, such as necrotizing enterocolitis or surgery. The proteins can be produced by the fifth week of gestation and are probably of primitive origin; their role in limiting infection is unknown.

C-reactive protein

Of the various serum acute-phase reactants that have been measured, C-reactive protein (CRP, named after the C-carbo-hydrate of pneumococcus with which it combines) has proved the most useful in the diagnosis of sepsis. It starts to rise within 12–24 hours of the onset of sepsis, earlier than the other acute-phase reactants. Tests for measuring CRP include qualitative latex tests and quantitative tests such as laser nephelometry, which are both cheap and rapid. In many laboratories, a quantitative serum CRP, measured by laser nephelometry, can be obtained within 1–2 hours. Serum CRP level is raised in 50% to over 95% of cases of sepsis and necrotizing enterocolitis but, as with all tests for sepsis, may be normal in some cases of true sepsis (Table 4.4). It returns to normal within 2–7 days of successful treatment, and a persistent increase in the serum CRP level may indicate persistent infection, as in bacterial meningitis [20] or abscess formation in necrotizing enterocolitis [21]. Serial CRP levels may also be useful in monitoring the response to treatment for osteomyelitis or septic arthritis.

An initial serum CRP level may be normal in early-onset sepsis, but abnormal 6–12 hours later. The sensitivity of CRP

	Sensitivity (%)	Specificity (%)	PPV (%)	NPV (%)	Refs
Early and late sepsis	47–100	81–94	6–83	71–99	3–6, 12, 16–19

Table 4.4 Serum CRP in neonatal sepsis

	Sensitivity (%)	Specificity (%)	PPV (%)	NPV (%)	Ref
Early and late sepsis	73	88	6	97	17

Table 4.5 Serum IL-6 in neonatal sepsis

is somewhat better for late-onset than for early-onset sepsis [12].

Levels of other acute-phase reactants such as orosomucoid (α_1-acid glycoprotein), fibrinogen and haptoglobin change more slowly than CRP during infection and their measurement has generally been far less useful [19].

CYTOKINES

Interleukin 6 (IL-6) is produced mainly by the macrophage–monocyte lineage and is an important inflammatory mediator produced in response to bacterial infection. IL-6 can be measured in serum by rapid, sensitive ELISA tests (Table 4.5). In one study, serum IL-6 was useful only in combination with serum CRP measurement, since IL-6 concentration was too often normal in septic babies, but was usually raised in septic babies with normal serum CRP levels [17].

Measurement of other cytokines has not been helpful in diagnosing neonatal sepsis.

SEPSIS SCREENS

Various research workers have described the combined use of several different techniques for identifying sepsis in order to improve the sensitivity for detecting infected babies. The haematological screen described by Rodwell *et al.* [10] has already been mentioned. Philip and Hewitt [3] showed that a panel of screening tests (white cell count, band/total neutrophil ratio, CRP, micro-ESR and haptoglobin), available within an hour, identified 93% of babies with sepsis. Nevertheless, their criterion of two or more positive tests indicating sepsis missed two of 30 cases of sepsis, and the authors stressed the importance of accurate clinical evaluation of each baby and stated that, if sepsis was strongly suspected, antibiotics should be started regardless of test results. These screens are expensive and none has 100% sensitivity. They can certainly reduce antibiotic use [3] but this must not be at the expense of delayed treatment of sepsis. It is best to make an individual clinical decision on each baby as to whether or not antibiotics should be prescribed, in conjunction with the guidelines on risk factors described in Chapter 6.

Serum C-reactive protein and I:T ratio are the most sensitive laboratory markers of late-onset sepsis.

RAPID MICROBIOLOGICAL TESTS

Several microbiological tests are available that qualify as rapid diagnostic tests. For example, Gram stains of tissue fluids may reveal potential pathogens: in CSF these are pathognomonic of infection, whereas positive Gram stains of surface swabs have a low specificity in neonatal sepsis. These will be considered in Chapter 5.

OTHER TESTS

A number of other rapid tests have been evaluated in the diagnosis of neonatal infection, but none has sufficient sensitivity and specificity to be used in practice. Examples are the serum fibronectin [4], serum lactate [22], plasma elastase α_1-proteinase [23,24], leukocyte alkaline phosphatase [25] and the nitro-blue tetrazolium (NBT) tests [5].

ACKNOWLEDGEMENT

The literature review and analysis of the sensitivity, specificity, positive and negative predictive values of tests were performed by Dr Joanne Ging of The New Children's Hospital, Sydney and are used with her kind permission.

SUMMARY

- The most useful rapid assay in early-onset sepsis is the immature to total neutrophil ratio, or I:T ratio.

- The most useful rapid assays in late-onset sepsis are the I:T ratio and the serum C-reactive protein.

- No test is abnormal in every case of sepsis; antibiotics should be started if there is a clinical suspicion of sepsis, regardless of any rapid test results.

References

1 Rodwell RL, Taylor KM, Tudehope DI & Gray PH. Hematologic scoring system in early diagnosis of sepsis in neutropenic newborns. *Pediatr Infect Dis J* 1993; **12**: 372–6.

2 Manroe BL, Weinberg AG, Rosenfeld CR *et al.* The neonatal blood count in health and disease. I. Reference values for neutrophilic cells. *J Pediatr* 1979; **95**: 89–98.

3 Philip AGS & Hewitt JR. Early diagnosis of neonatal sepsis. *Pediatrics* 1980; **65**: 1036–41.

4 Gerdes JS & Polin RA. Sepsis screen in neonates with evaluation of plasma fibronectin. *J Pediatr* 1987; **6**: 443–6.

5 Kite P, Millar MR, Gorham P & Congdon P. Comparison of five tests used in diagnosis of neonatal bacteraemia. *Arch Dis Child* 1988; **63**: 639–43.

6 Philip AGS. Detection of neonatal sepsis of late onset. *JAMA* 1982; **247**: 489–92.

7 Christensen RD, Bradley PP & Rothstein G. The leukocyte left shift in clinical and experimental neonatal sepsis. *J Pediatr* 1981; **98**: 101–5.

8 Engle WD & Rosenfeld CR. Neutropenia in high risk neonates. *J Pediatr* 1984; **105**: 982–5.

9 Leslie GI, Scurr RD & Barr PA. Early-onset bacterial pneumonia: a comparison with severe hyaline membrane disease. *Aust Paediatr J* 1981; **17**: 202–6.

10 Rodwell RL, Leslie AL & Tudehope DI. Early diagnosis of neonatal sepsis using a hematologic scoring system. *J Pediatr* 1988; **112**: 761–7.

11 Schelonka RL, Yoder BA, desJardins SE, Hall RB & Butler J. Peripheral leukocyte count and leukocyte indexes in healthy newborn term infants. *J Pediatr* 1994; **125**: 603–6.

12 Seibert K, Yu VYH, Dorey JCG & Embury D. The value of C-reactive protein measurement in the diagnosis of neonatal infection. *J Paediatr Child Health* 1990; **26**: 267–70.

13 Rozycki HJ, Stahl GE & Baumgart S. Impaired sensitivity of a single early leukocyte count in screening for neonatal sepsis. *Pediatr Infect Dis J* 1987; **6**: 440–2.

14 Dyke MP & Ott K. Severe thrombocytopenia in extremely low birthweight infants with systemic candidiasis. *J Paediatr Child Health* 1993; **29**: 298–301.

15 Philip AGS. Decreased use of antibiotics using a neonatal sepsis screening technique. *J Pediatr* 1981; **98**: 795–9.

16 Ainbender E, Cabatu EE, Guzman DM & Sweet AY. Serum C-reactive protein and problems of newborn infants. *J Pediatr* 1982; **101**: 438–40.

17 Buck C, Bundschu J, Gallati H, Bartmann P & Pohlandt F. Interleukin-6: a sensitive parameter for the early diagnosis of neonatal bacterial infection. *Pediatrics* 1994; **93**: 54–8.

18 Mathers NJ & Pohlandt F. Diagnostic audit of C-reactive protein in neonatal infection. *Eur J Pediatr* 1987; **146**: 147–51.

19 Sann L, Bienvenu F, Bienvenu J, Bourgeois J & Bethenod M. Evolution of serum pre-albumin, C-reactive protein and orosomucoid in neonates with bacterial infection. *J Pediatr* 1984; **105**: 977–81.

20 Sabel KG & Hanson LA. The clinical usefulness of C-reactive protein (CRP) determinations in bacterial meningitis and septicaemia in infancy. *Acta Paediatr Scand* 1974; **63**: 381–8.

21 Isaacs D, North J, Lindsell D & Wilkinson AR. Serum acute phase reactants in necrotizing enterocolitis. *Acta Paediatr Scand* 1987; **76**: 923–7.

22 Fitzgerald M, Goto M, Myers TF & Zeller WP. Early metabolic effects of sepsis in the preterm infant: lactic acidosis and increased glucose requirement. *J Pediatr* 1992; **121**: 951–5.

23 Rodwell RL, Taylor KM, Tudehope DI & Gray PH. Capillary plasma elastase α_1-proteinase inhibitor in infected and non-infected neonates. *Arch Dis Child* 1992; **67**: 436–9.

24 Speer C, Ninjo A & Gahr M. Elastase-alpha$_1$-proteinase inhibitor in early diagnosis of neonatal septicaemia. *J Pediatr* 1985; **108**: 987–9.

25 Paul RS & Kumar A. Value of leukocyte alkaline phosphatase and other leukocyte parameters in diagnosis of neonatal infection. *Biol Neonate* 1984; **45**: 275–9.

5 | **Microbiological diagnosis**

Some microbiological tests, such as lumbar puncture and CSF microscopy, are rapid diagnostic tests which provide immediate information. Others, such as blood culture, are slow and only provide later answers.

RAPID DIAGNOSTIC MICROBIOLOGICAL TESTS

GASTRIC ASPIRATES

Gram stains of gastric aspirates taken in the first few hours of life are frequently used to assess babies with respiratory distress for possible infection, particularly with group B streptococcus. However, the presence of polymorphonuclear leukocytes, which are maternal in origin, only indicates exposure to infection: less than 6% of babies born to mothers with clinical chorioamnionitis develop sepsis [1]. Ingram and co-workers performed Gram stains on gastric aspirates from 109 newborns with respiratory distress or suspected sepsis [2]. Of 13 babies with early-onset group B streptococcal sepsis, 10 had positive Gram stains, but 3 (23%) had false-negative smears.

This indicates that it would be unwise to place too much reliance on a negative gastric-aspirate Gram stain. Furthermore, there is a high rate of false positives, with bacteria and leukocytes identified in gastric aspirates from babies who are shown subsequently not to be septic.

In general, it is no longer recommended to obtain Gram stains of gastric aspirates in suspected sepsis both because too much reliance may be placed on a negative result and because the presence of pus cells and/or a scanty number of organisms is often overinterpreted as indicating probable sepsis.

TRACHEAL ASPIRATES

In early-onset neonatal sepsis, ascending infection is the commonest mode of infection, with the respiratory tract an important early site of bacterial replication, and early pneumonia is usual. Sherman and colleagues evaluated the use of Gram stains on smears of early tracheal aspirates in detecting congenital pneumonia [3]. They obtained tracheal aspirates, during or immediately following laryngoscopy, from 320 newborns with respiratory distress. Twenty-five babies had bacteria seen on the Gram stain; 14 of the 25 grew a compatible organism from blood cultures. The authors compared these babies with 25 of the babies with no organisms seen on tracheal aspirate smear: three of these 25 'controls' had positive blood cultures. The authors do not state how many of the remaining 270 babies with negative tracheal aspirate smears had positive blood cultures but, extrapolating from the 25 'control' babies, one might suppose that more than 30 had bacteraemia. Thus, for the total population of 320 babies, the sensitivity of early tracheal aspirate in detecting early sepsis may have been less than 30%. In a second study the same authors found that, of those babies who had organisms seen on Gram stain of the tracheal aspirates, 47% had early-onset bacteraemia, and 74% of all babies with early-onset bacteraemia had positive tracheal aspirate microscopy [4]. This is a much-improved sensitivity, although one-quarter of the babies with early-onset sepsis had negative tracheal aspirate microscopy.

Endotracheal aspirate cultures are frequently performed on babies requiring long-term artificial ventilation for surveillance purposes and to identify likely pathogens should sepsis be suspected. It is known that endotracheal suction frequently causes transient bacteraemia, and it seems likely that the upper respiratory tract is a common site of entry of invading pathogens in late sepsis, occurring as frequently as it does in artificially ventilated babies. Nevertheless, some studies have shown that endotracheal cultures are relatively insensitive in predicting the organisms causing late-onset septicaemia: either no organism is grown from the endotracheal aspirate when a baby is septicaemic (50–62% of cases) or the cultures yield many different organisms [5,6]. Furthermore, clinicians rarely pay any attention to the culture results, even when these are available [6]. Slagle and co-workers found that endotracheal cultures were insensitive in predicting the organisms causing late sepsis in ventilated babies and that in 42% of cases an antibiotic regimen based on the endotracheal culture would have resulted in inappropriate antibiotic therapy for the septicaemia [7].

The proportion of endotracheal tubes colonized with potential pathogens increases with time and colonization is almost inevitable in babies on long-term artificial ventilation [8]. Antibiotics should not be given merely because of growth of a potential pathogen, e.g. *Pseudomonas*, from the endotracheal aspirate.

SURFACE SWABS

Surface cultures and cultures from deep sites are commonly obtained when early- or late-onset sepsis is suspected. Evans and colleagues examined the sensitivity and specificity of cultures from the nasopharynx, external ear canal, axilla, rectum, umbilical cord, skin and eye [6]. They found the sensitivity of each of these tests to be <50% in predicting the organisms causing sepsis.

It is important to know whether a newborn with suspected early-onset sepsis is colonized, as blood cultures may be negative despite a strong clinical suspicion of sepsis. Thus a baby with heavy group B streptococcal (GBS) colonization and a clinical picture suggestive of early GBS sepsis should be treated for a full 7–10 days with antibiotics despite negative blood and CSF cultures. Similarly, babies with a clinical diagnosis of congenital listeriosis (rash, hepatosplenomegaly and respiratory distress) who are colonized with *Listeria monocytogenes* but have negative blood and CSF cultures should also be managed as for proven infection.

Increasing the number of surface cultures performed does not greatly alter reliability. Thus, it has been shown to be possible to reduce the number of surface swabs taken without impairing clinical care [9] and with considerable savings.

Ear swabs are most often used in the rapid diagnosis of early sepsis since liquor pools in the external ear canal. Gram stain of ear swabs has the same problems as gastric aspirate microscopy. Routine urgent microscopy of ear swabs in suspected early-onset sepsis is not recommended, but it is advisable to culture the ear swab along with an umbilical swab to detect colonization.

CSF: WHO NEEDS A LUMBAR PUNCTURE?

A lumbar puncture is effectively a 'biopsy' of the cerebrospinal fluid (CSF), allowing rapid diagnosis or exclusion of meningitis, and immediate identification of the likely causative organism. It is a simple, powerful test.

About 15–30% of babies with early-onset septicaemia and 10% of babies with late-onset septicaemia have concurrent meningitis [10,11], so the problem is not a trivial one. McIntyre and Isaacs reviewed the indications for neonatal lumbar puncture [12] and their arguments for immediate or delayed lumbar puncture are given in Table 5.1.

The organisms causing early- and late-onset sepsis are different. Empirical antibiotic therapy for early-onset sepsis with penicillin or ampicillin and an aminoglycoside will treat

Reasons for immediate LP	Reasons for delayed LP
Diagnosis If LP is only done on bacteraemic babies, the 15–40% of babies with meningitis who have negative blood cultures will be missed	**Trauma** Respiratory compromise from positioning of baby; particularly worrying in early respiratory distress syndrome (RDS)
LP is a 'biopsy': immediate diagnosis or exclusion of meningitis	Traumatic tap Introduction of infection Spinal epidermoid tumour
Treatment LP may alter empirical antibiotic therapy, e.g. if Gram-negative bacilli or fungi seen on Gram stain	**Dangers** Risk of cerebral herniation Might exacerbate intraventricular haemorrhage
CSF culture gives sensitivities	
Avoids confusion Interpretation of delayed LP often difficult	**Rarity of meningitis** In early RDS, need 320–1500 LPs to identify one case of meningitis

Table 5.1 Rationale for immediate or delayed lumbar puncture (LP) in the investigation of babies with suspected or possible sepsis

meningitis due to group B streptococcus, pneumococcus, *Listeria* and most *Haemophilus influenzae*, but not other Gram-negative bacilli such as *Escherichia coli*. Babies with early-onset meningitis usually have no signs referable to the central nervous system. On the other hand, an extremely large number of babies with early-onset respiratory distress are started on antibiotics for at least 48 hours until the results of cultures are known. Many authors have argued that, for these babies, the incidence of meningitis is extremely low and that lumbar puncture can be delayed and performed only if blood cultures are positive. Weiss and co-workers found that 0.3% of babies with RDS had bacterial meningitis and 1500 lumbar punctures would be needed to identify one baby with meningitis [13]. Others, on smaller samples, reported figures of 320 to over 900 lumbar punctures to identify one baby with meningitis [14–17].

The problem with using blood culture as a screening test for meningitis is that it is a very poor screening test. Wiswell and colleagues found that the incidence of early-onset meningitis in a large population was 0.25 per 1000 live births; using blood cultures alone, the diagnosis of bacterial meningitis would have been missed or delayed in 37% or 16 of 43 babies [18]. Delayed lumbar puncture would not have compromised the treatment of the 30 babies with GBS, one with *Listeria* and one with pneumococcus, since the empirical antibiotics used would have treated meningitis. In contrast, the other 11 babies with Gram-negative meningitis (10 with *E. coli*) would have received suboptimal antibiotic therapy for 24–48 hours. The rate of negative blood cultures in bacterial meningitis varies with the population studied, definitions, and with the use of maternal antepartum antibiotics: Wiswell quotes a range of rates in the literature varying from 15 to 55%.

Fielkow and co-workers [19] and Kumar and colleagues [20] examined the role of lumbar puncture in asymptomatic babies with maternal risk factors for sepsis. Fielkow *et al.* found that about 2% of babies with clinical signs had meningitis, whether or not there were maternal risk factors for sepsis, whereas none of 284 babies with risk factors but without signs at birth developed meningitis.

Very similar results were found by Kumar *et al.* in India: 3.3% of 148 babies with clinical signs, but none of 21 babies without signs, developed meningitis. The numbers of babies studied was not great and it is not known how many babies, if any, had more than one risk factor.

In late-onset sepsis there is much less of a problem with respiratory compromise, and the organisms causing meningitis are more varied and more likely to be resistant to the standard antibiotics in use. In addition, fungal meningitis may have an identical clinical presentation to bacterial meningitis. In general, lumbar puncture should be performed in babies with suspected late-onset sepsis, even in those who are thrombocytopenic. Thrombocytopenia is often given as a reason not to perform lumbar puncture, but is common in sepsis, and there is no evidence that lumbar puncture of thrombocytopenic babies is any more hazardous than venepuncture or insertion of central venous lines.

In practice, however, lumbar puncture is performed much less frequently than recommended: in an Australian study, only 55% of babies with proven late-onset septicaemia ever had a lumbar puncture [10]. This may reflect the number of times blood cultures are sent speculatively and grow coagulase-negative staphylococci. It does raise the interesting point of whether delayed lumbar puncture should be performed on babies with late-onset septicaemia already receiving antibiotics. Since this will affect the duration and perhaps the nature of antibiotic therapy for Gram-negative bacilli, streptococci, other bacteria and fungi, and the overall risk of meningitis in late septicaemia is about 10%, delayed lumbar puncture is clearly indicated for these babies with late-onset septicaemia. However, meningitis due to coagulase-negative staphylococci is extremely rare in babies without shunts: less than 1% in most studies [10,11]. It might reasonably be argued that lumbar puncture can be omitted in most babies with coagulase-negative staphylococcal bacteraemia, who did not have an initial lumbar puncture, if they are already receiving antibiotics.

The interpretation of CSF microscopy is considered in Chapter 8. Recommendations for lumbar puncture are summarized in Table 5.2.

BUFFY COAT MICROSCOPY

Because of the number of organisms present in neonatal septicaemia, organisms may be seen in neutrophils. These can be obtained by centrifuging a small volume of heparinized blood and aspirating the 'buffy coat' layer just above the red cells, or breaking a spun heparinized capillary tube full of blood at the buffy coat layer. The neutrophils are smeared on a slide and stained with Gram's iodine, methylene blue or acridine orange stains.

In expert hands, the sensitivity can be up to 80–90% [21–23] and some false negatives are due to neutropenia, itself

Clinical	All babies with suspected sepsis and with clinical signs suggestive of meningitis, e.g. severe apnoea, convulsions, irritability, bulging fontanelle, should have an immediate LP prior to commencing antibiotics
Late-onset sepsis	All babies with suspected late-onset sepsis should have an immediate LP prior to commencing antibiotics
Thrombocytopenia	Thrombocytopenia is not a contraindication to LP, unless profound and the baby is bleeding
Early-onset sepsis	*Babies with early-onset respiratory distress* LP should be delayed if there is danger of compromising cardiorespiratory status, but should be performed later if blood cultures are positive or there is clinical suspicion, and particularly if there was more than one maternal risk factor *Asymptomatic babies with risk factor(s) for sepsis* Do not routinely perform LP, unless two or more risk factors are present, when antibiotics should be started empirically after blood and CSF cultures
Bacteraemia	*Bacteraemic babies on antibiotics* Babies with early- or late-onset sepsis who were started on antibiotics without an LP and have positive blood cultures should always have a delayed LP to exclude meningitis. The only exception might be late-onset coagulase-negative staphylococcal bacteraemia, as meningitis is rare (<1%)

Table 5.2 Recommendations for lumbar puncture (LP)

strongly suggestive of sepsis. However, Rodwell and colleagues [24] found a sensitivity of only 17%. Buffy coat examination may occasionally reveal intracellular budding yeasts [25] and allow a rapid diagnosis of fungaemia.

URINE MICROSCOPY AND CULTURE

Urinary tract infection (UTI) may present acutely as a septicaemic illness or more insidiously with vomiting and/or jaundice. Urine collected in a sterile plastic bag ('bag urine') is easily contaminated by faeces, whereas a suprapubic aspirate of urine (SPA) is rarely contaminated unless the bowel is accidentally perforated. A catheter specimen of urine is occasionally used an an alternative. In investigating babies with prolonged jaundice or vomiting, a bag urine is appropriate initially because antibiotics need not be prescribed immediately and further urine samples can be obtained if necessary. In apparently septic babies, when antibiotics must be started immediately, consideration should be given to performing an SPA before starting treatment. Visser and Hall [26] have questioned the need for SPA urines, at least in early-onset sepsis. They analysed urine culture results in early- (<72 hours) and late-onset sepsis. In early sepsis a positive urine culture was rare: they only had three in a year; one baby also had positive blood cultures, while one of the urines was probably contaminated. In late-onset sepsis they had more positive urine cultures (14) but details of the organisms and the presence or absence of white cells in the urine were not reported and it is difficult to assess the likelihood of contamination.

Urinary tract infection is associated with pyuria (>10 WBCs per high-power field) in about 70–75% of cases [27]. Suprapubic aspiration can lead to complications, is traumatic (to babies, parents and medical staff) and may lead to hypoxaemia. At Oxford, we have seen no cases of early-onset UTI over 5 years (>25 000 live births) except in association with disseminated sepsis in which blood cultures were also positive. Late-onset UTI is more common but we still diagnose only one to two cases annually in our newborn nursery, which serves 5000 live births. This incidence is lower than that usually quoted for neonatal UTI. Our policy is to perform microscopy on a urine sample obtained from all babies with suspected late-onset sepsis, but we have elected not to culture routinely the urine of babies with suspected early-onset sepsis. We would obtain urine by SPA if there were one or more of the following: a strong clinical suspicion of UTI; persistent pyuria (>10 WBCs per high-power field); organisms seen on urine microscopy, or growth of organisms from two or more bag urines. The main problem with this approach is that a 'positive' urine culture (as defined by growth of $\geqslant 10^5$ organisms per ml of a single bacterial strain) does not necessarily indicate a true UTI, because bag specimens can be contaminated. In practice we find that this is rarely a problem, as bag specimens are usually either sterile or yield multiple organisms on culture, indicating probable contamination. In the occasional equivocal case, when antibiotics have already been started and there is a 'pure growth' of $\geqslant 10^5$ organisms per ml, with or without pyuria, from a bag urine specimen, we would treat and investigate as for UTI. We have seen only four such cases in over 5 years of a policy in which bag urine specimens were used to investigate possible UTI. As our initial radiological investigations of neonatal UTI are now relatively non-invasive (see Chapter 11), we think that the possibility of overdiagnosing a few children with UTI is offset by avoiding several hundred SPA procedures per year.

URINE GROUP B STREPTOCOCCAL ANTIGEN DETECTION

Group B streptococcal (GBS) antigen can be detected in the urine by latex particle agglutination, i.e. latex particles coated with specific anti-GBS antibody agglutinate in the presence of GBS antigen.

Urine GBS antigen detection has a reported sensitivity of 88–100% and specificity of 81–100% for detecting babies with early-onset GBS septicaemia [28]. Bag urine samples are easily contaminated by skin GBS, and positive antigen detection of a bag urine should be confirmed on a suprapubic sample. Even so, some authorities have queried the validity of using GBS antigen detection as a surrogate for septicaemia. Antigen detection may be most useful when the mother has been treated with intrapartum antibiotics. Blood cultures are negative in about half of those babies with early-onset GBS pneumonia defined as clinical and radiographic pneumonia plus heavy GBS colonization [29]. McIntosh and Jeffery [30] found that, in such babies, urine GBS antigen detection by latex particle agglutination had a sensitivity of 88%, specificity of 98%, positive predictive value of 79% and negative predictive value of 99%.

ANTIGEN DETECTION

Bacterial antigens may be detected using latex particle agglutination as described above, by enzyme-linked immunosorbent assay (ELISA), or by countercurrent immunoelectrophoresis (CIE). Of these, ELISA is the most sensitive and CIE the least. The tests are specific for a single microorganism, which limits their usefulness; for example, group B streptococcal antigen testing will not detect other organisms such as pneumococci.

Concentrated urine is the best sample, but antigen detection has been applied to serum, CSF, pleural and peritoneal fluid. Serum antigen detection is generally too insensitive (<50%) to be useful, but the sensitivity of GBS antigen detection in CSF is 67–88% [31].

POLYMERASE CHAIN REACTION

The polymerase chain reaction or PCR is a technique for detecting specific DNA or RNA in even minute quantities and amplifying nucleic acid to levels that can be easily detected [32]. At present, the only regular use of PCR in neonatal infection is to detect herpes simplex virus (HSV) DNA in CSF or serum from babies with suspected HSV encephalitis. PCR is extremely sensitive, although contamination can cause false positives. As PCR testing is increasingly automated it is likely to be used more widely in neonatal sepsis, for example to detect GBS, *Candida*, viruses, *Mycobacterium tuberculosis*, etc.

VIRAL DETECTION

Rapid detection of viral antigens is usually either by ELISA or by immunofluorescence. Immunofluorescence is either direct (a fluorescent-labelled specific antibody combines with antigen in the specimen) or indirect (specific antibody which combines with any antigen in the specimen is recognized by a second fluorescent antibody to the first antibody). Immunofluorescence is extremely important in diagnosing HSV in herpetic skin lesions and in nasopharyngeal aspirates in HSV pneumonitis. It can also be used for detecting respiratory syncytial virus (RSV) and *Chlamydia* in babies with late-onset respiratory distress.

OTHER MICROBIOLOGICAL INVESTIGATIONS

BLOOD CULTURES

Antibiotics should not be started without taking at least one blood culture. Preferably, blood should be taken from a peripheral vein or artery, after cleaning the overlying skin with an alcohol- or iodine-based solution which is first allowed to dry. Blood drawn through umbilical catheters that have just been inserted is unlikely to be contaminated; blood cultures taken through umbilical arterial or venous or peripheral arterial catheters that have been present for some time are less reliable, as growth of organisms not found in simultaneous peripheral venous blood cultures is a frequent finding. On the other hand, Pourcyrous and co-workers found that, of 318 paired simultaneous umbilical arterial catheter (UAC) and peripheral venous cultures, the same organism was grown in 13 episodes of sepsis [33]. Six UAC and five peripheral cultures grew organisms not found in the other blood culture pair. In the authors' opinion most of these were true episodes of sepsis and contamination rates of UAC cultures were actually marginally lower than those for peripheral blood cultures. Capillary blood cultures are easily contaminated by skin bacteria and should not be used.

Quantitative blood cultures may distinguish true sepsis from contamination when organisms such as *Staphylococcus epidermidis*, which may be pathogens or contaminants, are grown in blood cultures, but quantitative cultures are not usually routinely available.

Because of the large numbers of organisms generally present, only small volumes of blood may be needed to detect neonatal bacteraemia. As little as 0.2 ml of blood may detect *E. coli* bacteraemia [34]. It is, therefore, worth culturing blood even if only a small volume is obtained.

Because it is sometimes difficult to decide later about the validity of blood culture results, it is useful to record in the case notes the indications for blood culture, the site from which blood is taken and the quantity put in the bottles. Paired aerobic and anaerobic bottles are usually inoculated with blood. These are under vacuum and tend to suck in the whole specimen if the doctor is not careful.

VIRAL CULTURES

These will be addressed in Chapter 16 on viruses. If in doubt about the best specimen, always consult the virus laboratory.

SUMMARY

- The lumbar puncture is a 'biopsy' of the CSF, allowing rapid diagnosis or exclusion of meningitis and the causative organism; it should be performed whenever possible in suspected sepsis.

- Lumbar puncture is indicated in all babies with suspected late-onset sepsis.

- Lumbar puncture may be delayed in some babies with early-onset respiratory distress, but should be performed later if blood cultures prove positive.

- Ear and umbilical surface cultures are useful in early-onset sepsis, but Gram stain is often confusing as the sensitivity and specificity for diagnosing sepsis are too low.

- Urine group B streptococcal antigen detection is both sensitive and specific in the diagnosis of early-onset sepsis.

References

1 Siegel JD & McCracken GH. Sepsis neonatorum. *N Engl J Med* 1981; **304**: 642–7.

2 Ingram DL, Pengergrass EL, Bromberger PI *et al.* Group B streptococcal disease: its diagnosis with use of antigen detection, Gram's stain, and the presence of apnea, hypotension. *Am J Dis Child* 1980; **134**: 754–8.

3 Sherman MP, Goetzman BW, Ahlfors CE & Wennberg RP. Tracheal aspiration and its clinical correlates in the diagnosis of congenital pneumonia. *Pediatrics* 1980; **65**: 258–63.

4 Sherman MP, Chance KH & Goetzman BW. Gram's stains of tracheal secretions predict neonatal bacteremia. *Am J Dis Child* 1984; **138**: 848–50.

5 Isaacs D, Wilkinson AR & Moxon ER. Surveillance of colonisation and late-onset septicaemia in neonates. *J Hosp Infect* 1987; **10**: 114–19.

6 Evans ME, Schaffner W, Federspiel CF *et al.* Sensitivity, specificity and predictive value of body surface cultures in a neonatal intensive care unit. *JAMA* 1988; **259**: 248–52.

7 Slagle TA, Bifano EM, Wolf JW & Gross SJ. Routine endotracheal cultures for the prediction of sepsis in ventilated babies. *Arch Dis Child* 1989; **64**: 34–8.

8 Webber S, Lindsell D, Wilkinson AR *et al.* Neonatal pneumonia. *Arch Dis Child* 1990; **65**: 207–11.

9 Dobson S, Isaacs D, Wilkinson A *et al.* Reduced use of surface cultures for suspected neonatal sepsis and surveillance is safe. *Arch Dis Child* 1992; **67**: 44–7.

10 Isaacs D, Barfield C, Grimwood K *et al.* Systemic bacterial and fungal infections in infants in Australian neonatal units. *Med J Aust* 1995; **162**: 198–201.

11 Isaacs D, Barfield C, Clothier T *et al.* Late onset infections of infants in neonatal units. *J Paediatr Child Health* 1996; **32**: 158–61.

12 McIntyre P & Isaacs D. Lumbar puncture in suspected neonatal sepsis. *J Paediatr Child Health* 1995; **31**: 1–2.

13 Weiss MG, Ionides SP & Anderson CL. Meningitis in premature infants with respiratory distress: role of admission lumbar puncture. *J Pediatr* 1991; **119**: 973–5.

14 Visser VE & Hall RT. Lumbar puncture in the evaluation of suspected neonatal sepsis. *J Pediatr* 1980; **96**: 1063–7.

15 Eldadah M, Frenkel LD, Hiatt IM & Hegyi T. Evaluation of routine lumbar punctures in newborn infants with respiratory distress syndrome. *Pediatr Infect Dis J* 1987; **6**: 243–5.

16 Hendricks-Munoz KD & Shapiro DL. The role of the lumbar puncture in the admission sepsis evauation of the premature infant. *J Perinatol* 1990; **10**: 60–4.

17 Schwersenski J, McIntyre L & Bauer CR. Lumbar puncture frequency and cerebrospinal fluid analysis in the neonate. *Am J Dis Child* 1991; **145**: 54–8.

18 Wiswell TE, Baumgart S, Gannon CM & Spitzer AR. No lumbar puncture in the evaluation for early neonatal sepsis: will meningitis be missed? *Pediatrics* 1995; **95**: 803–6.

19 Fielkow S, Reuter S & Gotoff SP. Cerebrospinal fluid examination in symptom-free infants with risk factors for infection. *J Pediatr* 1991; **119**: 971–3.

20 Kumar P, Sarkar S, Narang A. Role of routine lumbar puncture in neonatal sepsis. *J Paediatr Child Health* 1995; **31**: 8–10.

21 Faden HS. Early diagnosis of neonatal bacteremia by buffy-coat examination. *J Pediatr* 1976; **88**: 1032–4.

22 Boyle RJ, Chandler BD, Stonestreet BS & Oh W. Early identification of sepsis in infants with respiratory distress. *Pediatrics* 1978; **62**: 744–50.

23 Kleiman MB, Reynolds JK, Schreiner RL *et al.* Rapid diagnosis of neonatal bacteremia with acridine orange-stained buffy coat smears. *J Pediatr* 1984; **105**: 419–21.

24 Rodwell RL, Leslie AL & Tudehope DI. Evaluation of direct and buffy coat films of peripheral blood for the early detection of bacteraemia. *Aust Paediatr J* 1989; **25**: 83–5.

25 Cattermole HEJ & Rivers RPA. Neonatal candida septicaemia: diagnosis on buffy coat smear. *Arch Dis Child* 1987; **62**: 302–4.

26 Visser VE & Hall RT. Urine culture in the evaluation of suspected neonatal sepsis. *J Pediatr* 1979; **94**: 635–8.

27 Ginsburg CM & McCracken GH. Urinary tract infections in young infants. *Pediatrics* 1982; **69**: 409–12.

28 Jeffery HE. Group B streptococcus infections. *Semin Perinatol* 1996; **1**: 77–89.

29 Webber S, Lindsell D, Wilkinson AR *et al.* Neonatal pneumonia. *Arch Dis Child* 1990; **65**: 207–11.

30 McIntosh EDG & Jeffery HE. Clinical application of urine antigen detection in early onset group B streptococcal disease. *Arch Dis Child* 1992; **67**: 1198–200.

31 Baker CJ & Edwards MS. Group B streptococcal infections. In: Remington JS & Klein JO (eds) *Infectious Diseases of the Fetus and Newborn Infant*, 3rd edn. Philadelphia: WB Saunders, 1990: 742–811.

32 Burgner D, Isaacs D & Givney R. New rapid microbiological tests. *J Paediatr Child Health* 1996; **32**: 83–5.

33 Pourcyrous M, Korones SB, Bada HS *et al.* Indwelling umbilical arterial catheter: a preferred sampling site for blood culture. *Pediatrics* 1988; **81**: 821–5.

34 Dietzman DE, Fischer GW & Schoenknecht FD. Neonatal *Escherichia coli* septicemia – bacterial counts in blood. *J Pediatr* 1974; **85**: 128–30.

6 | **A rational approach to antibiotic use**

WHICH BABIES TO TREAT

The risk factors for the development of early and late sepsis have already been discussed, as have possible adjuncts to the diagnosis of sepsis. However, some babies will develop sepsis, either early or late, with no known risk factors. Furthermore, no ancillary laboratory tests for sepsis have 100% sensitivity. If cases of sepsis are not to be missed, therefore, treatment should always be initiated if there is strong clinical suspicion of neonatal sepsis, regardless of whether there are risk factors or laboratory tests supporting sepsis. This inevitably means that far more babies receive antibiotics than ever have documented sepsis: approximately one baby has proven sepsis for every 10 babies treated for suspected sepsis. The effects of such widespread use of antibiotics can be minimized by using antibiotics for as short a duration as possible.

Certain clinical situations in which the use of antibiotics on a routine basis is often considered recur regularly in the newborn intensive care nursery. These situations and the policy we use to deal with them are discussed here.

PRETERM BABY WITH RESPIRATORY DISTRESS FROM BIRTH

It is the policy in Oxford (Table 6.1) that, for any preterm baby with early respiratory distress, an abnormal chest radiograph and one or more risk factors for sepsis, cultures are taken and antibiotics given. The risk factors in these babies are prolonged rupture of the membranes, maternal fever, and spontaneous preterm onset of labour with or without rupture of the membranes. These risk factors are known to be associated with sepsis attributable to group B streptococci [1], pneumococci [2] and enterococci [3], and probably apply to other organisms. Prolonged rupture of membranes is a continuum of increased risk: the greatest risk is after 18 hours, but the risk of sepsis increases when membranes are ruptured for >12 hours [1]. Smelly liquor has not been evaluated as a risk factor, but clinicians are unlikely not to treat a baby born through such liquor.

In our experience, the admitting doctor is highly likely to consider sepsis in the differential diagnosis of a baby with early respiratory distress and prolonged rupture of the membranes, maternal fever or smelly liquor. In contrast, respiratory distress in association with spontaneous preterm onset of labour is almost always called hyaline membrane disease and early pneumonia is rarely considered [4]. Nevertheless, in a series of babies with early-onset pneumonia, spontaneous preterm onset of labour was found to be by far the commonest risk factor (see Table 9.1) [4].

In practice, this means that the only preterm babies with respiratory distress who do not receive at least 48 hours of

1. Any toxic-looking baby
2. Baby with *one* risk factor for sepsis + respiratory distress
3. Baby with *one* risk factor + very preterm, e.g. 32 weeks' gestation or below, or needing i.v. fluids
4. Baby with *two* risk factors, even if asymptomatic
5. Baby with neutropenia (<1000 μL = <1 × 10⁹/L) for longer than 3 days, even if asymptomatic

Risk factors

- Spontaneous preterm onset of labour <37 weeks
- Prolonged rupture of membranes >18 hours
- Maternal fever >37.5°C
- Previous baby with group B streptococcal infection

Table 6.1 Babies who should be started on empirical antibiotics in the puerperium

antibiotics according to our practice are the small group of babies delivered by elective caesarean section or following induction of labour for maternal reasons.

We have specifically mentioned an abnormal chest radiograph in this context, usually a fine, generalized granularity identical to that in hyaline membrane disease (idiopathic respiratory distress syndrome, surfactant deficiency), but sometimes showing focal areas of consolidation. Where the radiograph is normal but there is respiratory distress, clinical suspicion of sepsis and one or more risk factors, we would nevertheless start antibiotics, because we have occasionally seen a normal chest radiograph early in severe GBS sepsis.

Some workers have suggested that it is possible to distinguish babies with early-onset bacterial pneumonia from those with hyaline membrane disease by the use of Gram stains of surface swabs, total neutrophil counts, and immature to total neutrophil count ratios [5]. However, up to 21% of babies with early-onset sepsis have completely normal haematological profiles [6] and there may be difficulties in obtaining these tests rapidly. Our view is that the decrease in the proportion of babies given antibiotics resulting from the use of sepsis screens (e.g. ref. 7) is outweighed by the danger of delay in administering antibiotics and the risk of placing too much reliance on a negative test.

BABY WITH RISK FACTORS FOR SEPSIS, BUT NO SYMPTOMS

The more risk factors present at birth, the more likely the baby is to be infected. Thus, if a baby is born with two or more risk factors for sepsis, e.g. a baby with spontaneous preterm onset of labour and prolonged rupture of membranes, a full septic screen should be performed and antibiotics started, even if the baby was asymptomatic, full-term, and there was no information on maternal vaginal cultures. On the other hand, if only one risk factor was present, e.g. preterm onset of labour, but the baby was clinically well, we would not necessarily start antibiotics. However, the more premature the baby the higher the risk of early sepsis. As a rough guide, if a baby needs an intravenous line for fluids from birth and has a single risk factor for sepsis, we would do a septic screen and start antibiotics. On the other hand, if a baby is mature enough to be fed enterally, we would usually wait and observe the baby. There is a paucity of data on the magnitude of the risk in these situations (see Table 6.1).

FULL-TERM BABY WITH RESPIRATORY DISTRESS

Hyaline membrane disease is rare in full-term babies, and respiratory distress at term should suggest the possibility of sepsis. Most full-term babies with respiratory distress will have a final diagnosis of transient tachypnoea of the newborn (TTN). In this condition the initial chest radiograph shows a 'wet lung' appearance with increased vascular markings and often fluid in the horizontal fissure. Unfortunately, an identical radiographic appearance has been described in about 10% of cases of early-onset GBS pneumonia [8]. Thus, although most cases of early pneumonia at term will have a generalized granularity mimicking hyaline membrane disease or areas of focal consolidation, a chest radiograph that is normal or shows 'wet lung' does not exclude pneumonia. Mifsud and colleagues have described tachypnoea, as monitored routinely in newborn babies at their hospital, as a useful early indicator of sepsis [9]. Early detection of infected babies in their study may have contributed to a fall in mortality from early sepsis.

Gram stains of gastric aspirates [10] and tracheal aspirates [11,12] are only moderately reliable, with sensitivities of 77% and 74% respectively, in predicting babies with early sepsis. Thus they may be used to aid diagnosis, but only in the knowledge that they will not identify all cases of early sepsis. For example, in the study by Ingram and co-workers, the gastric aspirate was negative in three of 16 (19%) babies with early-onset GBS pneumonia [10]. Another reason for not using gastric aspirates is the danger that junior staff may be falsely reassured by a negative Gram stain and may overinterpret if the Gram stain reveals a number of different organisms.

When assessing full-term babies with respiratory distress, additional laboratory tests such as total neutrophil count, ratio of immature to total neutrophil counts and serum CRP level may help to decide whether to treat or observe, but the clinical picture should always be the final arbiter.

POSITIVE URINE GROUP B STREPTOCOCCAL ANTIGEN TEST

Urine may be sent for a latex particle agglutination (LPA) test for group B streptococcal (GBS) antigen for a number of reasons. There are several variables when an LPA is performed. Maternal GBS carriage status may be known or unknown. There may be no, one or more maternal risk factors for neonatal sepsis (fever, prolonged membrane rupture, spontaneous preterm labour). Maternal antepartum antibiotics may or may not have been given. The baby may be asymptomatic or symptomatic. The baby may be anything from extremely premature to full term. The LPA may have been performed on a bag sample or a suprapubic sample. If a positive LPA was found on a bag specimen of urine, a suprapubic sample should be tested.

Some babies will require empirical antibiotic treatment regardless of the LPA test result. A positive LPA test is usually interpreted as meaning bacteraemia, but false positives occur due to contamination of bag urines by GBS on the skin and due to cross-reacting antigens from other bacteria. In general, antibiotics should be started after taking cultures on any symptomatic baby with a positive LPA test. A negative maternal GBS screening test at 28 weeks does not exclude neonatal GBS infection, since about 8% of women whose 28-week vaginal swab is negative, will acquire GBS carriage by term.

Asymptomatic babies with a positive LPA test are more of a problem. An empirical decision will need to be made in each case, based on the absence or presence of risk factors for sepsis and the baby's gestation. As with the discussion on babies with risk factors, the more immature babies are more likely to warrant immediate antibiotic treatment rather than observation.

MATERNAL INTRAPARTUM ANTIBIOTICS

Intrapartum antibiotics may be given to mothers who are known group B streptococcal vaginal carriers with one or more risk factors for neonatal sepsis, asymptomatic GBS carriers [13] or mothers who have not been screened for GBS, but have risk factors for neonatal sepsis [14]. There are no data on which to base decisions about which babies should start antibiotics if their mothers were given intrapartum antibiotics, and how long they should be continued.

In the original study of Boyer and Gotoff, all babies of GBS carrier mothers with one or more risk factors were treated with antibiotics from birth [15], but this would seem to be excessive. Asymptomatic babies who are born at or near term can probably be observed, with or without the aid (or complicating factor) of a urine LPA test for GBS antigen. For more premature babies it is advisable to start antibiotics empirically at birth. Empirical guidelines were published in 1996 by the Centers for Disease Control (Figure 6.1) for the management of babies whose mother received intrapartum antibiotics, and

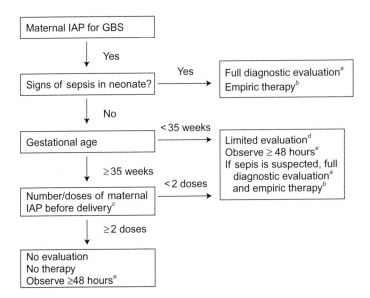

Figure 6.1 AAP 1997 algorithm for management of a neonate born to a mother who received intrapartum antimicrobial prophylaxis (IAP) for prevention of early-onset group B streptococcal (GBS) disease. Notes: [a]Includes a complete blood count (CBC) and differential, blood culture, and chest radiograph if neonate has respiratory symptoms. Lumbar puncture is performed at the discretion of the physician. [b]Duration of therapy will vary depending on blood culture and cerebrospinal fluid (CSF) results and the clinical course of the infant. If laboratory results and clinical course are unremarkable, duration of therapy may be as short as 48–72 hours. [c]Applies to penicillin or ampicillin chemoprophylaxis. [d]CBC and differential, and a blood culture. [e]Does not allow early discharge

were revised by the American Academy of Pediatrics [16]. These are based largely on consensus opinion rather than firm evidence, and are guidelines rather than rules. For example, it is assumed that two or more doses of maternal antibiotics will prevent all cases of sepsis in babies of 35 weeks' gestation or more. Nevertheless, the guidelines are practically useful as a basis for management of this clinically difficult situation.

SEVERE PERINATAL ASPHYXIA

Severe perinatal asphyxia may occasionally result from sepsis: up to 20% of babies with perinatal sepsis have respiratory depression requiring intubation [17]. On the other hand, most babies with perinatal asphyxia are not septic. If the baby is severely obtunded, then clinical signs of sepsis may be masked. Additionally, the haematological picture is often abnormal in severe asphyxia and neutropenia may occur [18]. As sepsis is a rare cause of asphyxia, the use of antibiotics should be determined on an individual basis for severely asphyxiated babies. Both asphyxia and infection may cause pulmonary hypertension ('persistent transitional circulation') and if this should supervene a full septic screen should be carried out and antibiotics started. Neutropenia is considered below.

MECONIUM ASPIRATION SYNDROME

Meconium aspiration may result from severe perinatal asphyxia. In addition, it has been argued that, although meconium is sterile, the plugging of airways resulting from meconium aspiration may predispose to secondary pneumonia. As is the case for severe perinatal asphyxia, it is not logical to prescribe antibiotics in case secondary pneumonia develops; each baby should be assessed for the likelihood of sepsis. Occasionally, sepsis may be the cause of the asphyxia that causes the aspiration. Meconium is unusual in preterm deliveries, and if present should alert the resuscitating doctor to the possibility of infection, particularly congenital listeriosis (see Chapter 14).

DIRTY PROCEDURES AROUND DELIVERY

In some babies, usually those with perinatal asphyxia or acute blood loss, intravascular catheters are inserted hurriedly, often in the delivery suite and under less than optimally sterile conditions. Antibiotics are often prescribed to cover such 'dirty' procedures. There is little evidence that sepsis occurs as a result of dirty procedures, nor that it can be prevented by giving antibiotics. Nevertheless, the practice of giving antibiotics under these conditions is likely to continue, whatever is argued, and is probably relatively harmless if antibiotics are stopped early when cultures are negative.

NEUTROPENIA

Neutropenia is a sinister sign in sepsis. However, most babies with neutropenia in the first 2 days after birth are not infected: Rodwell and colleagues found that only about one in six neutropenic babies had sepsis as a cause, while the rest had neutropenia due to maternal hypertension [19]. Neutropenia usually resolves by 3 days of age. Are babies with maternal hypertension-induced neutropenia at increased risk of sepsis, and if so how can this be prevented?

Koenig and Christensen found that 23% of maternal hypertension-associated neutropenic babies developed nosocomial infection aged 4–18 days, compared with 3% of non-neutropenic babies [20]. Mouzinho and co-workers [21] and Doron et al. [22] both found that about half of all infants born to mothers with severe pre-eclampsia developed neutropenia. Neutropenic babies were smaller and more preterm than non-neutropenic babies in the study of Mouzinho et al. [21], but there was no difference in incidence of sepsis between neutropenic babies and controls matched for birthweight and age.

Doron and colleagues also found that neutropenic babies born to pre-eclamptic mothers were more premature, lighter and more likely to be small for gestational age than non-neutropenic babies [22]. However, the rate of presumed or proven sepsis was 14% for neutropenic and 2% for non-neutropenic babies, which was significant even after correction for prematurity, while the respective rates for proven sepsis were 6% versus 0%.

Doron and colleagues [22] defined neutropenia as a total neutrophil count below 2.2×10^9/L in the first 12 hours after birth, as this was the lower limit of normal in Lloyd and Oto's study of very premature babies [23].

Early studies suggest that G-CSF or GM-CSF (granulocyte or granulocyte–macrophage colony-stimulating factor) administered daily in the first days of life can correct hypertension-induced neutropenia, and reduce the incidence of nosocomial sepsis (see Chapter 7). The use of colony-stimulating factors in neutropenia is promising, but not yet proven, and certainly not routine practice. An alternative would be to use prophylactic antibiotics for babies with neutropenia lasting longer than 3 days, until the neutropenia has resolved. Prophylactic antibiotics can hardly be said to be proven in this setting, but the rate of sepsis in neutropenic babies is high enough to warrant such an approach.

PROPHYLACTIC ANTIBIOTICS

Some neonatologists routinely prescribe antibiotics to babies with venous and arterial cannulas and to those requiring endotracheal intubation, as prophylaxis against infection. There is evidence that prophylactic antibiotics do *not* prevent sepsis from umbilical venous or arterial catheters, peripheral artery catheters (where the risk of sepsis is low) and indwelling peripheral or central venous catheters (summarized in ref. 24). Harris and colleagues found that antibiotics that were started at the time of endotracheal intubation and continued for a mean of 3–4 days protected against subsequent systemic infection, which invariably followed colonization of the endotracheal tube [25].

However, they also found that colonization was almost invariable after 72 hours of intubation. It may be that antibiotics decrease the number of colonizing organisms and hence the risk of sepsis. Other workers have not found such a clear correlation between the organisms causing endotracheal colonization and subsequent sepsis [4,26] and consider that the nature of late-onset sepsis may be changing since the time of Harris' study. We do not give prophylactic antibiotics to cover endotracheal intubation *per se* although, as stated previously, most artificially ventilated babies are given antibiotics in case they are already infected. The use of antibiotics in preterm babies with respiratory distress is often described as giving 'prophylactic' antibiotics. This is a misconception: antibiotics are being given to these babies to *treat* possible sepsis until culture results are obtained; a corollary of this is that antibiotics can be stopped when cultures are negative.

There are very few situations in which antibiotic prophylaxis has been shown to be effective in the neonatal period. Antibiotic use in neutropenic babies is discussed above. Babies with structural abnormalities of the urinary tract are at high risk for UTI. Although oral antibiotic prophylaxis is useful in preventing UTI in older children, its use is not proven in neonates. Many doctors continue to prescribe prophylactic oral antibiotics for babies with urinary tract abnormalities or with proven UTI. We are unaware of any formal studies on their efficacy in the newborn with urinary tract abnormalities.

Oral aminoglycosides prevent radiologically proven necrotizing enterocolitis (NEC), but do not reduce the number of NEC-like episodes nor mortality from NEC [27]. They are rarely used because of selection of resistant organisms. There is no evidence that antibiotics given at the time of insertion of cerebrospinal fluid shunts prevent shunt infections [28]. There is evidence that intravenous cefuroxime at induction for anaesthesia reduces the risk of subsequent sepsis in adult patients undergoing bowel surgery, but no such evidence exists for newborn infants.

Prophylactic oral nystatin is frequently used for infants and babies of very low birthweight, particularly those on antibiotics. The only placebo-controlled study of prophylactic oral nystatin was that of Sims *et al.* [29]. They randomized 77 babies under 1250 g to oral nystatin three times daily or placebo. The nystatin group had lower rates of both colonization (12% versus 44%) and infection (6% versus 35%) with fungi.

There have been a number of recent papers on the use of prophylactic vancomycin to prevent coagulase-negative staphylococcal infections. The rationale is that coagulase-negative staphylococcal infections prolong hospital stay and cause significant morbidity [30]. Schwartz and co-workers used a heparin–vancomycin solution to flush central venous lines in paediatric patients with cancer [31]. Prophylactic vancomycin has been used in preterm neonates as a twice-daily dose infused over 1 hour [32], as a continuous low-dose infusion [33], or added to parenteral nutrition [34,35]. Although these studies purport to show a reduction in staphylococcal bacteraemia without a 'compensatory' increase in sepsis due to other organisms, there are problems in definition. Using bacteraemia alone as the end-point will include many contaminants. These contaminants will be found in blood cultures from the control group, but blood cultures in the index group are likely to be sterilized by even low-dose vancomycin since only low levels of organisms will be present.

If vancomycin does prevent coagulase-negative staphylococcal infection, there are two dangers. One is that, as discussed in Chapter 1, preterm babies may be predestined by their degree of immunocompromise to develop septicaemia with any colonizing organism. Eradication of coagulase-negative staphylococci may merely allow more virulent organisms such as Gram-negative bacilli to colonize and invade. A second factor is the emergence of vancomycin-resistant organisms, notably vancomycin-resistant enterococci [36]. This worrying development should encourage us all to restrict vancomycin use as far as possible [37].

WHICH ANTIBIOTICS TO USE

The use of 'broad-spectrum' antibiotics selects for antibiotic-resistant organisms, 'broad-spectrum' resistance and for fungi. Ideally, 'narrow-spectrum' antibiotics should be used as much as possible, i.e. those that most narrowly cover the spectrum of organisms causing sepsis in the nursery and that have been shown to be effective in treating cases of sepsis. However, there may be great variation in the organisms causing sepsis, not only between regions, but also within one region and even within any one hospital over time. It is important to keep up-to-date records, therefore, on the organisms causing systemic sepsis in the newborn nursery and the outcome of episodes of sepsis, and to review these regularly. No antibiotic policy can be deemed wrong unless it patently fails to cover organisms causing significant sepsis, and infection with these organisms causes significantly morbidity or mortality (see Chapter 18).

EARLY-ONSET SEPSIS

Penicillin or ampicillin is generally used, together with an aminoglycoside (gentamicin, netilmicin or amikacin), as the empirical treatment of early sepsis. This is logical because in most industrialized countries group B streptococcus is currently the organism that most often causes early-onset sepsis and also causes the highest morbidity and mortality rates.

Group B streptococcus is rarely reported as causing sepsis in non-industrialized countries, although a report from Kingston, Jamaica showed it to be the commonest organism causing both early- and late-onset sepsis [38]. Aminoglycosides are used with a penicillin because Gram-negative organisms, particularly *Escherichia coli,* are a common cause of early sepsis. On the other hand *Listeria monocytogenes* is increasingly described as causing early sepsis, and in some European countries, such as France, it is one of the most common organisms. Ampicillin is preferred to penicillin for *Listeria* sepsis (with an aminoglycoside) on *in vitro* data, although treatment with penicillin and an aminoglycoside is generally effective (see Chapter 14). The third-generation cephalosporins, which have sometimes been advocated for monotherapy of neonatal sepsis, are ineffective against *Listeria* and also enterococci, and should not be used as sole agents to treat early (or late) neonatal sepsis.

The advantage of penicillin G over ampicillin is that widespread use of ampicillin is more likely to select for multiple drug resistance [39] and colonization with *Candida*. On the other hand, there are theoretical but unproven advantages of ampicillin over penicillin in treating infections with *Haemophilus influenzae,* enterococci and *Listeria monocytogenes*, all of which are increasing in the UK. The aminoglycoside of choice is again a moot point. Gentamicin is cheaper, there is more experience with its use and, consequently, potentially toxic drug levels are uncommon. On the other hand, netilmicin causes less ototoxity in adults [40] and is less likely to select for the emergence of resistant Gram-negative organisms [41]. Amikacin may be the most ototoxic of these three aminoglycosides, although because of confounding causes of deafness it has been difficult to show this in small studies on neonates [40,42].

In most cases of suspected early-onset sepsis, little additional information is available on which to base antibiotic treatment. If the culture results of a high vaginal swab from the mother before delivery are known, the antibiotics used should cover these organisms effectively. The results from Gram stains of surface swabs, gastric and tracheal aspirates are generally insufficiently reliable to form the basis for changing a tried and tested antibiotic regimen, although the presence of resistant organisms might suggest additional antibiotic cover in severe sepsis.

The mortality rate from early-onset sepsis is high and it is important that there is the minimum possible delay in giving the first doses of antibiotics. Ideally, the admitting doctor should take blood cultures and give intravenous antibiotics as soon as the decision is made to start treatment, usually within an hour of birth. Surface swabs and CSF can then be collected immediately after treatment has been started.

We are sceptical of the wisdom of attempts to introduce monotherapy with a ureidopenicillin or third-generation cephalosporin for early- and late-onset sepsis [43]. Such policies ignore the difference between the organisms causing early- and late-onset sepsis and do not sufficiently cover relatively common or increasing causes of sepsis such as *Listeria*.

Regardless of the antibiotic regimen for early-onset sepsis, the mortality and morbidity rates associated with proven sepsis are high. Delayed therapy or ineffective antibiotics are rarely responsible for the poor outcome; rather, the dissemination of a large microbial load, often in a compromised fetus without maternal antibody, has occurred before delivery. Efforts should be centred on prevention of severe early-onset sepsis by identifying and treating with intrapartum antibiotics those women at risk for delivery of a baby with early sepsis [15] and later by immunizing mothers once effective GBS vaccines become widely available (Chapter 19).

LATE-ONSET SEPSIS

Three possible approaches can be taken to the choice of antibiotics for late-onset sepsis, as outlined below.

Treat the baby according to a standard antibiotic policy

This is probably the best way of limiting the emergence of resistant organisms. If a large range of antibiotics is used simultaneously, multiple drug resistance may become a significant problem. Use of a standard regimen will usually result only in selection of organisms resistant to a single antibiotic. Furthermore, colonization with resistant organisms does not necessarily lead to sepsis with resistant organisms, which are sometimes less virulent than sensitive ones [44,45]. If episodes of systemic sepsis with resistant organisms occur, and particularly when those babies most at risk for sepsis (artificially ventilated, low birthweight) are also colonized with the resistant organisms, this can be used as an indication to change the antibiotic policy in order to withdraw the 'antibiotic pressure' [41], as discussed below.

There is no 'ideal' antibiotic regimen for treating suspected late-onset sepsis. When neonatal units in the UK were surveyed, it was found that a wide range of antibiotic regimens was being used. Such regimens must cover the organisms most likely to cause systemic sepsis, and this information is best obtained by reviewing the recent cases of sepsis, rather than from surface cultures [46]. Nevertheless, there may be rapid changes in the organisms causing sepsis in a single unit (Figure 1.3). At present, in most developed countries, late-onset sepsis is most commonly caused by coagulase-negative staphylococci such as *Staphylococcus epidermidis*, by Gram-negative enteric bacilli, enterococci (faecal streptococci) and *Staphylococcus aureus*.

The most commonly used regimens are:

- a penicillin and an aminoglycoside (the penicillin is usually a semi-synthetic penicillinase-resistant penicillin such as cloxacillin or methicillin since staphylococcal infection is a particular problem);
- a semi-synthetic anti-staphylococcal penicillin plus a third-generation cephalosporin;
- vancomycin plus an aminoglycoside or third-generation cephalosporin if methicillin-resistant *S. aureus* (MRSA) or coagulase-negative staphylococci are a problem;
- third-generation cephalosporin alone.

The disadvantages of using aminoglycosides are their potential to cause ototoxicity and nephrotoxicity and the consequent need to monitor drug levels. The third-generation cephalosporins do not need to be monitored and penetrate CSF well, but their use often leads to widespread colonization and sometimes sepsis with enterococci, while they provide relatively poor cover against staphylococci, so should not be used alone. Furthermore, widespread use of cephalosporins may lead rapidly to resistance [47], although this is not always the case [48]. The disadvantage of vancomycin use is the danger of vancomycin-resistant organisms, particularly enterococci. Although almost all coagulase-negative staphylococci are methicillin resistant [49], infections with these organisms are rarely fulminant and gentamicin has some anti-staphylococcal activity. If there is no MRSA colonization, cloxacillin may be preferred to vancomycin for initial empirical therapy, together with an aminoglycoside or third-generation cephalosporin, changing to vancomycin only if there is proven sepsis with a methicillin-resistant organism.

Since there are increasing problems with the introduction of multiresistant organisms, our preferred regimen in Oxford and Sydney in the absence of MRSA is cloxacillin (or equivalent) and gentamicin. In general, different antibiotics will be needed for treating babies with meningitis (see Chapter 8), so it is important, as discussed in Chapter 5, to do a lumbar puncture before starting antibiotics.

Treat according to the organisms colonizing the baby

Sprunt and colleagues [50] found that nasopharyngeal coloniization preceded the onset of systemic sepsis and that sepsis was almost always due to the colonizing organism. This has been used as one of the rationales for widespread and expensive surveillance of the organisms colonizing babies in the nursery. However, the value of surveillance cultures in this context has been questioned [45,46]. Isaacs and co-workers did not find any false-positive surface cultures in 26 babies with late-onset septicaemia (i.e. no babies were colonized *only* with organisms other than the invading one) but only 10 of the septic babies had positive surface cultures, giving a sensitivity of 39% for such cultures in predicting the organism causing sepsis, and 5 of the 10 were colonized with multiple organisms [45].

Evans and colleagues [46] showed that surface cultures taken on the day of sepsis had a sensitivity of 56% and that this fell to 50% for cultures taken 1 day before sepsis, 32% 2 days before and <30% for cultures taken earlier than this. Furthermore, they found a number of false-positive or misleading surveillance cultures.

Surveillance cultures are poor predictors of which babies will become infected, poor predictors of which organisms will cause systemic sepsis, and not infrequently will wrongly identify the organism causing sepsis.

Treat according to the prevalent organisms colonizing babies in the neonatal unit

It would be suspected that basing the choice of antibiotics for treating one baby on the organisms found to be colonizing other babies in the nursery would be even less sensitive and specific than if the decision were based on the baby's own colonizing organisms. Nevertheless, when there is widespread colonization with one organism, for example a gentamicin-resistant Gram-negative rod, it might be rational to treat all babies who develop suspected sepsis with an antibiotic that will cover this organism. White and colleagues, however, found substantial fluctuations in colonization rates of ampicillin- and gentamicin-resistant organisms and no correlation of patterns of colonization with episodes of sepsis [44]. Isaacs *et al.* reported similar fluctuations in the rates of colonization with gentamicin-resistant organisms. As these bacteria rarely caused systemic sepsis, we continued to use gentamicin until babies developed systemic sepsis with resistant organisms [45].

In Oxford and Sydney we regularly review the results of blood cultures and limited surveillance cultures (an endotracheal aspirate taken once weekly from each ventilated baby only) and change our antibiotic policy if widespread colonization with resistant organisms is accompanied by episodes of systemic sepsis with the resistant organism (see below). It could be argued that the surveillance endotracheal cultures are superfluous, but we prefer to know which organisms are colonizing the respiratory tract of our sickest babies. However, the most prevalent organisms may be gut-associated, e.g. Gramnegative enterics, in which case stool cultures would be more relevant.

WHEN TO CHANGE THE UNIT ANTIBIOTIC POLICY

The unit antibiotic policy will need changing when babies develop systemic sepsis with a resistant organism. Colonization with resistant organisms alone is not sufficient to warrant changing the antibiotic policy, although if the sickest, highest risk babies are all heavily colonized with a resistant organism, this is certainly a worrying situation.

Although routine surveillance cultures are advocated far less than before, they may be indicated in special circumstances. In Oxford in 1988 there was widespread colonization with a gentamicin-resistant strain of *Klebsiella*. It was known that all the intubated babies had endotracheal tube colonization with this organism. When two babies developed systemic sepsis with the *Klebsiella*, the aminoglycoside for treating suspected late sepsis was changed from gentamicin to netilmicin until the problem resolved, then promptly changed back to gentamicin.

In Sydney in 1996 there was an outbreak of systemic sepsis with a multiresistant *Klebsiella* which was gut-associated, and five of the six patients had underlying bowel abnormalities. In this outbreak, stool cultures were used to screen for colonized babies (see Chapter 18). The regimen for late sepsis was changed to imipenem and vancomycin until the outbreak resolved. In an MRSA outbreak, vancomycin will need to be used.

HOW MANY CASES CONSTITUTE AN OUTBREAK?

The first case of sepsis with a resistant organism should be a warning. A decision has to be made whether to screen other babies for colonization of respiratory or gastrointestinal tract. It may not be appropriate to screen immediately, but a second case certainly indicates that widespread colonization is likely. Babies should be screened for colonization with the resistant organism, or the unit antibiotic policy should be changed to a regimen that is effective against the resistant organism.

WHEN TO CHANGE BACK TO THE OLD POLICY

Changing the unit antibiotic policy reduces 'antibiotic pressure' and the resistant organism often disappears within weeks. The antibiotic policy can be changed back to the previously favoured one when there have been no cases of sepsis with the resistant organism for at least, say, 2 weeks. The policy on isolation of colonized babies and screening will be discussed in detail in Chapter 18.

DURATION OF ANTIBIOTICS

An important corollary of the liberal use of antibiotics for suspected sepsis is that they should be stopped as early as possible if cultures prove negative. It used to be argued that stopping antibiotics before completing a 'full course' would select for antibiotic-resistant organisms; on the contrary, there is evidence that resistant organisms are selected by long courses of antibiotics [51]. Furthermore, babies who receive antibiotics for longer than 72 hours are more likely to become colonized with Gram-negative enteric organisms [52]. As 96% of positive blood cultures have grown within 48 hours and 98% within 72 hours [53], it is advisable to stop antibiotics after 2–3 days' treatment if cultures are sterile. This policy has proved to be practical and not associated with missed cases of sepsis or clinical deterioration [54].

The advantages of this approach are that antibiotics are used for a short duration, thereby reducing selection of resistant organisms, colonization with abnormal oropharyngeal and bowel flora [52] and the risks of systemic candidiasis and aminoglycoside toxicity.

In addition, there are cost savings [54] both from using fewer antibiotics and from rarely having to measure drug levels; aminoglycoside levels are not usually measured unless antibiotics are continued beyond 72 hours. This approach has led to a 25–40% reduction in the average duration of antibiotic therapy (see Figure 18.1).

COMMON PROBLEMS

Some frequently encountered problems regarding the use of antibiotics in different situations are discussed below.

BABY LOOKED SEPTIC, BUT CULTURES WERE NEGATIVE

It is not known how often false-negative blood cultures occur in the neonatal period, i.e. no growth from blood cultures despite bacteraemia. Neonatal bacteraemia is characterized by relatively large numbers of circulating organisms and therefore only small volumes of blood are needed to obtain a positive blood culture, which might suggest that false-negative cultures would be rare.

Nevertheless, negative blood cultures where the circumstantial evidence for sepsis is strong are common. In one study, blood cultures pre-mortem were negative in seven of 39 babies

(18%) who died from infection [55]. In a study of babies with early-onset pneumonia, 11 were identified who had blood cultures which grew group B streptococci, and also nine babies who were heavily colonized with group B streptococci, and had sterile blood cultures [4]; this latter group almost certainly had pneumonia. Most of them would probably have had GBS antigen detected in concentrated urine [8], but that test was not performed. Thus, the sensitivity of blood culture in GBS pneumonia is only 55%. We have also seen two babies with the clinical features of congenital listeriosis who were heavily colonized with *Listeria monocytogenes*, but whose blood cultures were negative. In babies with neonatal meningitis, 15–55% have negative (presumably false negative) blood cultures [56,57].

Early-onset sepsis arises as a result of ascending or transplacental infection and heavy colonization almost invariably occurs concomitantly with septicaemia. If a baby with strongly suspected early-onset sepsis but negative systemic cultures (blood, urine, CSF) is heavily colonized with a probable pathogen such as group B streptococcus, *Listeria* or *E. coli,* it seems reasonable to continue a full course of antibiotics as if for proven sepsis. Conversely, if surface cultures as well as systemic cultures are negative, early-onset sepsis is unlikely and antibiotics can be stopped after 48–72 hours [54].

In suspected late-onset sepsis, colonization with potential pathogens is a poor indicator of sepsis because colonization is extremely common in asymptomatic babies [46]. It has been shown that stopping antibiotics after 48–72 hours is safe in late-onset sepsis and that babies do not subsequently need to be restarted on antibiotics [54]. Far too often, antibiotics are continued despite negative cultures because the baby 'looked septic'. Since the signs of sepsis are non-specific, this seems irrational, and antibiotics could be stopped after 2–3 days.

CULTURES NEGATIVE, MOTHER HAD INTRAPARTUM ANTIBIOTICS

Increasingly, women in labour are being treated with intrapartum antibiotics. We have discussed the problems of deciding which of their babies should be treated, without reaching any firm conclusions, since there are no data. Similarly, once antibiotics have been started, it is often difficult to decide how long to continue them. Intrapartum antibiotics prevent GBS septicaemia, but also reduce the proportion of babies colonized from 50% to 10% [15]. The worry is that they may increase the number of false-negative blood cultures. If superficial and systemic cultures (ear, blood) are sterile after 48–72 hours and GBS antigenuria is not detected, it seems reasonable to stop antibiotics. They should be continued for 7–10 days if GBS antigenuria is present, and probably also if the superficial cultures show heavy colonization and the clinical picture was suggestive of sepsis.

The Centers for Disease Control consider that babies under 35 weeks' gestation born after maternal intrapartum antibiotics for GBS should be treated empirically (Figure 6.1).

POSITIVE BLOOD CULTURES, DUBIOUS ORGANISM

A common scenario is that the doctor has to decide whether or not a baby with a doubtful blood culture result requires a full course of antibiotics. Certain organisms are relatively common contaminants of blood cultures, contamination occurring either in taking blood from the baby or subsequently in the laboratory. Common, relatively common and rare contaminants are shown in Table 6.2 and, as might be expected, the commonest are organisms that colonize skin. Multiple organisms in blood cultures are usually, but not always, contaminants. As septicaemia is generally associated with large numbers of bacteria and contamination of blood cultures is generally associated with small numbers, rapid growth of an organism in both aerobic and anaerobic blood culture bottles is more likely to indicate true

Significance	Organisms
Almost always significant	Group B streptococcus
	Streptococcus pneumoniae
	Listeria monocytogenes
	Haemophilus influenzae
	Group A streptococcus
	Group C/G streptococci
	Neisseria meningitidis
	Neisseria gonorrhoeae
	Gram-negative bacilli
	Candida and other fungi
Sometimes significant (about 50%)	*Staphylococcus aureus*
	Coagulase-negative staphylococci
	(*S. epidermidis*, etc.)
	Enterococci (*Streptococcus faecalis*,
	S. faecium, S. bovis, etc.)
	Streptococcus viridans group
	(including *S. mitis, S. mitior,*
	S. milleri, S. sanguis, etc.)
	Multiple isolates (polymicrobial)
Almost always contaminants	Diphtheroids
	Propionibacterium
	Bacillus species

Table 6.2 Significance of blood culture isolates

septicaemia, whereas delayed growth in a single bottle is more likely to be due to contamination. Nevertheless, contaminants may grow in both bottles, and only one bottle may grow up in true sepsis. Some laboratories can perform quantitative or semi-quantitative blood cultures, which are the best way to distinguish contamination from sepsis. As quantitative cultures are time-consuming and expensive, they are scarcely ever available except as part of a research project.

It is always important to interpret blood culture results in the context of the clinical picture, and additional tests such as total and differential white cell count, platelet count and serum CRP can be helpful. It should be noted that certain organisms are rare contaminants and should generally be taken seriously;

for example, in disseminated candidiasis it is common to find that there has been earlier growth of *Candida* from a blood culture, which has been dismissed as a probable contaminant [58].

It is always helpful to know, and preferably for the doctor taking the blood cultures to record in the notes, from whence the blood was drawn (vein, artery, through an umbilical or peripheral cannula) and the indications for taking blood. We have seen a baby whose blood culture taken 1 hour after birth grew *Staphylococcus aureus*, an unlikely early-onset pathogen. On questioning, the doctor was honest enough to admit to having aspirated blood that leaked out of the vein onto the baby's skin after a difficult venepuncture. Polymicrobial bacteraemia is suspicious of contamination; after one such example it was discovered that junior doctors were using a 'broken needle' (a 23-gauge metal needle with the plastic hub broken off) to collect blood, which was dripped into specimen bottles. This useful technique for taking blood samples was also being used to take blood cultures by dripping the blood into the barrel of a syringe and needle from which the plunger had been removed. The plunger was then replaced to inject the blood into blood culture bottles.

Sometimes a syringeful of blood is collected and some of the sample is injected into the porthole of a blood gas machine, which is often heavily contaminated, before filling blood culture bottles (which, because of their vacuum tend to suck in the whole sample). Similarly, if blood is first injected into fluid-containing bottles such as ESR, clotting or urea and electrolyte bottles, even if the needle is changed before filling the blood culture bottles, water-loving organisms such as *Pseudomonas maltophilia* or *Acinetobacter* may grow. If this technique is repeated often, there can be an apparent outbreak of sepsis or 'pseudo-bacteraemia'.

If it is decided that the blood culture isolate is a contaminant, antibiotics should be stopped or, in the rare cases in which antibiotics have not been started, the blood cultures repeated. It is always wise to repeat the blood cultures, even if the baby seems well, because cases have been described of asymptomatic but persistent bacteraemia [59]. It should be remembered that neonates are extremely susceptible to infection and may become infected with organisms of low virulence. *Staphylococcus epidermidis*, which used to be considered only a contaminant, is increasingly recognized as a neonatal pathogen and babies may be infected with anaerobes secondary to chorioamnionitis. Thus, blood culture results must always be interpreted with care and in the appropriate clinical context.

SEPTICAEMIA

If the baby is clinically septic and has positive blood cultures or a positive urine GBS antigen test, a full 'course' of antibiotics should be prescribed. There are no firm data on the correct duration of antibiotics for proven sepsis, as recurrence is rare. In the opinion of most authors, 7–10 days of antibiotics is appropriate, although it would be advisable to continue longer if the baby remained ill. *Listeria* septicaemia should be treated for 14 days because it is an intracellular pathogen, and meningitis requires longer antibiotic therapy (see Chapter 8).

Most antibiotic regimens incorporate a penicillin (penicillin G, ampicillin or a semi-synthetic penicillin such as cloxacillin) and an aminoglycoside. Even if a baby is shown to have, say, GBS sepsis, the aminoglycoside is often continued because of the theoretical advantage, rather than any proven clinical benefits, of synergy between penicillin and aminoglycoside.

The toxic effects of aminoglycosides are cumulative, particularly after 7 days of treatment, and it is important to stop the aminoglycoside if a baby is infected with a penicillin-sensitive organism (group B streptococcus, *Listeria*, etc.) as soon as there is sustained clinical improvement, usually after 2 or 3 days.

In approximately 30% of episodes of neonatal septicaemia, there is concurrent bacterial meningitis. If a lumbar puncture was not performed in the initial investigations of sepsis because the baby's respiratory status was too unstable, or because that is the unit's policy, and blood cultures are positive, it is imperative to perform one as soon as possible. Even if this will not alter the antibiotics used, or the dose, it will affect the duration of antibiotics (see Chapter 8), and the earlier the lumbar puncture can be done, the easier it will be to interpret the CSF findings.

SUMMARY

- Start antibiotics early; stop them early.
- Babies with early-onset respiratory distress should receive antibiotics if they have one or more maternal risk factors: spontaneous onset of preterm labour (<37 weeks), maternal fever (>37.5°C), prolonged rupture of membranes (>18 hours).
- Spontaneous onset of preterm labour is the commonest risk factor for sepsis, and the one most often forgotten by junior doctors.
- Antibiotic use should be as narrow spectrum as possible to cover likely organisms, not broad spectrum.
- Penicillin or ampicillin and an aminoglycoside is preferred for early-onset sepsis.
- Cloxacillin or methicillin and an aminoglycoside is preferred for late-onset sepsis, unless there is widespread colonization with MRSA (use vancomycin and an aminoglycoside) or with other resistant organisms.
- Antibiotics should be stopped after 2–3 days if blood cultures are negative, even if the baby 'looked septic'; the exception would be if early-onset sepsis seemed likely and the baby was heavily colonized with a likely pathogen (GBS, *Listeria*) or GBS antigenuria was present.

   Antibiotics should be continued for 7–10 days for proven septicaemia with most organisms (blood culture positive or GBS antigenuria), 14 days for *Listeria* septicaemia,

2–3 weeks for GBS meningitis and at least 21 days for Gram-negative meningitis.

- Prophylactic nystatin reduces fungal colonization and infection in babies under 1250 g birthweight.
- Prophylactic antibiotics are rarely indicated, but possible indications are maternal hypertension-induced neutropenia and urinary tract abnormalities.

References

1 Boyer KM, Gadzala CA, Burd LI et al. Selective intrapartum chemoprophylaxis of group B streptococcal early-onset disease. I. Epidemiologic rationale. J Infect Dis 1983; **148**: 795–801.

2 Bortolussi R, Thompson TR & Ferrieri, P. Early-onset pneumococcal sepsis in newborn infants. Pediatrics 1977; **60**: 352–5.

3 Dobson SRM & Baker CJ. Enterococcal sepsis in neonates: features by age at onset and occurrence of focal infection. Pediatrics 1990; **85**: 165–71.

4 Webber S, Lindsell D, Wilkinson AR et al. Neonatal pneumonia. Arch Dis Child 1990; **65**: 207–11.

5 Leslie GI, Scurr RD & Barr PA. Early-onset bacterial pneumonia: a comparison with severe hyaline membrane disease. Aust Paediatr J 1981; **17**: 202–6.

6 Rozycki HJ, Stahl GE & Baumgart S. Impaired sensitivity of a single early leukocyte count in screening for neonatal sepsis. Pediatr Infect Dis J 1987; **6**: 440–2.

7 Philip AGS & Hewitt JR. Early diagnosis of neonatal sepsis. Pediatrics 1980; **65**: 1036–41.

8 Baker CJ & Edwards MS. Group B streptococcal infections. In: Remington JS & Klein JO (eds) Infectious Diseases of the Fetus and Newborn Infant, 3rd edn. Philadelphia: WB Saunders, 1990: 742–811.

9 Mifsud A, Seal D, Wall R & Valman B. Reduced neonatal mortality from infection after introduction of respiratory monitoring. BMJ 1988; **296**: 17–18.

10 Ingram DL, Pengergrass EL, Bromberger PI et al. Group B streptococcal disease: its diagnosis with use of antigen detection, Gram's stain, and the presence of apnea, hypotension. Am J Dis Child 1980; **134**: 754–8.

11 Sherman MP, Goetzman BW, Ahlfors CE & Wennberg RP. Tracheal aspiration and its clinical correlates in the diagnosis of congenital pneumonia. *Pediatrics* 1980; **65**: 258–63.

12 Sherman MP, Chance KH & Goetzman BW. Gram's stains of tracheal secretions predict neonatal bacteremia. *Am J Dis Child* 1984; **138**: 848–50.

13 Jeffery HE & McIntosh EDG. Antenatal sereening and non-selective intrapartum chemoprophylaxis for group B streptococcus. *Aust NZ J Obstet Gynaecol* 1994; **34**: 14–19.

14 Gilbert GL, Isaacs D, Burgess MA et al. Prevention of neonatal group B streptococcal sepsis: Is routine antenatal screening appropriate? *Aust NZ J Obstet Gynaecol* 1995; **35**: 120–6.

15 Boyer KM & Gotoff SP. Prevention of early-onset neonatal group B streptococcal disease with selective intrapartum chemoprophylaxis. *N Engl J Med* 1986; **314**: 1665–9.

16 American Academy of Pediatrics. Revised guidelines for prevention of early-onset group B streptococcal (GBS) infection. *Pediatrics* 1997; **99**: 489–96.

17 Gluck L, Wood HF & Fousek MD. Septicemia of the newborn. *Pediatr Clin North Am* 1966; **13**: 1131–48.

18 Manroe BL, Weinberg AG, Rosenfeld CR et al. The neonatal blood count in health and disease. I. Reference values for neutrophilic cells. *J Pediatr* 1979; **95**: 89–98.

19 Rodwell RL, Taylor KM, Tudehope DI & Gray PH. Hematologic scoring system in early diagnosis of sepsis in neutropenic newborns. *Pediatr Infect Dis J* 1993; **12**: 372–6.

20 Koenig JM & Christensen RD. Incidence, neutrophil kinetics, and natural history of neonatal neutropenia associated with maternal hypertension. *N Engl J Med* 1989; **321**: 557–62.

21 Mouzinho A, Rosenfeld CR, Sancher PJ & Risser R. Effect of maternal hypertension on neonatal neutropenia and risk of nosocomial infection. *Pediatrics* 1992; **90**: 430–5.

22 Doron MW, Makhlouf RA, Katz VL, Lawson EE & Stiles AD. Increased incidence of sepsis at birth in neutropenic infants of mothers with preeclampsia. *J Pediatr* 1994; **125**: 452–8.

23 Lloyd BW & Oto A. Normal values for mature and immature neutrophils in very preterm babies. *Arch Dis Child* 1982; **57**: 233–5.

24 Nelson JD. Control of infection acquired in the nursery. In: Remington JS & Klein JO (eds) *Infectious Diseases of the Fetus and Newborn Infant*, 2nd edn. Philadelphia: WB Saunders, 1983: 1035–52.

25 Harris H, Wirtshaffer D & Cassady G. Endotracheal intubation and its relationship to bacterial colonization and systemic infection of newborn infants. *Pediatrics* 1976; **58**: 816–23.

26 Slagle TA, Bifano EM, Wolf JW & Gross SJ. Routine endotracheal cultures for the prediction of sepsis in ventilated babies. *Arch Dis Child* 1989; **64**: 34–8.

27 Baley JE & Fanaroff AA. Neonatal infections. In: Sinclair JC & Bracken MB (eds) *Effective Care of the Newborn Infant*. Oxford: Oxford University Press, 1992: 454–75.

28 Editorial. Cerebrospinal fluid shunt infections. *Lancet* 1989; **i**: 1304–5.

29 Sims ME, Yoo Y, You H *et al*. Prophylactic oral nystatin and fungal infections in very-low-birth weight infants. *Am J Perinatol* 1988; **5**: 33–6.

30 Gray JE, Richardson DK, McCormick MC & Goldmann DA. Coagulase-negative staphylococcal bacteremia among very low birthweight infants: relation to admission illness severity, resource use and outcome. *Pediatrics* 1995; **95**: 225–30.

31 Schwartz C, Henrickson KJ, Roghman K & Powell K. Prevention of bacteraemia attributed to luminal colonisation of tunnelled central venous catheters with vancomycin-susceptible organisms. *J Clin Oncol* 1990; **8**: 1591–7.

32 Moller JC, Nachtrodt G, Richter A & Tegtmeyer FK. Prophylactic vancomycin to prevent staphylococcal septicaemia in very low birth weight infants. *Lancet* 1992; **340**: 424.

33 Kacica MA, Morgan MJ, Venezia RA, Yocum RA, Ochoa L & Lepon M. Prevention of Gram positive bacteraemia with low dose vancomycin infusion. *Pediatr Res* 1992; **32**: 278.

34 Kacica MA, Morgan MJ, Sandler R, Leplow ML & Venezia RA. Prevention of Gram positive sepsis in neonates weighing less than 1500 grams. *J Pediatr* 1994; **125**: 253–8.

35 Spafford PS, Sinkin RA, Cox C, Reubens L & Powell KR. Prevention of central venous catheter related coagulase negative staphylococcal sepsis in neonates. *J Pediatr* 1994; **125**: 259–63.

36 Gin AS & Zhanel GG. Vancomycin-resistant enterococci. *Ann Pharmacother* 1996; **30**: 615–24.

37 Barefield ES & Philips JB. Vancomycin prophylaxis for coagulase-negative staphylococcal bacteremia. *J Pediatr* 1994; **125**: 230–2.

38 Macfarlane DE. Neonatal group B streptococcal septicaemia in a developing country. *Acta Paediatr Scand* 1987; **76**: 470–3.

39 Tullus K & Burman LG. Ecological impact of ampicillin and cefuroxime in neonatal units. *Lancet* 1989; **i**: 1405–7.

40 Davey P. Aminoglycosides and neonatal deafness. *Lancet* 1985; **ii**: 612.

41 Isaacs D, Catterson J, Hope PL *et al*. Factors influencing colonisation with gentamicin resistant Gram negative organisms in the neonatal unit. *Arch Dis Child* 1988; **63**: 533–5.

42 Finitzo-Heiber T, McCracken GH & Brown KC. Prospective controlled evaluation of auditory function in neonates given netilmicin or amikacin. *J Pediatr* 1985; **106**: 129–36.

43 Isaacs D & Wilkinson AR. Antibiotic use in the neonatal unit. *Arch Dis Child* 1987; **62**: 204–8.

44 White RD, Townsend TR, Stephens MA & Moxon ER. Are surveillance of resistant enteric bacilli and antimicrobial usage among neonates in a newborn intensive care unit useful? *Pediatrics* 1981; **68**: 1–4.

45 Isaacs D, Wilkinson AR & Moxon ER. Surveillance of colonisation and late-onset septicaemia in neonates. *J Hosp Infect* 1987; **10**: 114–19.

46 Evans ME, Schaffner W, Federspiel CF *et al.* Sensitivity, specificity and predictive value of body surface cultures in a neonatal intensive care unit. *JAMA* 1988; **259**: 248–52.

47 Modi N, Damjanovic V & Cooke RW. Outbreak of cephalosporin resistant *Enterobacter cloacae* infection in a neonatal intensive care unit. *Arch Dis Child* 1987; **62**: 148–51.

48 Spritzer R, Kamp HJVD, Dzolvic G & Sauer PJJ. Five years of cefotaxime use in a neonatal intensive care unit. *Pediatr Infect Dis J* 1990; **9**: 92–6.

49 Isaacs D, Barfield C, Clothier T *et al.* Late onset infections of infants in neonatal units. *J Paediatr Child Health* 1996; **32**: 158–61.

50 Sprunt K, Redman W & Leidy G. Antibacterial effectiveness of routine hand-washing. *Pediatrics* 1973; **52**: 264–7.

51 Lacey RW. Evolution of microorganisms and antibiotic resistance. *Lancet* 1984; **ii**: 1022–5.

52 Goldmann DA, Leclair J & Macone A. Bacterial colonization of neonates admitted to an intensive care unit. *J Pediatr* 1978; **69**: 193–7.

53 Pichichero MD & Todd JK. Detection of neonatal bacteremia. *J Pediatr* 1979; **94**: 958–60.

54 Isaacs D, Wilkinson AR & Moxon ER. Duration of antibiotic courses for neonates. *Arch Dis Child* 1987; **62**: 727–8.

55 Squire E, Favara B & Todd J. Diagnosis of neonatal bacterial infection: hematologic and pathologic findings in fatal and non-fatal cases. *Pediatrics* 1979; **64**: 60–4.

56 McIntyre P & Isaacs D. Lumbar puncture in suspected neonatal sepsis. *J Paediatr Child Health* 1995; **31**: 1–2.

57 Wiswell TE, Baumgart S, Gannon CM & Spitzer AR. No lumbar puncture in the evaluation for early neonatal sepsis: will meningitis be missed? *Pediatrics* 1995; **95**: 803–6.

58 Weese-Mayer DE, Fondriest DW, Brouillette RT & Shulman ST. Risk factors associated with candidemia in the neonatal intensive care unit: a case–control study. *Pediatr Infect Dis J* 1987; **6**: 190–6.
59 Albers WH, Tyler CW & Boxerbaum B. Asymptomatic bacteremia in the newborn infant. *J Pediatr* 1966; **69**: 193–7.

7 | Supportive therapy for septic babies

INTRODUCTION

Despite the undoubted importance of specific antimicrobial therapy against pathogenic microbes, the role of other facets of the management of sepsis should not be underestimated: antimicrobials are only one aspect of the treatment of the septic baby. Because of real or perceived difficulties in recruiting sufficient babies and organizing controlled trials, many of the possible adjunctive therapies have not been critically evaluated and their use remains controversial.

TREATMENT OF SHOCK

It is necessary to assess whether a septic baby is shocked and, if it is, to take immediate steps to reverse this. The diagnosis of shock is based on a clinical picture of pallor, paucity of movement, poor peripheral perfusion (as shown, for example, by slow return of colour when a digit is pressed) and tachycardia with poorly palpable pulses. Hypotension is not necessarily present, as peripheral vasoconstriction may maintain an adequate blood pressure despite hypovolaemia. There is oliguria or anuria. The rectal temperature is often low (<35.5°C) [1]. The peripheral core temperature gradient is a less useful indicator of shock in neonates than in older children [1].

The immediate use of fresh frozen plasma, 10–20 ml/kg given i.v. and repeated until shock is reversed, employs a physiological fluid that contains immunoglobulins and clotting factors. Plasma substitutes can be used until the fresh frozen plasma is thawed or if none is available. If there is significant bleeding, as for example in association with disseminated intravascular coagulopathy (DIC), it is more appropriate to use fresh blood for volume replacement.

If the baby remains shocked despite adequate fluid replacement, or if cardiac output is profoundly depressed, it may be beneficial to use a continuous infusion of dopamine at 2–10 µg/kg per hour to improve myocardial function and renal perfusion. Infusion rates higher than 10 µg/kg per hour divert blood from the kidneys and are counterproductive. Central venous pressure monitoring is important in determining whether or not fluid replacement has been adequate, before using dopamine.

Echocardiography, if available, can be used to evaluate left ventricular function and, if myocardial contractility is depressed, can indicate the need for dopamine.

ARTIFICIAL VENTILATORY SUPPORT

Babies with severe sepsis, if not already shocked, are often in imminent danger of cardiovascular collapse, which may be prevented by initiating artificial ventilation. Early elective intubation and ventilation of septic babies is an important supportive measure that is often neglected. Too often, severely ill babies are given antimicrobials and watched in the hope that they will not need artificial ventilation; some recover, but others collapse and need emergency resuscitation for mixed metabolic and respiratory acidosis.

CORRECTION OF METABOLIC ACIDOSIS

Metabolic acidosis commonly accompanies systemic sepsis. When this is severe, many neonatal units use sodium bicarbonate to correct the acidosis, which impairs normal cell metabolism. The policy in the John Radcliffe Hospital, Oxford is to use the buffered alkali tris-hydroxymethyl aminomethane (THAM) as part of the management of metabolic acidosis if the base deficit exceeds 10, because $PaCO_2$ rises less with THAM than when sodium bicarbonate is used. If sodium bicarbonate is used, it should be with caution because of its hypertonicity; we use it diluted 1:1 with 5% dextrose. Excessive use can cause hypernatraemia and hypercarbia. The latter may precipitate respiratory failure by depressing respiratory drive and can lead to the need for urgent respiratory support.

HYPOGLYCAEMIA

Hypoglycaemia may accompany sepsis, particularly in babies who have also had perinatal asphyxia, and should be urgently corrected. Intravenous dextrose should be given if the blood glucose concentration falls below 2.6 mmol/L.

THROMBOCYTOPENIA

Significant thrombocytopenia may accompany sepsis. Thrombocytopenia may be caused by bone marrow suppression or by peripheral destruction of platelets. The latter may be due to the toxic effect of bacterial factors such as lipopolysaccharide (endotoxin), to peripheral immune platelet destruction or to DIC. Platelet transfusions are needed if significant bleeding accompanies thrombocytopenia or if thrombocytopenia is severe enough (usually $<20 \times 10^9$/L) to threaten haemorrhage.

CONVULSIONS

Convulsions accompany about one-half of all cases of meningitis, but may also occur in severe sepsis without meningitis. Convulsions are often subclinical or difficult to diagnose. Where these are a strong possibility, and particularly if the baby is receiving muscle relaxants, continuous EEG monitoring if available, or serial EEGs may enable the diagnosis to be made and allow monitoring of the response to anticonvulsants.

NEUTROPHIL TRANSFUSIONS

Christensen has been the keenest advocate of neutrophil transfusions for those babies with severe sepsis who are neutropenic and who have depleted bone marrow neutrophil reserves, as shown by bone marrow examination. He has shown that transfusions of fresh neutrophils to septic neutropenic puppies can improve their survival rate. In a study in which neutropenic septic babies were randomly assigned to treatment with neutrophil transfusions or no neutrophil transfusions, all seven treated babies, but only one of nine untreated babies, survived [2]. Two other studies have shown improved survival of septic infants given neutrophil transfusions, even in the absence of neutropenia [3,4]. In a trial comparing neutrophil transfusions with intravenous immunoglobulin, the mortality rate was 0 of 21 neutrophil transfusion babies, but 5 of 14 babies receiving i.v. immunoglobulin [5]. On the other hand, Baley and colleagues found no improvement in a small randomized controlled trial of buffy coat neutrophil transfusions to neutropenic neonates, some of whom were septic [6].

The number of babies studied has been small and, although no adverse effects have been reported, there are a number of theoretical risks such as sensitization, graft-versus-host reactions and transmission of viruses such as cytomegalovirus (CMV). In addition, there are considerable logistical problems. Neutrophils for transfusion have to be obtained fresh by leucophoresis of one of an identified panel of donors who have to be screened regularly for CMV and HIV antibodies and who are available to be called at short notice. The process of leucophoresis is also time-consuming, causing several hours' delay before neutrophils are available. In our experience, neutropenic sepsis is so rare (one or two cases a year) that the Blood Transfusion Service in Oxford, which does not prepare neutrophil transfusions for other patients, is, quite reasonably, not prepared to offer such a service. There is insufficient evidence to recommend the use of neutrophil transfusions for all babies with suspected sepsis.

COLONY-STIMULATING FACTORS

Colony-stimulating factors which promote granulocyte (G-CSF) or granulocyte and macrophage (GM-CSF) development can now be made by recombinant technology. Recombinant preparations are available. Their use is increasingly accepted for neutropenic oncology patients, and studies of colony-stimulating factors in neonates are being reported.

Three small studies have reported the use of G-CSF to treat babies with neutropenia (see Table 7.1) [7–9]. These studies were uncontrolled and showed improvements in neutropenia, but could not examine rates of sepsis or mortality. One study found exacerbation of thrombocytopenia in babies given G-CSF.

Gillan and co-workers randomized 42 babies with possible sepsis to G-CSF or placebo [10]. G-CSF was associated with a dose-dependent increase in the neutrophil storage pool and in neutrophil counts, but the rate of proven sepsis was much too low to examine the possible benefit of G-CSF in treating sepsis.

Cairo and colleagues used GM-CSF prophylactically in babies of 500–1000 g birthweight and their published abstract shows a significant ($P = 0.04$) reduction in nosocomial sepsis [11].

Overall, the role of G-CSF remains unproven, although it looks promising in the treatment of babies with neutropenia and possibly to prevent nosocomial sepsis in very small babies.

EXCHANGE TRANSFUSION

Exchange transfusion is performed fairly frequently for severe sepsis, but has never been subjected to a satisfactory randomized controlled trial, so its efficacy is difficult to evaluate.

Nature of study	Study	n	Babies	Control	Duration of CSF	Beneficial effects	Adverse effects
Treatment of neutropenia	[7]	12	Neutropenic, preterm	No	1–8 days G-CSF	Rise in neutrophil counts	Exacerbation of thrombocytopenia (two deaths from sepsis)
Treatment of neutropenia	[8]	4	Neutropenia for >3 days due to maternal hypertension	No	3 days G-CSF	Rise in neutrophil counts	None
Treatment of neutropenia	[9]	9	Neutropenia, low birthweight, maternal hypertension	No	1–3 days G-CSF	Rise in neutrophils within 6 hours in 8 of 9 babies. One dose gave sustained neutrophilia for >72 hours	
Treatment of sepsis	[10]	42	Babies <3 days old, 26–40 weeks' gestation, possible sepsis	Yes	3 days G-CSF	Dose-dependent increase in neutrophil storage pool and neutrophil count	None
Prophylaxis	[11]	29	Birthweight 500–1000 g	Yes	28 days GM-CSF	Reduction in nosocomial sepsis 4/29 (14%) vs 11/31 (35%) $P = 0.04$	None reported (abstract only)

Table 7.1 Studies of the use of recombinant human granulocyte colony-stimulating factors

There are reports of its use in treating septic neonates [12–15], but none included controls. In one uncontrolled study, seven of ten babies with severe sepsis and sclerema improved immediately after exchange transfusion, and survived [16]. Mathur *et al.* found an increase in neutrophil counts and function in septic, neutropenic babies treated with exchange transfusion [17].

Blood transfusion is less effective than exchange transfusion [14], presumably due to removal of toxins in the latter process, and the blood used for exchange should ideally be less than 24 hours old to optimize benefit from transfused neutrophils. In theory, there are many potential advantages to exchange transfusion: improvement of circulatory status; replacement of clotting factors and immunoglobulins (although these may be equally well served by plasma infusions); better oxygenation of the tissues by improving the oxygen-carrying capacity of the blood; and the removal of toxic bacterial products, such as endotoxin. Exchange transfusion may, however, cause untoward haemodynamic changes and it is probably best used only as a last resort.

IMMUNOGLOBULIN THERAPY

The prophylactic use of intravenous immunoglobulin preparations is discussed in Chapter 19. The relatively low serum levels of IgG in the neonate, particularly before 32 weeks' gestational age, suggest that there might be a role for immunoglobulin **therapy** to improve serum opsonic capacity, particularly in preterm babies [18].

Animal studies have suggested that intravenous immunoglobulins (IVIG), used as an adjunct to antibiotics, might have a role in treating established infection [19]. The role of IVIG in prophylaxis against infection is discussed in Chapter 19.

There have been surprisingly few studies of the therapeutic use of IVIG in human neonates. Sidiropoulos and co-workers randomized 35 neonates with proven infection to IVIG

(1 g daily × 6 days for full-term babies; 0.5 g daily × 6 days for preterm babies). Four of 15 babies (27%) in the control group died, compared with 2 of 20 IVIG-treated babies; this was not significant, but 4 of 9 preterm babies in the control group died, compared with 1 of 13 treated with IVIG ($P = 0.04$) [20]. Haque and colleagues randomized 60 preterm babies with suspected sepsis to antibiotics alone, or plus IgM-enriched IVIG [21]. This study, which was not blinded, showed a significant reduction in mortality rate, from 4 of 23 (17%) to 1 of 21 (5%) in the treatment group. In a small study of 22 septic preterm babies given 750 mg/kg IVIG in a single dose as an adjunct to antibiotics, no babies died, but IVIG therapy was often associated with immature cells being released from the bone marrow, rapid resolution of neutropenia and improvement in pulmonary function [22]. Cairo *et al.* compared granulocyte transfusions with 1 g/kg IVIG daily × 3 days for septic babies [5]. Nine of 14 (64%) of the IVIG group survived, but all 21 of the granulocyte transfusion babies survived. It is possible, however, that the dose of IVIG was too high: in experimental animals doses higher than 2 g/kg IVIG are detrimental [19].

Weisman *et al.* examined the effect of a single dose of 500 mg/kg IVIG in the treatment of early-onset sepsis in preterm neonates [23]. The IVIG was being given as part of a prophylaxis study, but 31 babies already had sepsis. Five of 17 placebo babies (29%), but none of 14 IVIG-treated babies had died within 7 days of birth ($P < 0.05$). However, there was no reduction in final mortality due to sepsis (5 of 30 placebo versus 2 of 14 IVIG).

A meta-analysis of the efficacy of IVIG in the treatment of sepsis in preterm babies considered that only the studies of Haque *et al.* [21] and Weisman *et al.* [23] met the inclusion criteria for randomized, controlled trials [24]. The relative risk of mortality from sepsis was 0.38 (95% confidence interval 0.12–1.19) in the IVIG groups in the two trials combined. Lacy and Ohlsson's conclusion [24] was that there was no proven benefit from IVIG treatment, but another conclusion could be that the two small studies lacked the numbers to have sufficient power. A relative risk of 0.38 means a 62% reduction in mortality rate, but the wide confidence intervals spanning unity means that the results are statistically non-significant.

Hill interprets the data more optimistically and recommends a single dose of IVIG 750 mg/kg in the septic-appearing neonate, especially if the baby has shock and severe neutropenia, perhaps repeated once 5–7 days later [19]. However, he acknowledges that this approach has little more scientific basis than giving the baby a kiss on the forehead.

REMOVAL OF INDWELLING CANNULAS

The incidence of sepsis with coagulase-negative staphylococci such as *Staphylococcus epidermidis* is rising in most neonatal units in the UK and elsewhere. In the neonatal units in Sydney, about one-half of the cases are associated with an indwelling umbilical arterial catheter (UAC) or a percutaneous intravenous silicone catheter ('central line'). A decision frequently must be made as to whether or not to remove an important line from a baby with suspected sepsis, who has poor vascular access. The two commonest scenarios are the *acute* presentation, in which the baby appears acutely septic with a UAC or silicone 'central line' *in situ*, and the *subacute* presentation in which the baby with such a line still in place has remained moderately unwell after 2 days on antibiotics and blood cultures are reported to be growing *S. epidermidis*. An individual assessment of the baby must be made, with particular reference to the degree of illness, changes in the white cell and platelet counts, and the necessity for the UAC or silicone intravenous catheter.

If the baby is shocked, neutropenic and thrombocytopenic, it is probably necessary to remove the vascular catheter and to treat the baby with antibiotics through peripheral venous cannulas. It should be remembered that, although *S. epidermidis* is the commonest cause of catheter-associated sepsis and generally causes a relatively mild illness, *Staphylococcus aureus* can also infect catheters and tends to cause a much more fulminating illness [25]. Gram-negative organisms and fungi less commonly infect catheters, but infections with fungi seldom resolve without catheter removal.

As *S. epidermidis* infection is rarely fulminant, several attempts have been made to treat babies who are only moderately unwell, and whose catheter is particularly vital for feeding and vascular access, by using antibiotics and leaving the catheter in place. Sadiq and colleagues described the management of catheter-associated infections in neonates who predominantly were preterm and often were of very low birthweight [26]; their experience is summarized in Table 7.2. In general, they were successful in managing *S. epidermidis* septicaemia without catheter removal, but only half the babies with methicillin-resistant *S. aureus* (MRSA) sepsis were successfully managed in this way.

Our current approach to suspected line-associated sepsis is as follows. If it is decided to treat a baby with antibiotics and to leave the catheter in place, the baby is constantly reviewed and, if there is any clinical deterioration, the catheter is

Organism cultured from blood	No. of cases	No. managed without catheter removal	No. managed successfully without catheter removal
Staphylococcus epidermidis	8	6	5
Methicillin-resistant *Staphylococcus aureus*	8	6	3
Candida albicans	4	0	0
Escherichia coli	2	2	2
Miscellaneous streptococci	4	4	4
Total	26	18	14
After ref. [26].			

Table 7.2 Management of catheter-associated infections in neonates

removed. If, after 48–72 hours, the blood cultures grow *S. epidermidis*, the baby is reassessed; if the baby is well, the catheter is left in place, antibiotics are continued and repeat blood cultures performed. The further management depends on the clinical picture and repeat blood culture results. If there is anything to suggest continuing sepsis, either clinically or in the form of decreasing white cell or platelet counts (the latter is a particularly useful indicator of continuing sepsis with *S. epidermidis*), and the organism is sensitive to the antibiotics being used, the catheter is removed. Vancomycin is used for babies infected with methicillin-resistant staphylococci who have continuing clinical evidence of infection. The catheter is removed if fungi are cultured (Chapter 15).

REMOVAL OF CSF SHUNT

CSF shunt infections in older children and adults will not resolve unless the shunt is removed [27]. Although this has not been formally confirmed in neonatal CSF shunt infections, it is generally accepted that the same principle applies, and that the infected shunt must be removed before the infection can be cured (see also Chapter 8).

SUMMARY

- Correction of shock is a priority.
- Hypoglycaemia should be sought and urgently corrected.
- Neutrophil transfusions may be helpful in babies with neutropenic sepsis, but are difficult to arrange.
- Exchange transfusion has not been proven to be of benefit in sepsis.
- There is some evidence that adjunctive therapy with intravenous immunoglobulin may be beneficial in sepsis.

References

1 Messaritakis J, Anagnostakis D, Laskari H & Katerelos C. Rectal-skin temperature difference in septicaemic newborn infants. *Arch Dis Child* 1990; **65**: 380–2.

2 Christensen RD, Rothstein G, Anstall HB & Bybee B. Granulocyte transfusions in newborns with bacterial infection, neutropenia and depletion of mature marrow neutrophils. *Pediatrics* 1982; **70**: 1–6.

3 Laurenti F, Ferro R, Isacchi G *et al.* Polymorphonuclear leukocyte transfusion for the treatment of sepsis in the newborn infant. *J Pediatr* 1981; **98**: 118–23.

4 Cairo MS, Rucker R, Bennetts GA *et al.* Improved survival of newborns receiving leukocyte transfusions for sepsis. *Pediatrics* 1984; **74**: 887–92.

5 Cairo MS, Worcester CC, Rucker RW *et al.* Randomized trial of granulocyte transfusions versus intravenous immune globulin therapy for neonatal neutropenia and sepsis. *J Pediatr* 1992; **120**: 281–5.

6 Baley JE, Stork EK, Warkentin PI & Shurin SB. Buffy coat transfusions in neutropenic neonates with presumed sepsis: a prospective, randomized trial. *Pediatrics* 1987; **80**: 712–20.

7 Russell AR, Davies EG, Ball SE & Gordon-Smith E. Granulocyte colony stimulating factor and treatment for neonatal neutropenia. *Arch Dis Child* 1995; **72**: F53.

8 La Gamma EF, Alpan O & Kocherlakota P. Effect of granulocyte colony-stimulating factor on preeclampsia-associated neonatal neutropenia. *J Pediatr* 1995; **126**: 457.

9 Makhlouf RA, Doron MW, Bose CL, Price WA & Stiles AD. Administration of granulocyte colony-stimulating factor to neu-tropenic low birthweight infants of mothers with preeclampsia. *J Pediatr* 1995; **126**: 454–6.

10 Gillan ER, Christensen RD, Suen Y, Ellis R, van de Ven C & Cairo MS. A randomized, placebo-controlled trial of recombinant human granulocyte colony-stimulating factor administration in newborn infants with presumed sepsis: significant induction of peripheral and bone marrow neutrophilia. *Blood* 1994; **84**: 1427–33.

11 Cairo MS, Seth T & Fanaroff A. A double blinded, randomized placebo controlled pilot study of RhGM-CSF in low birth weight neonates. *Pediatr Res* 1996; **39**: 294A.

12 Prodhom LS, Choffat JM, Frenck N, Relier JP & Torrado A. Care of the seriously ill neonate with hyaline membrane disease and with sepsis. *Pediatrics* 1964; **53**: 170–81.

13 Tollner F, Pohlandt F, Heinze F & Henrichs I. Treatment of septi-caemia in the newborn infant: choice of initial antimicrobial drugs and the role of exchange transfusions. *Acta Paediatr Scand* 1977; **66**: 605–10.

14 Narayanan I, Mitter A & Gujral VV. A comparative study on the value of exchange and blood transfusion in the management of severe neonatal septicaemia with sclerema. *Indian J Pediatr* 1982; **49**: 519–23.

15 Gottuso MA, Williams ML & Oski FA. The role of exchange transfusion in the management of low birth weight infants with and without severe respiratory distress syndrome. *J Pediatr* 1976; **89**: 279–85.

16 Vain ND, Mazlumian, JR, Swarner OW *et al.* Role of exchange transfusion in the treatment of severe septicemia. *Pediatrics* 1980; **66**: 693–7.

17 Mathur NB, Subramanian BKM, Sharma VK & Puri RK. Exchange transfusion in neutropenic septicemic neonates: effect on granulocyte functions. *Acta Paediatr* 1993; **82**: 939–43.

18 Whitelaw A. Treatment of sepsis with IgG in very low birth weight infants. *Arch Dis Child* 1990; **65**: 347–8.

19 Hill HR. Intravenous immunoglobulin use in the neonate: role in prophylaxis and therapy of infection. *Pediatr Infect Dis J* 1993; **12**: 549–58.

20 Sidiropoulos D, Boehme U, von Muralt G *et al.* Immunoglobulin-substitution bei der Behandling der neonatalen sepsis. *Schweiz Med Wochenschr* 1981; **111**: 1649–55.

21 Haque KN, Zaidi MH & Bahakim H. IgM-enriched intravenous immunoglobulin therapy in neonatal sepsis. *Am J Dis Child* 1988; **142**: 1293–6.

22 Christensen RD, Brown MS, Hall DC, Lassiter HA & Hill HR. Effect on neutrophil kinetics and serum opsonic activity of intravenous administration of immune globulin to neonates with clinical signs of early-onset sepsis. *J Pediatr* 1991; **118**: 606–14.

23 Weisman LE, Stoll BJ, Kueser TJ *et al.* Intravenous immune globulin therapy for early-onset sepsis in premature neonates. *J Pediatr* 1992; **121**: 434–43.

24 Lacy JB & Ohlsson A. Administration of intravenous immunoglobulins for prophylaxis or treatment of infection in preterm infants: meta-analyses. *Arch Dis Child* 1995; **72**: F151–5.

25 Decker MD & Edwards KM. Central venous catheter infections. *Pediatr Clin North Am* 1988; **35**: 579–612.

26 Sadiq HF, Devaskar S, Keenan WJ & Weber TR. Broviac catheterisation in low birth weight infants: incidence and treatment of associated complications. *Crit Care Med* 1987; **15**: 47–50.

27 Schoenbaum SC, Gardner P & Shillito J. Infections of cerebrospinal fluid shunts: epidemiology, clinical manifestations and therapy. *J Infect Dis* 1975; **131**: 543–52.

8 | Meningitis

INCIDENCE

Meningitis is more common in the first month postnatally than at any other age, and more common in the first week than later [1]. About 10–30% of cases of early-onset neonatal septicaemia and about 10% of late-onset cases are complicated by bacterial meningitis. In addition, viruses may cause meningitis or meningo-encephalitis, and fungal meningitis can occur in babies of very low birthweight. The incidence of neonatal bacterial meningitis is higher in infants of low birthweight; the reported incidence will therefore vary according to the population being studied. Whole population-based studies in the United States have consistently shown 0.2–0.5 cases of bacterial meningitis per 1000 live births [2]. The incidence of neonatal bacterial meningitis has remained constant in England and Wales at 0.25–0.32 cases per 1000 live births from 1969 until the early 1990s [3,4], while the minimum incidence in Australia was reported by Francis and Gilbert as 0.17 per 1000 [5]. In Oxford, the incidence of neonatal bacterial meningitis was 0.25 per 1000, viral meningitis was 0.11 per 1000, and fungal meningitis 0.02 per 1000 live births [4]. A study from Sweden suggests that, unlike other countries, the incidence of neonatal meningitis there may be falling [6].

In non-industrialized countries, the incidence of neonatal bacterial meningitis is usually higher than in industrialized countries. In Nigeria, the incidence was 1.9 per 1000 [7], it was 2.9 per 1000 in Trinidad, West Indies [8], while in Durban, South Africa the incidence fell from 1.3 per 1000 in 1981 to 0.95 per 1000 in 1981–86 and 0.22 per 1000 in 1987 [9].

Certain groups of babies are at greatly increased risk of meningitis irrespective of birthweight. Babies with open myelomeningoceles are particularly likely to develop bacterial meningitis, especially that attributable to Gram-negative enteric bacilli. CSF shunts are highly likely to become infected.

Dermal sinuses overlying the CSF anywhere from the bridge of the nose, over the skull and down the back to the sacrum may penetrate through to the dura and give rise to meningitis. If a dermal sinus is missed (and they can be very small and hidden under the hair), then recurrent meningitis can occur.

ORGANISMS

In Britain, group B streptococcus is now the commonest cause of neonatal bacterial meningitis (about one-third of all cases), having overtaken *Escherichia coli*, which is easily the second commonest (approximately 30%). *Listeria monocytogenes* is the third most prevalent, causing <10% of cases, but with the frequency rising [3,10]. These are followed by various Gram-negative bacilli (*Pseudomonas, Proteus, Klebsiella, Enterobacter, Neisseria meningitidis* and *Haemophilus influenzae*) and Gram-positive cocci (*Streptococcus pneumoniae* and other streptococci). Anaerobic meningitis is rare. Table 8.1 lists organisms causing bacterial meningitis based on the studies of de Louvois *et al.* [3] and Synnott and co-workers [10], in the approximate order of frequency for the UK (approximate because bacterial meningitis is under-reported).

Typically, the pattern of organisms causing bacterial

Group B streptococcus
Escherichia coli
Listeria monocytogenes
Streptococcus pneumoniae
Enterococci
Other streptococci
Proteus species
Neisseria meningitidis
Staphylococcus aureus
Klebsiella species
Haemophilus influenzae
Pseudomonas species
Enterobacter species
Citrobacter species
Serratia species
Salmonella species
Other Gram-negative bacilli
Anaerobes
Mycobacterium tuberculosis
Campylobacter species
Coagulase-negative staphylococci (shunt infections)

Table 8.1 Organisms causing neonatal bacterial meningitis in approximate order of frequency for the UK

meningitis in non-industrialized countries is very different from that in industrialized countries. For example, group B streptococcal (GBS) infection is generally rare in non-industrialized countries, although this may be changing. There were no cases of GBS meningitis over 3 years in Nigeria [7] where the most common organisms were *S. aureus* and *Klebsiella*. GBS caused 11.7% of cases in Thailand between 1980 and 1990 [11]; the other main organisms were the Gram negatives *Pseudomonas aeruginosa* (16.9%), *Klebsiella pneumoniae* (13.0%), *E. coli* (10.4%) and *Enterobacter* species (10.4%). In the 1980s, *Klebsiella* was the commonest cause in Durban, South Africa, followed by *E. coli* and GBS, but more recently in South Africa [12] GBS has caused more cases (35%) than *Klebsiella* (28%) and *E. coli* (17%) [9]; GBS is now the predominant organism in Trinidad, West Indies, with a mean age at presentation of 4 days [8]. *Shigella* meningitis is rare, but almost only ever occurs in the newborn period.

Shunt infections are most commonly due to coagulase-negative staphylococci. A specimen of CSF should always be obtained in suspected shunt infections because these may also be caused by *S. aureus*, Gram-negative bacilli or fungi.

Meningitis due to myelomeningocele is usually caused by Gram-negative enteric bacilli.

The isolation of certain organisms should alert the physician to special problems. For example, *Citrobacter* meningitis is frequently associated with brain abscess, although abscess may occur with other organisms such as *Proteus*.

Enteroviruses are increasingly recognized as a cause of neonatal aseptic meningitis. In Galveston, Texas, in 1984–88, enterovirus was the most common cause of meningitis in babies aged 8–28 days and, accounted for one-third of all cases of neonatal meningitis [13]. Enteroviral infection is considered in Chapter 16.

Fungal meningitis almost exclusively affects babies <1500 g birthweight, and, as survival of this group increases with improved neonatal care, the incidence of fungal meningitis is increasing (see Chapter 17). It is still extremely rare compared with bacterial meningitis: one-tenth as common in Oxford [4].

PATHOGENESIS

When infant rats are inoculated intranasally with *Haemophilus influenzae*, organisms colonize and invade the nasopharyngeal epithelium, resulting in bacteraemia [14]. In this animal model of meningitis, the magnitude of bacteraemia correlates strongly with the probability of meningitis; bacterial concentrations of $>10^3$/mL of blood were found to be necessary, but not always sufficient, to result in meningitis [15]. These observations are consistent with observations in human neonates [16], also showing an association between the magnitude of bacteraemia and the occurrence of Gram-negative meningitis.

Less commonly, meningitis can be due to direct spread, either from an infected scalp lesion with spread through skull sutures and thrombosed veins [17] or from otitis media [18].

Certain organisms are far more likely to cause bacterial meningitis than others, so that the virulence of the invading organism as well as host factors are important in determining whether or not meningitis occurs. The K1 capsular antigen of *E. coli*, which is similar to the capsular polysaccharide of group B *Neisseria meningitidis*, is important in facilitating bloodstream survival. More than 80% of cases of neonatal *E. coli* meningitis are caused by strains carrying the K1 antigen [19]. Tullus and colleagues looked at the relative pathogenetic importance of predisposing *host* factors and virulence-associated *bacterial* characteristics of *E. coli*, such as possession of P-fimbriae, O and K antigens and haemolysins [20]. Bacterial factors were more important in neonatal meningitis and urinary tract infection (UTI), whereas host factors contributed to septicaemia or bacteraemia.

The type III capsular polysaccharide of group B streptococcus is an important virulence factor for late-onset meningitis has already been emphasized. Group III GBS strains are disproportionately likely to cause late-onset meningitis (>80% of cases), compared with early-onset sepsis when strains I, II and III are equally common. In experimental GBS meningitis in infant rats, early meningitis involved acute inflammation of the subarachnoid space and ventricles, vascular engorgement and neuronal injury, mainly in the cortex, which often followed a vascular pattern. Within days, injured areas became demarcated and showed new cellular infiltrates [21].

Other organisms that are common causes of neonatal septicaemia virtually never cause meningitis. Coagulase-negative staphylococci are the commonest cause of late-onset septicaemia in industrialized countries, but meningitis virtually only occurs if there is a CSF shunt. *Staphylococcus aureus* is another common cause of septicaemia, but a rare cause of meningitis unless there has been surgery, a shunt or seeding from bacterial endocarditis.

Clearly, these organisms lack factors that allow them to survive in the CSF or cross the blood–brain barrier. Exactly what these factors are is not obvious, although a polysaccharide capsule is one characteristic of most organisms causing meningitis which is lacking in staphylococci.

Despite earlier diagnosis and more effective antimicrobial therapy, the mortality and morbidity from neonatal meningitis remain extremely high. Various reasons can be advanced for this. Neonatal meningitis occurs at an age when host defences are poor and the brain is at its most susceptible to damage. The high bacterial load in neonatal meningitis means that toxic products of the bacterial cell wall, peptidoglycans and teichoic acid from Gram-positive and lipopolysaccharide (endotoxin) from Gram-negative organisms, cause substantial damage to the endothelial cells of the cerebral capillaries which form the so-called 'blood–brain barrier'. Disruption of the tight junctions between the endothelial cells increases the permeability and allows entry of bacteria and white cells, and leakage of protein. Indeed, the introduction of more than a critical number of killed bacteria, either Gram-positive or Gram-negative, into the CSF of an experimental animal is lethal. However, it is increasingly clear that it is not merely the toxic effects of bacterial products, but also the host immune response, which causes damage to the central nervous system (see Figure 8.1). Infection results in the release of substances such as tumour necrosis factor (also called cachectin) and interleukin 1 (IL-1) from mononuclear cells, which may damage endothelial cells and lead to raised intracranial pressure and cerebral oedema. Arachidonic acid metabolites from platelets are also probably important in pathogenesis. Levels of prostaglandin E_2 – a potent vasoactive substance – rise in the CSF in experimental meningitis, and this contributes to cerebral oedema; both the increased levels and cerebral oedema can be blocked by indomethacin [22]. Complement may be important in opsonizing organisms, but can also lyse host cells if bacterial cell wall products are incorporated into them [23].

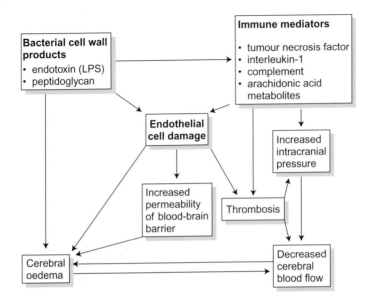

Figure 8.1 Mechanisms in the pathophysiology of bacterial meningitis. LPS, lipopolysaccharide

Cerebral blood flow is reduced in animal models of bacterial meningitis [22]; this may be due to focal vasculitis, to raised intracranial pressure or to vasoconstriction. Autoregulation of cerebral blood flow is frequently impaired in meningitis. Thus, cerebral blood flow varies with blood pressure, and hypotension or hypertension will result in cerebral hypoperfusion or intracranial hypertension, respectively. The degree of impairment of cerebral blood flow correlates with CSF levels of bacteria and lipopolysaccharide. Reduced cerebral blood flow produces regional hypoxaemia, increased metabolism of arachidonic acid, and anaerobic glycolysis with increased production of lactate. There is also decreased carrier-mediated transport of glucose into CSF, and this is probably the main cause of the characteristically low CSF level of glucose (hypoglycorrhachia) seen in bacterial meningitis. Consumption of glucose by bacteria or white cells is unlikely to be a major cause of low CSF glucose concentration, since the CSF sugar level can be low, even zero, for weeks after acute bacterial meningitis, without causing any symptoms.

Intracranial pressure (ICP) is always raised in bacterial meningitis; the possible mechanisms include cerebral oedema, vasodilatation of cerebral veins and capillaries, loss of auto-regulation of cerebral blood flow and impaired circulation of CSF. In a rabbit model of pneumococcal meningitis, methyl-prednisolone reduces cerebral oedema but not raised intra-cranial pressure, whereas dexamethasone reduces both [24]; this suggests that raised ICP is not due to cerebral oedema alone.

The outcome in neonatal meningitis is generally worse than that in older children. The relatively poor neonatal immune response, permitting rapid bacterial multiplication, is one possible reason. Severe ventriculitis, a hallmark of neona-tal meningitis is rarely seen outside the newborn period. Fever is relatively uncommon in neonatal meningitis, and this may contribute to the poor outcome, since CSF bacterial multiplica-tion in experimental pneumococcal meningitis is far more rapid at normal body temperatures than when animals are febrile [25].

PATHOLOGY

Ventriculitis is common in neonatal bacterial meningitis, particularly Gram-negative meningitis, and there may be collections of pus in the ventricles and subarachnoid space. Subdural effusions are rarely of a sufficient size to cause raised intracranial pressure. Hydrocephalus may develop secondary to purulent exudate obstructing the arachnoid granulations over the surface of the brain, or as a result of exudate in the ventri-cles obstructing the foramina of Magendie and Luschka or the aqueduct. Intraventricular haemorrhage may occur, and con-tribute to hydrocephalus. Vasculitis is common and may lead to venous thrombosis; there may be infarcts and focal necrosis. In severe cases there is often widespread neuronal damage which leads to necrotic liquefaction or cerebral atrophy. If abscesses develop they often lack the capsule seen in older children and are multiple.

The most common associated site of infection outside the CNS is the lung (pneumonia or empyema). There may also be otitis or omphalitis (which have occasionally been the original source of sepsis), peritonitis, pyelonephritis, enterocolitis, osteomyelitis, septic arthritis and abscesses in other organs (skin, liver, etc.).

CLINICAL FEATURES

The classic clinical features of bacterial meningitis are frequently absent and there may be no apparent distinction between the newborn with sepsis with or without meningitis. Klein and Marcy summarized the clinical signs in 255 neonates with bacterial meningitis in six centres: fever was present in 61%, lethargy in one-half, abdominal signs (anorexia, vomiting, abdominal distension) in one-half, respiratory distress in 47%, convulsions in 40%, irritability in 32%, jaundice in 28%, and apnoea in 7%; 28% had a full or bulging fontanelle, and only 15% had neck stiffness [2]. A high-pitched cry may accompany cerebral irritation from any cause, including meningitis.

DIAGNOSIS

Because of the difficulty in making a clinical diagnosis of meningitis, it is vital that if sepsis is suspected either a lumbar puncture (LP) is performed or, if the LP is delayed because of the baby's unstable condition, blood cultures are taken and antibiotics started that will adequately cover the organisms likely to cause bacterial meningitis. We have already discussed in Chapter 5 the reasons for performing an LP in all but the most compromised babies. This is particularly true for late-onset infection, in which a far wider range of organisms may cause infection (including enterococci, *Listeria* and fungi as well as group B streptococci and Gram-negative enteric bacteria).

This wide range makes empirical antimicrobial therapy without an LP far more difficult. Up to one-third of all cases of early-onset meningitis are associated with negative blood cultures [26], so if antibiotics are started for suspected early-onset sepsis without performing a lumbar puncture, LP should be done later, particularly if blood cultures are positive. However, occasionally meningitis may be present with normal CSF microscopy, while an intraventricular haemorrhage may complicate the later interpretation of the CSF white cell count.

INTERPRETATION OF CSF FINDINGS

Information on normal CSF findings in term and preterm infants comes from a number of different studies [2]. In general, CSF white cell count and protein levels are higher and CSF glucose levels lower in normal neonates than in older children and adults. These differences are even more marked in preterm infants.

In normal preterm infants the mean CSF white cell count is up to 27 per μL, about one-half neutrophils, with a range of 0–112 [27]. In normal term infants the mean white cell count is lower (5–10 per μL) in most studies, but again the range is up to 130 [28]. Sarff and colleagues found no difference in CSF findings between term and preterm infants at high risk of infection but without meningitis [29]. The mean CSF white cell counts were 8 and 9 per μL and the ranges 0–32 and 0–29 for term and preterm babies, respectively. Sixteen babies with septicaemia without meningitis had a mean CSF white count of 20 per μL (range 0–112).

Of 21 babies with proven group B streptococcal meningitis and of 98 babies with Gram-negative enteric meningitis, 29% and 4%, respectively, had CSF white counts <32 per μL [29]. This shows that there is considerable overlap between the CSF white cell count in babies with and without meningitis.

Bacteria may sometimes be cultured from the CSF of babies with normal CSF microscopy (no white cells and no organisms seen). Ahmed and co-workers closely examined a cohort of 108 full-term neonates, and excluded meningitis using the most stringent criteria, including performing a polymerase chain reaction for enteroviruses [28]. The mean CSF white blood cell count was 7.3 per μL (95% confidence interval 6.6–8.0). The SD was 14, so 2 SD above the mean would be 35. The median was 4, and most babies had CSF white counts between 0 and 20 (90% had <11). However, there was one baby with a CSF white count of 130 and one with a count of 62. Clearly, this degree of overlap between apparently uninfected babies and babies with meningitis makes interpretation of white counts in the 20–130 range problematic.

A summary of the CSF characteristics of full-term babies without meningitis is shown in Table 8.2. The values for two standard deviations above the mean CSF white cell count and/or the highest normal count are given.

The mean CSF protein in preterm babies without meningitis is about 100 mg/dL (1.0 g/L) with the normal range approx 50–290 mg/dL (0.5–2.9 g/L). For term babies the mean is approx. 60 mg/dL (0.6 g/L) and the range 30–240 mg/dL (0.3–2.4 g/L).

The CSF protein level is often raised in bacterial meningitis, but in one study was within the normal range of 20–170 mg/dl (0.2–1.7 g/L) in 47% of babies with group B streptococcal meningitis and 23% with Gram-negative enteric bacillary meningitis [29]. Raised CSF protein levels in the absence of pleocytosis may be seen in parameningeal infections, congenital infections and intracranial haemorrhage.

Mean absolute CSF glucose concentrations in normal babies have varied from 50 to 80 mg/dL (2.7–4.4 mmol/L) with a range of 24–100 mg/dL (1.5–5.5 mmol). The CSF glucose level is generally low in bacterial meningitis, and may be zero, but in some cases may be higher than the lower limit of the 'normal range'. As CSF and blood glucose concentrations are both lower in healthy newborn infants than in older children, it

Study	Age days	n	Mean WBC count (mm³/μL)	Mean + 2SD CSF WBC count (mm³/μL)	Highest WBC count (mm³/μL)	Mean glucose (mg/dL)	Lower limit CSF glucose (mg/dL)	Mean protein (g/L)	Upper limit of protein (g/L)
Naidoo (1968) [30]	1	135	12	–	42	48	38	0.73	1.48
Naidoo (1968) [30]	7	20	3	–	9	55	48	0.47	0.65
Sarff et al. (1976) [29]	Most <7	87	8.2	22	32	52	34	0.90	1.70
Pappu et al. (1982) [31]	0–32	24	11	–	38	–	–	–	–
Bonadio et al. (1992) [32]	0–28	35	11	32	–	46	26	0.84	1.74
Ahmed et al. (1996) [28]	0–30	108	7.3	35	130	51	27	0.64	1.12

Table 8.2 Cerebrospinal fluid in uninfected full-term neonates

has been suggested that the ratio of CSF to blood glucose is a useful indicator of neonatal meningitis. In the study by Sarff and colleagues the mean CSF:blood glucose ratio was 81 (range 44–248) in preterm infants without meningitis and 74 (range 55–105) in term infants [29]. However, 45% of infants with group B streptococcal meningitis and 15% with Gram-negative bacillary meningitis had CSF:blood glucose ratios >44, showing that the CSF:blood glucose ratio is relatively poor at discriminating babies with and without meningitis.

Of the 119 babies with neonatal meningitis reviewed by Sarff *et al.*, only one had completely normal CSF microscopy and biochemistry [29]. The Gram stain reveals organisms in about 80% of cases of meningitis. The CSF white cell count is generally higher in Gram-negative enteric bacillary than in group B streptococcal meningitis (median number 2000 and 100 respectively). Although neutrophils usually predominate in bacterial meningitis, CSF neutrophilia often occurs in early viral meningitis.

In brain abscess there may be a moderate increase in CSF white cell count, with up to a few hundred cells, mostly mononuclear, and raised CSF protein levels. Organisms are not usually seen on Gram stain nor grown from the CSF.

Ventriculitis is present in most babies with Gram-negative enteric meningitis and many with group B streptococcal meningitis. The diagnosis can be made by finding >100 white cells/µL in ventricular CSF obtained by ventricular tap. On the other hand, ventricular taps can result in intracerebral cysts, and ventriculitis is so common that it can almost be assumed to be present, particularly in Gram-negative bacillary meningitis. Ventriculitis can sometimes be diagnosed on cerebral ultrasonography by seeing unusual fibrin strands in the ventricles.

In viral meningitis the CSF glucose level is usually normal, although low glucose levels may occur; the protein level is often raised and the mean CSF white cell count is usually <1000/µL, although it may be up to 4500 with a neutrophil predominance. Thus, in the absence of organisms on Gram staining, it can be extremely difficult to distinguish viral from bacterial meningitis.

MANAGEMENT

CLINICAL ASSESSMENT

When meningitis is 'proven' (organisms seen on CSF Gram staining) or probable (raised CSF white cell count, but no organisms seen), a careful clinical assessment is the first priority. The baby should be examined for a source of infection, notably otitis, omphalitis and osteomyelitis of the skull, and also for midline CNS anomalies such as congenital dermal sinuses. These can occur anywhere in the midline from the bridge of the nose, on the scalp under the hairline and down the spine to the sacrum.

Skin rashes – erythematous, maculopapular or purpuric – may accompany bacterial meningitis, while a fine, macular rash may occur in enteroviral meningitis. The eyes should be examined for the characteristic retinal or vitreous lesions of fungal meningitis.

The head circumference should be measured, both to see whether there has been a marked increase from the last measurement and to act as a baseline for serial measurements during treatment.

A full clinical examination is, of course, essential, both to look for other foci of infection and to assess the overall clinical state. The blood pressure should be measured, but may be artificially maintained due to raised intracranial pressure and peripheral vasoconstriction. Thus, an assessment for shock should also include an assessment of peripheral perfusion (capillary return and core–peripheral temperature difference), of pulse character and heart rate, and of urinary output.

ANTIBIOTIC THERAPY

The choice of antibiotic therapy will depend on which organisms are seen on Gram staining, either Gram-positive cocci (most probably group B streptococcus, enterococcus or pneumococcus), Gram-positive bacilli (*Listeria*) or Gram-negative bacilli (most likely *E. coli*, *Pseudomonas*, coliforms or *Haemophilus influenzae*), or no bacteria at all. The situation is completely different for infected ventricular shunts and is considered later in this chapter.

It is generally acknowledged that all antibiotics should be given parenterally for the entire duration of therapy of neonatal meningitis. Oral absorption of antibiotics is extremely erratic in the neonatal period. Aminoglycosides are sometimes given intramuscularly because intravenous boluses can give rise to high serum peak levels, but recent evidence suggests that high peak levels do not cause toxicity, and intravenous therapy is safe and kinder. All antibiotics used for treating bacterial meningitis should be given intravenously because muscle perfusion may be poor.

For GBS or pneumococcal meningitis, penicillin or ampicillin and an aminoglycoside is the treatment of choice. The recommended dose of penicillin G for treating GBS meningitis is 250 000 units (150 mg) per kg per day [33], because of the relatively high minimum inhibitory concentration (MIC) of some isolates and the poor penetration of penicillin into CSF. Ampicillin should be used at 300–400 mg/kg per day for meningitis. The dose frequency varies with gestational age; the dose and frequency of aminoglycoside is as for systemic sepsis (see Appendix 2).

For meningitis attributable to *Listeria monocytogenes*, ampicillin and an aminoglycoside is the regimen for which there are most data. *Listeria* is susceptible to penicillin *in vitro*, and, although there have been a few reports of treatment failures using penicillin G and an aminoglycoside, ampicillin is not always successful either. Penicillin and an aminoglycoside is, therefore, a reasonable alternative regimen. The doses of these two regimens are as for GBS meningitis. The third-generation cephalosporins are inactive against *Listeria*. There are no data on which antibiotics to use if *Listeria* meningitis is not responding to ampicillin and an aminoglycoside. *In vitro* data suggest rifampicin, cotrimoxazole or ciprofloxacin might be effective.

Cefotaxime is now the preferred antibiotic therapy for Gram-negative bacillary meningitis. Although this choice is that of the majority of experts polled in the USA in 1992 [34], cefotaxime has never been compared to previous antibiotic regimens, such as ampicillin and gentamicin, in controlled trials. However, cefotaxime achieves good CSF levels, whereas aminoglycosides only ever penetrate inflamed meninges. Cefotaxime is effective against all Gram-negative enteric bacilli except *Pseudomonas*; for proven or suspected *Pseudomonas* meningitis, ceftazidime should be used. The addition of an aminoglycoside to cefotaxime or ceftazidime may improve outcome.

Studies from McCracken's group showed that ampicillin and gentamicin sterilized the CSF of most cases of Gram-negative meningitis, even when due to ampicillin-resistant *E. coli* [35,36]. Clearance of septicaemia plus some CSF penetration of inflamed meninges are the probable mechanisms. Cephalosporins and aminoglycosides act by different mechanisms and synergy might be expected. As prognosis depends on speed of sterilization of CSF, it is advisable to use both a third-generation cephalosporin and an aminoglycoside for Gram-negative bacillary meningitis, unless the latter is contraindicated.

One exception to the above recommendation is if the baby with meningitis is known to be infected with a cefotaxime-resistant Gram-negative bacillus or if there is widespread colonization of other babies with resistant organisms (see Chapters 6 and 18). In such a case, the baby should be treated with an antibiotic with good CSF penetration to which the organism is sensitive, e.g. imipenem.

Cefotaxime is completely ineffective against *Listeria* and against enterococci (faecal streptococci), both of which can cause early- or late-onset meningitis. Cefotaxime is inappropriate, therefore, for empirical monotherapy for meningitis.

If a baby has presumed bacterial meningitis with CSF pleocytosis, but no organisms seen on Gram stain, the most appropriate empirical antibiotic therapy is with ampicillin (to cover *Listeria* and enterococci) and a third-generation cephalosporin (to cover Gram-negative enteric organisms). The possibility of other diagnoses, such as herpes simplex virus (HSV) encephalitis, should also be considered in the baby with CSF pleocytosis and negative Gram stain.

The history of the antibiotic treatment of neonatal meningitis is interesting and instructive. For many years, ampicillin and an aminoglycoside was the preferred regimen. In 1971–75, the mortality rate for Gram-negative enteric meningitis was 30% and half the survivors were believed to be normal [35]. In order to improve CSF delivery of antibiotics, McCracken studied intrathecal administration of aminoglycosides, which did not improve the outcome [35]. He then studied intraventricular administration of aminoglycosides, which actually increased the mortality rate [36].

The advent of the third-generation cephalosporins was heralded as solving the problem of CSF penetration of antibiotics, although there was no difference when the combination of ampicillin and moxalactam was compared with ampicillin and gentamicin for Gram-negative meningitis [37]. Moxalactam sometimes caused a bleeding tendency and is no longer used. Ceftriaxone has been used in the USA [38], but caution is needed in the neonatal period because it can displace bilirubin bound to albumin and aggravate hyperbilirubinaemia [39]. The usual dose of either cefotaxime or ceftazidime, the most widely used third-generation cephalosporins for neonatal meningitis, is 150 mg/kg per day in three divided doses.

Historically, chloramphenicol was widely used in the UK. The mortality rate of babies treated with chloramphenicol varied from 36% to 61% [40,41], and morbidity was high. This may reflect the fact that chloramphenicol is bacteriostatic for most Gram-negative enteric bacilli. However, the toxicity was also very high. In a study of 64 neonates treated with chloramphenicol in ten UK hospitals, five developed 'grey baby syndrome', four of whom had cardiovascular collapse, one baby became 'very grey', and four more had reversible haematological abnormalities [40]. There are virtually no indications for using chloramphenicol nowadays, except perhaps in non-industrialized countries, where the cheap cost and oral bioavailability may override safety considerations.

Other antibiotics which may be needed in special circumstances include vancomycin for the unusual event of primary meningitis with methicillin-resistant staphylococci (MRSA or coagulase-negative staphylococci), although shunt infections with these organisms are now uncommon. Trimethroprim–sulphamethoxazole (cotrimoxazole) can be very useful against multiresistant Gram-negative bacilli. Imipenem has good CSF penetration, but causes convulsions in older children with meningitis, so should be used only if there are strong microbiological grounds.

DURATION OF THERAPY

The duration of therapy for neonatal meningitis has not been well studied, is ignored in some textbooks, and is largely empirical. Relapses are not uncommon from Gram-negative and, more rarely, Gram-positive meningitis; however, the histories of those babies who have more than one relapse suggest the relapses are not due to inadequate duration of therapy, but rather to sequestration of organisms.

Ventriculitis is almost invariable in Gram-negative enteric meningitis. It may be diagnosed by showing a pleocytosis in CSF obtained by ventricular tap, or less invasively by showing fibrin strands on cerebral ultrasonography. Gram-negative enteric meningitis should be treated for at least 3 weeks because of the difficulty of treating ventriculitis. It is usually stated that GBS meningitis can be treated for 2 weeks. As ventriculitis rarely complicates GBS meningitis, at the John Radcliffe Hospital we prefer to obtain an ultrasonographic image. We treat for 2 weeks if there is no evidence of ventriculitis, but for at least 3 weeks if fibrin strands are seen.

SUPPORTIVE THERAPY

The same basic principles for supportive therapy apply as described for systemic sepsis in Chapter 7. Although inappropriate secretion of antidiuretic hormone (ADH) is common in bacterial meningitis, the first priority is to support the systemic circulation with fresh frozen plasma and, if necessary, inotropic agents. Only when the circulation is adequate should babies be fluid-restricted.

STEROIDS

Although there is some evidence that dexamethasone may be of value in childhood meningitis in preventing hearing loss and possibly other neurological sequelae, this has not been studied in neonates. The rationale for steroids is to diminish a harmful inflammatory response. In newborns it seems likely that a poor immune response and rapid bacterial multiplication are the major problems and there seems little justification at present for using steroids.

MONITORING

Close monitoring of vital parameters is essential in order to minimize morbidity and mortality, and newborns with bacterial meningitis should ideally be looked after in a tertiary referral centre. In shocked babies, continual monitoring of arterial and central venous pressure allows better fluid balance management. Urine output, urine and serum osmolality, and serum electrolytes should be monitored to permit anticipation of problems with inappropriate ADH secretion. Haematological parameters, including clotting, should be regularly measured. Sabel and Hanson found serial serum C-reactive protein (CRP) measurements to be a useful indicator of progress, low levels showing resolution and raised levels suggesting continuing infection [42]. Drug levels of antibiotics and anticonvulsants may need to be measured. Head circumference should be measured at least daily, as should the baby's weight.

Regular neurological examination is, of course, essential. Intracranial pressure (ICP) is rarely monitored in the newborn period, but cerebral perfusion pressure (arterial blood pressure minus ICP) may be an important determinant of outcome. The measurement of fontanelle pressure by fontanometer, although non-invasive, is less reliable than invasive ICP monitoring. Invasive monitoring of ICP by subdural catheter or intraventricular catheter is rarely performed in newborns, but might be indicated when there is evidence (e.g. rising blood pressure, falling heart rate) of significantly raised ICP. Continuous EEG monitoring, particularly of comatose babies and those receiving muscle relaxants, may reveal clinically unrecognized convulsions which can impair cerebral perfusion. Where this facility is not available, serial EEGs can be helpful.

REPEAT LUMBAR PUNCTURES

In neonatal meningitis, unlike meningitis in older children, it is usual to repeat a lumbar puncture within 48 hours of starting antibiotics and often every day until the CSF is sterile, to monitor the response to treatment. CSF cultures remain positive in Gram-negative bacillary meningitis (mean 6 days, range 2–11 days) for longer than in GBS meningitis, in which CSF cultures are usually sterile within 2–3 days of starting treatment [43].

It has not been shown to be useful to do a lumbar puncture just before stopping therapy. Babies with no cells may relapse, while babies with persistent CSF pleocytosis may recover if therapy is stopped.

COMPLICATIONS

Small subdural effusions are often seen in bacterial meningitis and very rarely need any intervention. Larger effusions may cause persistent fever and midline shift of the brain with symptoms of raised intracranial pressure. Such effusions may show up on transillumination of the skull.

Seizures may be clinically evident, they may present insidiously with apnoeic attacks or episodes of hypoxia, or may be subclinical and only diagnosed by EEG. In general, the presence of seizures is a poor prognostic feature, particularly if they are not controlled by anticonvulsants. Hydrocephalus is more likely after neonatal meningitis than after meningitis in infancy or in childhood. Similarly, brain abscess, although still rare, is commoner in the neonatal period, particularly in association with *Citrobacter* and *Proteus* meningitis.

Persisting or recurrent fever may be due to persistence of meningitis, to subdural or intracerebral abscess, to infection in other sites (pleural empyema, septic arthritis, osteomyelitis) or to intercurrent infection.

Recurrences of both Gram-positive and Gram-negative meningitis may occur after stopping apparently successful treatment. A careful search, both clinical and radiographic, should be made for persisting foci of infection, but these are rarely found.

In Oxford, we have seen a baby with two recurrences of *E. coli* meningitis despite apparently adequate and successful treatment with cefotaxime; no underlying cause was found and the baby was finally cured using intravenous trimethoprim–sulphamethoxazole. In one small study from Australia, Anderson and Gilbert reported that five (21%) of 24 babies with Gram-negative meningitis relapsed when treatment with chloramphenicol and gentamicin (three babies) or cefotaxime (two) was stopped [44]. However, in a national study, only two (5%) of 40 Gram-negative and one (2%) of 41 GBS meningitis relapsed [5]. Mulder and Zanen reported an 8% relapse rate [45].

MORTALITY AND MORBIDITY

The mortality rate of neonatal meningitis has fallen from greater than 30%, but still remains high at 20–25%, whether the meningitis is of early or late onset [2]. The mortality rate increases with prematurity. Brain abscess is associated with a mortality rate of around 50%, and a high rate of long-term sequelae such as hydrocephalus and neurodevelopmental problems.

Although it is not always clear to what extent meningitis and other predisposing factors such as extreme prematurity have contributed to the outcome, significant neurological sequelae develop in 20–60% of all survivors of neonatal bacterial meningitis caused by any organism [2]. These sequelae include major neurodevelopmental handicap, hemiparesis, spastic paraparesis, cranial nerve palsies, hydrocephalus, hearing loss, visual handicap, convulsions, and speech and hearing disorders.

SHUNT INFECTIONS

Infections of ventriculoperitoneal (VP) or ventriculoatrial (VA) shunts should be considered separately from bacterial meningitis. These occur in between 3 and 27% of shunts, with a mean of 11% [46]. Although shunt infections may present like classic bacterial meningitis, they commonly present more insidiously. VP shunt infections cause vomiting, lethargy and irritability with or without fever, whereas VA shunt infections may cause low-grade fever, progressive anaemia, and haematuria and hypertension secondary to shunt nephritis. Infection of a newly placed shunt is highly likely if there is significant infection of the skin overlying the reservoir, a situation that readily occurs in small preterm neonates when the skin of the scalp is stretched over the reservoir.

Coagulase-negative staphylococci, such as *Staphylococcus epidermidis*, are the commonest cause of shunt infections, but these may also be caused by *Staphylococcus aureus* and, particularly in babies of low birthweight, by Gram-negative bacilli (e.g. *Pseudomonas*), by low-grade pathogens such as diphtheroids and by fungi [46].

The first priority in suspected shunt infection is to obtain a specimen of CSF for microscopic examination by tapping the shunt reservoir. Measurement of serum CRP concentration has been helpful in identifying whether babies with non-specific symptoms have shunt infections.

If shunt infection is confirmed, the entire shunt must be removed, as the infection will not resolve on antibiotics alone [47]. The appropriate antibiotics can be given intravenously. As an intraventricular reservoir or external ventricular drain is usually inserted to drain CSF until the shunt infection is cleared, antibiotics can be given directly into the ventricles (e.g. vancomycin, gentamicin) if there is a problem with severe infection or infection with a multiply resistant organism. Intraventricular antibiotics can themselves cause a chemical meningitis, so, when the CSF is sterile and organisms are no longer seen, intraventricular antibiotics should not be continued merely because of a raised CSF white cell count and protein concentration.

Although one-half of our isolates of coagulase-negative staphylococci are cloxacillin (methicillin) resistant, we start empirical antibiotic therapy of shunt infections in which Gram-positive cocci are seen on the Gram stain of the CSF, using cloxacillin and aminoglycoside rather than vancomycin, because these infections are rarely fulminant and symptoms often resolve simply with removal of the shunt.

There is no evidence that administration of prophylactic antibiotics at the time of shunt insertion reduces the incidence of shunt infections [46].

SUMMARY

- Bacterial meningitis is more common in the first month than at any other age.
- Bacterial meningitis has a mortality rate of 20–25%, and 20–60% of survivors have major neurodevelopmental sequelae.
- About 10–30% of babies with early-onset septicaemia, and 10% with late-onset septicaemia, have meningitis.
- Group B streptococcus is the commonest cause of early-onset meningitis in industrialized countries.
- Gram-negative enteric bacilli are the commonest cause of late-onset meningitis.
- Treatment of early-onset meningitis should be with penicillin or ampicillin and an aminoglycoside (unless Gram-negative bacilli are seen on Gram stain).

- Treatment of Gram-negative meningitis should be with cefotaxime (or ceftazidime for *Pseudomonas*) and an aminoglycoside.
- Empirical therapy for neonatal meningitis (organism unknown) should be with ampicillin and cefotaxime.
- Repeat lumbar puncture is indicated for Gram-negative meningitis until cultures are sterile.
- Lumbar puncture before stopping antibiotics is not necessary.
- Gram-negative meningitis should be treated for at least 3 weeks.
- Babies with GBS meningitis should have cerebral ultrasonography; treat with antibiotics for at least 2 weeks, but at least 3 weeks if ventriculitis is present.

References

1 Goldacre MJ. Acute bacterial meningitis in childhood: incidence and mortality in a defined population. *Lancet* 1976; **i**: 28–31.

2 Klein JO & Marcy SM. Bacterial sepsis and meningitis. In: Remington JS & Klein JO (eds) *Infectious Diseases of the Fetus and Newborn Infant*, 4th edn. Philadelphia: WB Saunders, 1995: 835–90.

3 de Louvois J, Blackbourn J, Hurley R & Harvey D. Infantile meningitis in England and Wales: a two year study. *Arch Dis Child* 1991; **66**: 603–7.

4 Hristeva L, Booy R, Bowler I & Willeinson AR. Prospective surveillance of neonatal meningitis. *Arch Dis Child* 1993; **69**: 14–18.

5 Francis BM & Gilbert GL. Survey of neonatal meningitis in Australia: 1987–1989. *Med J Aust* 1992; **156**, 240–3.

6 Bennhagen R, Svenningsen NW & Bekassy AN. Changing pattern of neonatal meningitis in Sweden. *Scand J Infect Dis* 1987; **19**: 587–93.

7 Airede AI. Neonatal bacterial meningitis in the middle belt of Nigeria. *Dev Med Child Neurol* 1993; **35**: 424–30.

8 Ali Z. Neonatal meningitis: a 3 year retrospective study at the Mount Hope Women's Hospital, Trinidad, West Indies. *J Trop Pediatr* 1995; **41**: 109–11.

9 Coovadia YM, Mayosi B, Adhikari M, Solwa Z & van den Ende J.

Hospital-acquired neonatal bacterial meningitis: the impacts of cefotaxime usage on mortality and of amikacin use on incidence. *Ann Trop Paediatr* 1989; **9**: 233–9.

10 Synnott MB, Morse DL & Hall SM. Neonatal meningitis in England and Wales: a review of routine national data. *Arch Dis Child* 1994; **71**: F75–F80.

11 Chotpitaya sunondh T. Bacterial meningitis in children: etiology and clinical features, an 11-year review of 618 cases. *Southeast Asian J Trop Med Public Health* 1994; **25**: 107–15.

12 Adhikari M, Coovadia YM & Singh D. A 4 year study of neonatal meningitis: clinical and microbiological findings. *J Trop Pediatr* 1995; **41**: 81–5.

13 Shattuck KE & Chonmaitree T. The changing spectrum of neonatal meningitis over a fifteen year period. *Clin Pediatr (Phila)* 1992; **31**: 130–6.

14 Moxon ER, Smith AL, Averill DR & Smith DH. *Haemophilus influenzae* meningitis in infant rats after intranasal inoculation. *J Infect Dis* 1974; **129**: 154–62.

15 Moxon ER & Ostrow PT. *Haemophilus influenzae* meningitis in infant rats: role of bacteremia in pathogenesis of age-dependent inflammatory responses in cerebrospinal fluid. *J Infect Dis* 1977; **135**: 303–7.

16 Dietzman DE, Fischer GW & Schoenknecht FD. Neonatal *Escherichia coli* septicemia – bacterial counts in blood. *J Pediatr* 1974; **85**: 128–30.

17 Morrison JE. *Foetal and Neonatal Pathology*, 3rd edn. Washington, DC: Butterworth, 1970.

18 Ermocilla R, Cassady G & Ceballos R. Otitis media in the pathogenesis of neonatal meningitis with group B beta-hemolytic streptococcus. *Pediatrics* 1974; **54**: 643–4.

19 Robbins JB, McCracken GH, Gotschlich EC *et al. Escherichia coli* K1 capsular polysaccharide associated with neonatal meningitis. *N Engl J Med* 1974; **290**: 1216–20.

20 Tullus K, Brauner A, Fryklund B *et al.* Host factors versus virulence-associated bacterial characteristics in neonatal and infantile bacteraemia and meningitis caused by *Escherichia coli. J Med Microbiol* 1992; **36**: 203.

21 Kim YS, Sheldon RA, Elliott BR, Liu Q, Ferriero DM & Tauber MG. Brain injury in experimental neonatal meningitis due to group B streptococci. *J Neuropathol Exp Neurol* 1995; **54**: 531–9.

22 Sande MA, Scheld WM, McCracken GH *et al.* Report of a workshop: pathophysiology of bacterial meningitis – implications for new management strategies. *Pediatr Infect Dis J* 1987; **6** (Suppl): 1143–71.

23 Hummell DS, Swift AJ, Tomasz A *et al.* Activation of the alternative pathway of complement pathway by pneumococcal lipoteichoic acid. *Infect Immun* 1985; **47**: 384–7.

24 Tauber MG, Khayam-Bashi H & Sande MA. Effects of ampicillin and corticosteroids on brain water content, cerebrospinal fluid pressure, and cerebrospinal fluid lactate levels in experimental pneumococcal meningitis. *J Infect Dis* 1985; **151**: 528–34.

25 Small PM, Tauber MG, Hackbarth CJ *et al.* Influence of body temperature on bacterial growth rates in experimental pneumococcal meningitis in rabbits. *Infect Immun* 1986; **52**: 484–7.

26 Visser VE & Hall RT. Lumbar puncture in the evaluation of suspected neonatal sepsis. *J Pediatr* 1980; **96**: 1063–7.

27 Gyllensward A & Malmstrom S. The cerebrospinal fluid in immature infants. *Acta Paediatr Scand* 1962; **51** (Suppl 35): 54–62.

28 Ahmed A, Hickey SM, Ehrett S *et al.* Cerebrospinal fluid values in the term neonate. *Pediatr Infect Dis J* 1996; **15**: 298–303.

29 Sarff LD, Platt LH & McCracken GH. Cerebrospinal fluid evaluation in neonates: comparison of high-risk infants with and without meningitis. *J Pediatr* 1976; **88**: 473–7.

30 Naidoo BT. The cerebrospinal fluid in the newborn infant. *South Afr Med J* 1968; **42**: 933–5.

31 Pappu LD, Purohit DM, Levkoff AH & Kaplan B. CSF cytology in the neonate. *Am J Dis Child* 1982; **136**: 297–8.

32 Bonadio WA, Stanco L, Bruce R, Barry D & Smith E. Reference values of normal cerebrospinal fluid composition in infants aged 0 to 8 weeks. *Pediatr Infect Dis J* 1992; **11**: 589–91.

33 McCracken GH & Feldman WE. Editorial comment. *J Pediatr* 1976; **89**: 203–4.

34 Klass PE & Klein JO. Therapy of bacterial sepsis, meningitis and otitis media in infants and children: 1992 poll of directors of programs in pediatric infectious diseases. *Pediatr Infect Dis J* 1992; **11**: 702–5.

35 McCracken GH & Mize SG. A controlled study of intrathecal antibiotic therapy in Gram-negative enteric meningitis of infancy. *J Pediatr* 1976; **89**: 66–72.

36 McCracken GH, Mize SG & Threlkeld N. Intraventricular gentamicin therapy in gram-negative bacillary meningitis of infancy. *Lancet* 1980; **i**: 787–91.

37 McCracken GH, Threlkeld N, Mize S *et al.* Moxalactam therapy for neonatal meningitis due to Gram-negative enteric bacilli. A prospective controlled evaluation. *JAMA* 1984; **252**: 1427–32.

38 Steele RW. Ceftriaxone therapy of meningitis and serious infections. *Am J Med* 1984; **77**: 50–3.

39 Robertson A, Fink S & Karp W. Effect of cephalosporins on bilirubin–albumin binding. *J Pediatr* 1988; **112**: 291–4.

40 Mulhall A, de Louvois J & Hurley R. Efficacy of chloramphenicol in the treatment of neonatal and infantile meningitis: a study of 70 cases. *Lancet* 1983; **i**: 284–7.

41 Heckmatt JZ. Coliform meningitis in the newborn. *Arch Dis Child* 1976; **51**: 569–73.

42 Sabel KG & Hanson LA. The clinical usefulness of C-reactive protein. CRP; determinations in bacterial meningitis and septicaemia in infancy. *Acta Paediatr Scand* 1974; **63**: 381–8.

43 McCracken GH. The rate of bacteriologic response to antimicrobial therapy in neonatal meningitis. *Am J Dis Child* 1972; **123**: 547–53.

44 Anderson SG & Gilbert GL. Neonatal Gram-negative meningitis; a ten year review; with reference to outcome and relapse of infection. *J Paediatr Child Health* 1990; **26**: 212–16.

45 Mulder CJ & Zanen HC. Neonatal group B streptococcal meningitis. *Arch Dis Child* 1984; **59**: 439–43.

46 Editorial. Cerebrospinal fluid shunt infections. *Lancet* 1989; **i**: 1304–5.

47 Schoenbaum SC, Gardner P & Shillito J. Infections of cerebrospinal fluid shunts: epidemiology, clinical manifestations and therapy. *J Infect Dis* 1975; **131**: 543–52.

9 | **Pneumonia**

INTRODUCTION

Neonatal pneumonia may be subdivided into four categories, although there is some overlap between them:

1. Congenital pneumonia (transplacentally acquired): as a result of congenital infection with rubella, cytomegalovirus (CMV), *Toxoplasma*, *Listeria* and *Treponema pallidum*.
2. Intrauterine pneumonia: autopsy finding of lung inflammation associated with asphyxia and/or infection.
3. Early-onset pneumonia: pneumonia present at birth or soon after, due to infection of amniotic fluid via the maternal genital tract (ascending infection).
4. Late-onset pneumonia: pneumonia presenting at least 48 hours after delivery, due to organisms acquired either around delivery or nosocomially or in the community.

DEFINITION

Pneumonia is probably the most difficult infection to define [1]. Even when histological studies are obtained at autopsy, it may be difficult to distinguish between true infection and inhalation of infected amniotic fluid without endogenous infection of the lungs [2]. This emphasizes the inadequacy of the usual autopsy definition of pneumonia as 'the presence of alveolar and/or interstitial neutrophils'.

In liveborn infants, the radiological appearance of early-onset pneumonia may be identical to that of idiopathic respiratory distress syndrome (hyaline membrane disease). In babies on long-term artificial ventilation, particularly those with bronchopulmonary dysplasia, there may be fluctuating consolidation which can be due to pulmonary oedema, haemorrhage, atelectasis or infection.

In Oxford, we use a working definition of pneumonia in liveborn babies as follows: a clinical picture of respiratory distress associated with chest radiographic changes, suggesting pneumonia, that persist for at least 48 hours. These changes include nodular or coarse patchy infiltrates, diffuse haziness or granularity with air bronchogram, perihilar interstitial streaking, and lobar or sublobar consolidation. When there is difficulty distinguishing between pneumonia and hyaline membrane disease, additional evidence of sepsis is looked for, such as neutropenia, abnormal immature to total white cell ratio, or chest radiographic appearances not completely typical of hyaline membrane disease. If blood cultures are positive, this is described as 'definite pneumonia'; if negative, as 'probable pneumonia' with the probable causative organism (particularly in early pneumonia) being the organism cultured from the tracheal aspirate or nasopharyngeal aspirate at the onset of symptoms [3].

PATHOGENESIS

CONGENITAL PNEUMONIA

In congenital pneumonia, the lung infection is part of a generalized fetal infection which has been acquired transplacentally. This infection may have been acquired in the first trimester of pregnancy, as with toxoplasmosis, rubella and congenital CMV infection, or near delivery, as seen in congenital listeriosis and congenital syphilis. Unfortunately, the term congenital pneumonia is often used imprecisely so that there is confusion with intrauterine pneumonia or early-onset pneumonia.

INTRAUTERINE PNEUMONIA

By definition, intrauterine pneumonia occurs in babies who are stillborn or die within 24 hours, but there is overlap with early-onset pneumonia. The former is a pathological diagnosis made on the basis of diffuse lung inflammation with infiltration of alveoli by polymorphs, and often round-cell infiltrates of the interstitium of small bronchioles and interalveolar septa [2,4]. In many ways, however, it is unlike classic bacterial pneumonia in that there is no pleural reaction, little or no infiltration of bronchopulmonary tissue and no fibrinous exudate in the alveoli [2].

The possible causes of intrauterine pneumonia include asphyxia and ascending infection of the amniotic fluid. Asphyxia may encourage fetal gasping and aspiration of infected amniotic fluid, with the result that the fetal alveolar neutrophils are from aspirated amniotic fluid [2]. Naeye and his colleagues have often found histological evidence of chorioamnionitis in cases of intrauterine pneumonia [5–7], but others have found this correlation far less clear-cut and frequently no bacteria are isolated from cases of intrauterine pneumonia [8]. Benirschke and Driscoll found histological evidence of chorioamnionitis in 11% of a series of unselected pregnancies [9], and Siegel and McCracken have estimated that only 1–6% of infants of mothers with clinical chorioamnionitis become infected [10]. Thus, it is not clear whether intrauterine pneumonia is a true pneumonia or whether it often represents terminal aspiration of infected amniotic fluid in a pregnancy complicated by chorioamnionitis, which itself may have precipitated preterm labour.

EARLY-ONSET PNEUMONIA

The pathogenesis of early-onset pneumonia is similar to that for early-onset sepsis. The disease is more likely to occur in association with maternal risk factors such as spontaneous

Risk factor	n	Solitary risk factor
Spontaneous onset of preterm labour	23	17
Prolonged rupture of membranes (> 18 hours)	9	2
Maternal fever (> 37°C)	3	1
Offensive liquor	2	0
No risk factors	8	–
Total		20 (57%)
From ref. [3]		

Table 9.1 Risk factors for sepsis in 35 babies with early-onset pneumonia; Oxford, 1 May 1984 to 30 September 1987

preterm onset of labour, prolonged rupture of the membranes and maternal fever (see Table 9.1). The route of infection is by ascending infection from the maternal vaginal tract or perineum which causes a clinical or subclinical chorioamnionitis.

Histologically, the appearance of early-onset pneumonia is unlike that of intrauterine pneumonia and more closely resembles pneumonia of children or adults. There is a dense cellular exudate with congestion, haemorrhage and necrosis, and bacteria are usually seen. Alveolar hyaline membranes are seen in about one-half of all cases of early-onset pneumonia and, although these have been best described in group B streptococcal (GBS) pneumonia, they occur with equal frequency in pneumonia due to other streptococci and Gram-negative organisms [11]. Although it has been suggested that this represents pneumonia complicating idiopathic respiratory distress syndrome (hyaline membrane disease), it seems more likely that bacterial pneumonia can actually induce hyaline membranes. This picture is seen in term infants with GBS pneumonia and the hyaline membrane may comprise densely packed bacteria [12].

LATE-ONSET PNEUMONIA

Most cases of nosocomial pneumonia occurring after 48 hours of age in hospitalized babies are in babies receiving artificial ventilation. The endotracheal tubes of such babies rapidly become colonized with potential pathogens, and the tubes by-pass the mucociliary escalator which is an important defence mechanism against bacteria entering the lower respiratory tract. Aspiration pneumonia is particularly likely to occur in babies with neurological deficit, and those with oesophageal atresia, tracheo-oesophageal fistula or diaphragmatic hernia.

More rarely, organisms acquired at birth can cause pneumonia of later onset. This is more likely with viruses, such as CMV, herpes simplex virus and enteroviruses, or allied organisms such as *Chlamydia*, than with bacteria.

The aetiology of community-acquired pneumonia in neonates in non-industrialized countries is unknown [13].

EPIDEMIOLOGY

Intrauterine and early-onset pneumonia have been diagnosed at autopsy in 15–38% of stillborn and 20–32% of liveborn babies who died [14]. This may be an overestimate of the true incidence of pneumonia because of the problems of definition already outlined. The incidence of early-onset pneumonia over a 41-month period in Oxford, using the definition stated in the earlier section, was 1.78 per 1000 live births [3].

In the Collaborative Study of the National Institutes of Health, the incidence of pneumonia in babies who died within 48 hours of birth was 27.7% for black babies, but 11.3% for white babies, and this difference was consistent at different birthweights [15]. In a study of 1044 autopsies of babies, the incidence of pneumonia was higher in black (38%) than in Puerto Rican (22%) or white babies (20%) [6].

Late-onset pneumonia is commonest in preterm babies who required prolonged artificial ventilation. In the neonatal unit in Oxford, there were 41 episodes of late-onset pneumonia affecting 39 babies over a 41-month period: 36 of the babies were preterm and 34 were being artificially ventilated. The mean gestational age at birth was 27.8 weeks (range 23–41) and the mean time to onset of pneumonia was 35 days (range

3–150 days). Of all babies ventilated for more than 24 hours, 10% developed late-onset pneumonia [3].

In the 1950s and 1960s, outbreaks of *Staphylococcus aureus* infection in neonatal units resulted in many cases of severe staphylococcal pneumonia. Although *S. aureus* pneumonia is now uncommon, outbreaks with other bacteria and with viruses, such as respiratory syncytial virus (RSV) and enteroviruses, may still occur and cause pneumonia.

Neonatal pneumonia is an enormous problem in non-industrialized countries, and has been estimated to kill about 2 million babies a year worldwide [16]. In a field trial of community-based management of childhood pneumonia in Indian villages, more than half the deaths were of neonates [17]. Parents of babies with severe neonatal pneumonia often refused hospital referral, necessitating home management with oral cotrimoxazole. The case fatality rate was 15% (10 of 65) for all community-acquired neonatal pneumonia and 6% (3 of 52) for babies without defined high-risk or referral indications [16].

MICROBIOLOGY

Most microbiological data on pneumonia come from autopsy studies. In a study of neonatal pneumonia, blood cultures were positive in 44% of early-onset cases [3]. About one-half of the babies with negative blood cultures were heavily colonized with a bacterial pathogen (Table 9.2). Sherman and colleagues cultured tracheal aspirates taken within 8 hours of birth from 320 babies with early respiratory distress and non-specific radiographic changes: 25 had bacteria seen on Gram staining and cultured from the aspirate (Table 9.3), and 14 (56%) were bacteraemic [18]. In a further study, the same authors found a similar spectrum of organisms with and without bacteraemia, but also *Bacteroides* species [19]. *Staphylococcus aureus* is a relatively unusual early-onset pathogen, and the organisms causing early-onset pneumonia are generally covered by the combination of penicillin G or ampicillin with an aminoglycoside.

Pneumonia with bacteraemia			Pneumonia with negative blood cultures		
Blood culture	n	Deaths	Endotracheal, nasopharyngeal or surface culture	n	Deaths
Group B streptococcus	11	5	Group B streptococcus	9	2
Streptococcus pneumoniae	3	2	Group F streptococcus	1	0
Haemophilus influenzae	2	1	No organism	9	0
Total	16	8	Total	19	2

From ref. [3]

Table 9.2 Bacterial isolates from 35 cases of early-onset pneumonia (presenting before 48 hours of age), Oxford, 1 May 1984 to 30 September 1987

Organism	n	Bacteraemic
Group B streptococcus	14	7
Haemophilus influenzae	3	2
Streptococcus viridans	2	0
Escherichia coli	2	1
Listeria monocytogenes	2	2
Staphylococcus aureus	1	1
Pseudomonas aeruginosa	1	1
Streptococcus pneumoniae	1	–
From ref. [18], with permission.		

Table 9.3 Organisms isolated from tracheal aspirate in 25 babies with probable early-onset pneumonia, Sacramento, 1975–77

There has been increasing interest in the role of fastidious organisms that will not grow using conventional bacterial culture techniques. *Ureaplasma urealyticum* colonization of the maternal genital tract is associated with preterm labour. Rudd and co-workers examined the evidence that *U. urealyticum* might cause pneumonia and found it to be unconvincing [20]. Nevertheless, there are occasional cases of babies dying with pneumonia from whom this is the only organism that can be cultured. The isolation of *U. urealyticum* from endotracheal aspirates was associated with an increased risk of chronic lung disease in a study by Cassell *et al.*, and they suggested that this might be due to pneumonia leading to iatrogenic damage from increased ventilatory requirements [21]. Waites and colleagues described three babies with persistent pulmonary hypertension associated with *Ureaplasma urealyticum* [22]. There have been no controlled studies using antibiotic treatment effective against *Ureaplasma*, such as erythromycin, so it remains doubtful whether the organism is a true pathogen or a commensal (see Chapter 14).

Earlier studies suggested that the organisms that caused late-onset sepsis in artificially ventilated babies could be predicted from the organisms colonizing the pharynx or endotracheal tube [23,24]. However, recent studies have found such cultures to be poorly predictive [25,26] and even misleading [27]. Concurrent bacteraemia is far less common in late-onset than in early-onset pneumonia: in the Oxford study, seven (17%) of 41 episodes of late-onset pneumonia were bacteraemic compared with 16 (46%) of 35 early-onset episodes [3]. Furthermore, different organisms from those in the blood were found in the endotracheal or nasopharyngeal aspirate cultures in four of the seven late-onset cases, no organisms in two cases and the same organism in only one case (see Table 9.4). Thus, there must be some doubt that the organisms cultured from the nasopharynx or endotracheal tube are truly those causing late-onset pneumonia.

In the absence of pneumonia, the mere isolation of a potential pathogen from endotracheal tube aspirate cultures is clearly not an indication for antibiotics. Although babies with late-onset pneumonia have positive endotracheal tube cultures more often than those without pneumonia, such babies are often very low birthweight and receiving prolonged ventilatory support. When they are matched with babies of the same birthweight who have been ventilated for an equal period, the same proportion of babies are colonized, and colonization of the endotracheal tube occurs at the same rate (Table 9.5). Barter and Hudson found bacteria almost as frequently in the lungs of babies dying without pneumonia as in those dying with pneumonia [8].

If there is a pleural effusion, aspiration of this will often give a microbiological cause of the pneumonia. Needle aspiration of the lung has been suggested for the critically ill child with pneumonia, or one who has not responded to antibiotics [14]. The mortality rate from late-onset pneumonia is now very low, however, and needle aspiration is hazardous, while in early-onset pneumonia there is usually less problem in determining the aetiology.

In an Indian study of neonates with pneumonia, Gram-negative bacilli and *Streptococcus pneumoniae* were the commonest organisms detected [28].

It is not clear how often organisms not cultured by

(a) Definite late-onset pneumonia (7 babies) = pneumonia with positive blood culture		
Case	Blood culture	Culture from nasopharynx or endotracheal tube
1	*Pseudomonas aeruginosa* *Achromobacter xylosoxidans*	No growth
2[a]	*Pseudomonas aeruginosa* *Streptococcus faecalis*	No growth
3	*Staphylococcus epidermidis*	*Staphycoccus aureus*
4	*Staphylococcus epidermidis*	Coliform species *Streptococcus faecalis*
5	*Pseudomonas aeruginosa*	*Pseudomonas aeruginosa*
6	*Staphylococcus epidermidis*	*Pseudomonas aeruginosa* Coliform species
7	*Staphylococcus epidermidis*	Coliform species

[a]Baby had cystic fibrosis; died.

(b) Probable late-onset pneumonia (32 babies, 34 episodes) = negative blood culture	
Cultures of nasopharyngeal or endotracheal secretions	*n*
Gram-negative bacilli (30)	
Coliform species	15
Pseudomonas aeruginosa	12
Escherichia coli	2
Proteus mirabilis	1
Staphylococcus aureus	5
Staphylococcus epidermidis	2
Group B streptococcus	1
Haemophilus influenzae	1
No organism	4
Total isolates[a]	39

[a]Multiple isolates common.
From ref. [3].

Table 9.4 Bacterial isolates from 39 babies with late-onset nosocomial pneumonia (presenting after 48 hours of age), Oxford, 1 May 1984 to 30 September 1987

Colonization rate		Significance
Pneumonia present	Pneumonia absent	
Before controlling for gestational age and duration of artificial ventilation:		
34/36 (94%)	80/194 (41%)	$P < 0.001$
After controlling for gestational age and duration of artificial ventilation:		
28/30 (93%)[a]	25/30 (83%)[b]	NS[c]

[a]Mean time to colonization of endotracheal tube 8 days (range 1–15 days).
[b]Mean time to colonization of endotracheal tube 10 days (range 2–39 days); difference not significant.
[c]NS, not significant.

Table 9.5 Endotracheal tube colonization patterns in babies with and without late-onset pneumonia artificially ventilated for > 24 hours, Oxford, 1 May 1984 to 30 September 1987

conventional bacterial techniques are responsible for pneumonia or pneumonitis in older babies. In Wilson–Mikity syndrome, babies without initial chest signs or radiographic changes develop these after a few days; an infectious cause or causes has been suspected, but not proven. Babies with chronic lung disease often develop exacerbations with increased pulmonary shadowing which might be due to bacteria, viruses (such as CMV which can be acquired perinatally or from blood transfusion) or organisms like *Ureaplasma urealyticum*, *Mycoplasma hominis*, *Mycoplasma pneumoniae*, *Chlamydia trachomatis* or *Pneumocystis carinii*. Stagno and colleagues found evidence of infection with *C. trachomatis* (25%), *U. urealyticum* (21%), CMV (20%) and *P. carinii* (18%) in 104 infants in Alabama aged 1–3 months with pneumonitis, but not in controls [29]. However, Rudd and Carrington could find little evidence of infection with viruses or *Mycoplasma* in a prospective survey of babies in the neonatal unit of the Hammersmith Hospital, London [30]. *C. trachomatis* is an occasional cause of afebrile neonatal pneumonitis which can be severe enough for the baby to require ventilatory support. The role of mycoplasmas and ureaplasmas is discussed in more detail in Chapter 14.

CLINICAL FEATURES

Babies with early-onset pneumonia often present with respiratory distress at or very soon after birth and usually within 24 hours. A smaller proportion develop respiratory distress on the second day of life. The signs are identical to hyaline membrane disease with grunting, tachypnoea, tachycardia, flaring of the alar nasi, intercostal recession, sternal retraction and cyanosis. Pulmonary hypertension (persistent transitional or persistent fetal circulation) may mean that cyanosis persists in 100% oxygen; such babies often have a barrel or hyperexpanded chest. If there is associated septicaemia, the baby may be shocked and become apnoeic or even have convulsions. Fever occurs in only about half of the babies.

Babies with late-onset pneumonia usually present more insidiously. Most babies who acquire pneumonia while on a neonatal unit are already receiving ventilatory support and develop increased oxygen requirements, apnoea or tachypnoea if they are on a low rate of ventilation, and may develop abdominal distension and stop tolerating enteral feeds.

Those not on ventilatory support may present with grunting, dyspnoea, tachypnoea or apnoea, cyanosis, tachycardia and intercostal recession. If pneumonia is unilateral and particularly if there is a large effusion, chest movements may be asymmetrical.

Community-acquired neonatal pneumonia in non-industrialized countries is harder to identify and treat in the community than pneumonia in older children [16]. A clinical diagnosis of pneumonia based on cough and tachypnoea was more applicable to older children than to newborns [17]. Singhi and Singhi advocated that a clinical definition of neonatal pneumonia be widened to include babies with 'cough and chest wall retraction' and 'history of rapid breathing and chest wall retraction' [31].

Staphylococcal pneumonia, due to *S. aureus*, is now rare but, when it occurs, babies are extremely ill and usually septicaemic. They may rapidly develop pneumatoceles (Figure 9.1) which can rupture and cause pneumothorax or empyema; ileus is common and there may be staphylococcal enterocolitis with bloody diarrhoea.

About one-half of the babies with chlamydial pneumonitis have a maternal history of vaginal discharge and one-half have, or have had, conjunctivitis. Most babies present between 4 and 11 weeks of age, but sometimes as early as 2 weeks, and symptoms may even start within 1–2 days of birth [32]. There is little

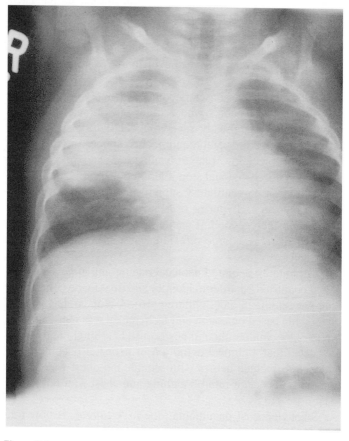

Figure 9.1a

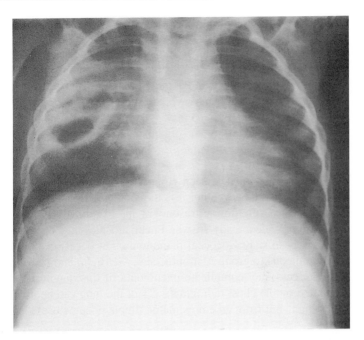

Figure 9.1b

Figure 9.1 Staphylococcal pneumonia. (a) Initial radiograph shows right upper lobe consolidation. (b) Pneumatocele formation 12 hours later

or no fever. Nasal congestion without discharge, tachypnoea, sometimes apnoea, and a paroxysmal, staccato cough are typical. Crepitations may be heard, but wheezing is rare. In up to one-half of the babies, the tympanic membrane has a pearly white appearance. There is hyperexpansion of the chest, which is barrel-shaped and associated with bilateral, perihilar, interstitial infiltrates on the chest radiograph [32–34] (see Figure 9.5).

RADIOLOGY

The chest radiograph in early pneumonia is very variable. In GBS pneumonia, more than one-half of the radiographs resemble hyaline membrane disease (Figure 9.2a), but pneumonic infiltrates occur in about one-third and most of the rest have radiographs mimicking transient tachypnoea or pulmonary oedema. In babies with pulmonary hypertension, the radiograph may show hyperexpanded, hypertranslucent lungs with little or no added shadowing (Figure 9.2b), and it may very occasionally be normal early in the illness [35]. A similar pattern is found with other organisms causing early-onset pneumonia, such as *Haemophilus influenzae*, pneumococcus and *Listeria* (Figure 9.3).

Pleural fluid may be seen (Figure 9.4). If there is doubt about its presence or whether it is too loculated to take a sample by needle aspiration, ultrasonographic examination of the chest can provide a ready answer. Pneumatoceles may be seen, particularly in staphylococcal pneumonia, but occasionally in pneumonia due to group A streptococci, *Klebsiella* and *E. coli*. Lung abscess may complicate pneumonia; if this diagnosis is suspected on the chest radiograph, CT of the lung can be used to distinguish it from an empyema or simple pneumatocele.

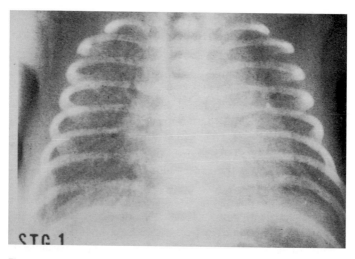

Figure 9.2a

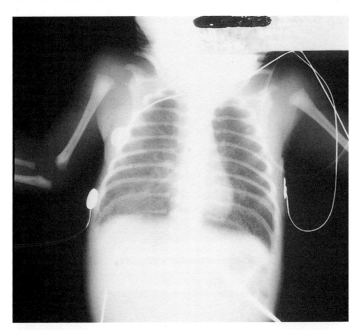

Figure 9.2b

Figure 9.2 Group B streptococcal pneumonia. (a) Appearance resembling hyaline membrane disease. (b) Hypertranslucent lungs, minimal added shadowing

A pattern of perihilar interstitial shadowing is seen in *Chlamydia* pneumonitis (Figure 9.5), which is caused by *Chlamydia trachomatis* (Figure 9.6).

DIAGNOSIS

It can be extremely difficult to distinguish early-onset pneumonia from hyaline membrane disease and late-onset pneumonia from pulmonary oedema secondary to a patent ductus arteriosus or other heart lesion, pulmonary haemorrhage (although usually there is tracheal blood) or pulmonary infarct. Not only may the clinical picture be identical, but so may the chest

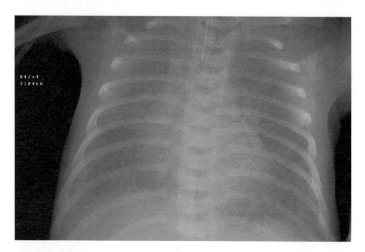

Figure 9.3 Pneumonia due to *Listeria monocytogenes*

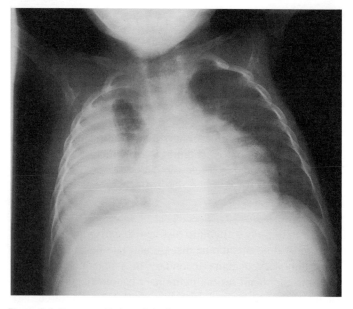

Figure 9.4 Empyema. D-shaped shadow

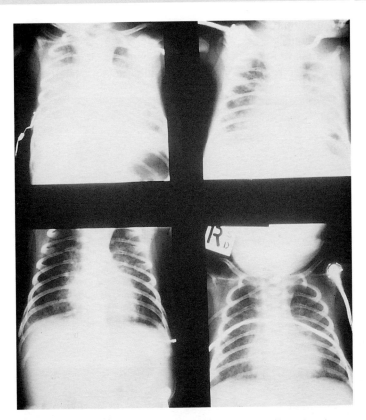

Figure 9.5 *Chlamydia trachomatis* pneumonitis. Resolution with treatment

radiograph. Often, treatment for pneumonia has to be initiated without any certainty of the diagnosis, and time may resolve best whether the condition was or was not pneumonia. Rapid resolution of pulmonary shadowing within 24–48 hours makes a diagnosis of pneumonia highly unlikely since pneumonic shadowing usually persists for several days. The clinical response to a bolus dose of a diuretic in babies with chronic lung disease and new added shadowing may differentiate pulmonary oedema from pneumonia: babies with pulmonary oedema improve rapidly and the chest radiograph improves within hours.

We have found in Oxford that, when assessing babies with early-onset respiratory distress, junior doctors tend not to

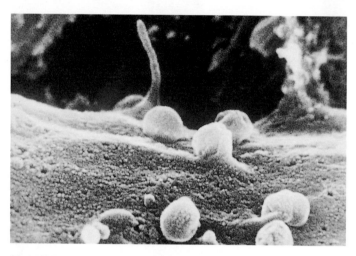

Figure 9.6a

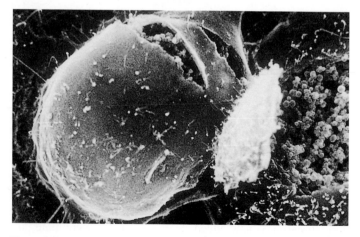

Figure 9.6b

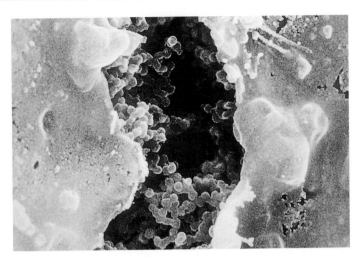

Figure 9.6c

Figure 9.6 Scanning electron micrographs of *Chlamydia trachomatis*. (a) Elementary bodies on cell surface. (b,c) Cell ruptures to release organisms. (Courtesy of Dr Ian Allan)

recognize spontaneous preterm onset of labour as a risk factor for neonatal pneumonia. Yet this was the commonest risk factor for sepsis in a study of babies with early-onset pneumonia, and in 49% it was the solitary risk factor (Table 9.1; [3]).

Some workers [36], but not others [37], have found that microscopy of gastric aspirates is useful in the diagnosis of late-onset pneumonia by showing a raised neutrophil count. The limitations of gastric aspirates in early-onset pneumonia and sepsis have been discussed in Chapter 5.

Serology is of very limited value in pneumonia. Immunoglobulin M (IgM) antibodies can be measured against the TORCH agents (*Toxoplasma*, rubella, CMV and herpes simplex virus) and against *Chlamydia trachomatis*. Antigen-detection tests are widely used for RSV, and increasingly are available for other organisms such as *C. trachomatis*, group B streptococcus and *Streptococcus pneumoniae*.

ANTIBIOTIC TREATMENT

The antibiotic treatment of early-onset bacterial pneumonia is as for early-onset sepsis. Penicillin or ampicillin and an aminoglycoside provide good antibiotic cover against the common early-onset pathogens; in most countries, this means not only group B streptococcus, pneumococcus, untypable *Haemophilus influenzae* and *Listeria monocytogenes*, but also Gram-negative enteric bacilli such as *Escherichia. coli*. Staphylococci, both coagulase positive (*S. aureus*) and coagulase negative (*S. epidermidis*), are occasionally reported as early-onset pathogens, although only one case occurred in 5 years in Oxford (Table 9.3).

For late-onset nosocomial pneumonia, we have already argued that antibiotic treatment based on the organisms known to be colonizing an individual baby can be misleading. We, therefore, treat babies in Oxford with late-onset pneumonia according to a unit antibiotic policy, which is based on the organisms causing infections (Table 9.4) and the outcome of these infections.

In the John Radcliffe Hospital and in Sydney, penicillin and gentamicin are used for early-onset pneumonia and flucloxacillin and gentamicin for late-onset pneumonia. These are not presented as the correct antibiotic regimens, but merely represent antibiotics that have proved appropriate for our population. Different antibiotic regimens will be appropriate for different populations. Pneumonia is treated, whether or not bacteraemia is also present, with antibiotics for 7–10 days, although proven *S. aureus* pneumonia should probably be treated for at least 3 weeks.

SUPPORTIVE TREATMENT

The critical supportive treatment of pneumonia will involve an assessment of whether increased ambient oxygen and ventilatory support are required (or need to be increased) for respiratory failure. Continual monitoring of arterial PaO_2 by skin electrode or arterial saturation by pulse oximeter together with intermittent arterial sampling (preferably via an umbilical or peripheral artery cannula) to monitor pH and PaO_2 allows an assessment of whether ventilatory and metabolic status is satisfactory.

Most babies with pneumonia will not tolerate enteral fluids, which anyway can distend the abdomen, impairing respiration, and are in danger of being aspirated if the baby is not intubated. Intravenous fluids are given, therefore, and nothing is given enterally; a nasogastric or orogastric tube is passed to aspirate air and stomach contents. Electrolytes need to be monitored; inappropriate secretion of antidiuretic hormone has been described in older children with pneumonia, although not in newborns. Supportive therapy for sepsis, as described in Chapter 7, may be needed if the baby is shocked.

Persistent pulmonary hypertension (sometimes called persistent transientional or persistent fetal circulation) may complicate early-onset pneumonia, particularly that due to group B streptococcus, but also *Streptococcus pneumoniae* and *Haemophilus influenzae*. It is important to maintain a good blood pressure, because if this is lower than the pulmonary pressure right-to-left shunting will persist. Thus, fresh frozen plasma or blood as appropriate and inotropic support such as a dopamine infusion may be needed. The arterial PaO_2 should be kept relatively high and not allowed to dip, as this exacerbates pulmonary vasoconstriction. Pulmonary vasodilators such as tolazoline or prostacycline may need to be infused, but the systemic circulation must first be adequately supported or profound hypotension can occur. Inhaled nitric oxide is increasingly being used in this situation.

Significant pleural effusions should be aspirated for diagnostic purposes. If these are infected, either they will need to be repeatedly aspirated for therapeutic reasons or a wide-bore intercostal drain should be inserted. Staphylococcal empyema virtually always requires a wide-bore chest drain because the pus is thick with necrotic debris. It is usual to connect the chest drain to a suction pump with underwater drain (closed suction), as pus may be thick. If this fails to drain the empyema adequately, the chest drain may need to be cut short (open drainage) or chest surgery may be needed. For large empyemas, it is often necessary to place two wide-bore chest drains, one anterior and one low posterolaterally.

PROGNOSIS

The contribution made by pneumonia to stillbirths and early neonatal deaths is obscure because of the difficulties in defining intrauterine pneumonia and the contribution of other factors. In various autopsy studies from 1922 to 1964, summarized by Klein, evidence of pneumonia was found in 15–38% of stillbirths and 20–32% of liveborn infants [14].

Mortality and morbidity rates in liveborn babies will depend on the population being studied. The mortality rate is far higher for early-onset than for late-onset pneumonia. In the Oxford study, ten of 35 babies (29%) with early-onset pneumonia died, but only one of 39 babies experiencing 41 episodes of late-onset pneumonia (2%) died – a baby with cystic fibrosis [3]. The mortality rate of early-onset pneumonia is higher in preterm than in term babies: in Oxford, 10 of 23 preterm babies (43%) died, including two with negative blood cultures, but none of the 12 term babies with early-onset pneumonia died.

There is little information about long-term morbidity from pneumonia. It seems likely that the morbidity caused by early-onset pneumonia is greater than that from late-onset pneumonia. The outcome in the very small babies requiring prolonged ventilatory support who develop late-onset pneumonia is mainly influenced by other antenatal and perinatal factors, which confound the results of follow-up studies. Infantile pneumonitis due to *Chlamydia trachomatis* and other organisms results in recurrent wheezing in almost one-half of the cases, and in lung function evidence of persistent obstructive airway disease [38,39].

SUMMARY

- Neonatal pneumonia may be: congenital (transplacentally acquired), intrauterine, early-onset, late-onset nosocomial, or late-onset community-acquired.

- Early-onset pneumonia is mainly due to group B streptococcus in industrialized countries.

- Late-onset nosocomial pneumonia is mainly due to staphylococci and Gram-negative bacilli.

- Endotracheal tube cultures will grow organisms whether or not the baby has pneumonia; treat infection, not colonization.

- Community-acquired neonatal pneumonia kills about 2 million babies in the world each year.

References

1 Campbell JR. Neonatal pneumonia. *Semin Respir Infect* 1996; **11**: 155–62.

2 Davies PA & Aherne W. Congenital pneumonia. *Arch Dis Child* 1962; **37**: 598–602.

3 Webber S, Lindsell D, Wilkinson AR *et al.* Neonatal pneumonia. *Arch Dis Child* 1990; **65**: 207–11.

4 Barter R. The histopathology of congenital pneumonia. A clinical and experimental study. *J Pathol Bacteriol* 1953; **66**: 407–15.

5 Naeye RL & Peters EC. Amniotic fluid infections with intact membranes leading to perinatal death: a prospective study. *Pediatrics* 1978; **61**: 171–7.

6 Naeye RL, Dellinger WS & Blanc WA. Fetal and maternal features of antenatal bacterial infections. *J Pediatr* 1971; **79**: 733–9.

7 Naeye RL, Tafari N, Judge D *et al.* Amniotic fluid infections in an African city. *J Pediatr* 1977; **90**: 965–70.

8 Barter RA & Hudson JA. Bacteriological findings in perinatal pneumonia. *Pathology* 1974; **6**: 223–30.

9 Benirschke K & Driscoll SG. *The Pathology of the Human Placenta*. Berlin: Springer, 1967.

10 Siegel JD & McCracken GH. Sepsis neonatorum. *N Engl J Med* 1981; **304**: 642–7.

11 Jeffery H, Mitchinson R, Wigglesworth JS & Davies PA. Early neonatal bacteraemia. *Arch Dis Child* 1977; **52**: 683–6.

12 Katzenstein A-L, Davis C & Braude A. Pulmonary changes in neonatal sepsis due to group B beta-haemolytic streptococcus: relation to hyaline membrane disease. *J Infect Dis* 1976; **133**: 430–5.

13 World Health Organization. *Clinical Signs and Etiological Agents of Pneumonia in Young Infants*. Report of meeting, Geneva, 21–24 November 1989. WHO/ARI/90.14. Programme for Control of Acute Respiratory Infections. Geneva: WHO, 1990.

14 Klein JO. Bacterial infections of the respiratory tract. In: Remington JS & Klein JO (eds) *Infectious Diseases of the Fetus and Newborn Infant*, 3rd edn. Philadelphia: WB Saunders, 1990: 657–73.

15 Fujikura T & Froehlich LA. Intrauterine pneumonia in relation to birth, weight and race. *Am J Obstet Gynecol* 1967; **97**: 81–4.

16 Bang AT, Bang RA, Morankar VP, Sontakke PG & Solanki JM. Pneumonia in neonates: can it be managed in the community? *Arch Dis Child* 1993; **68**: 550–6.

17 Bang AT, Bang RA, Tale O *et al.* Reduction in pneumonia mortality and total childhood mortality by means of community based intervention trial in Gadchireli, India. *Lancet* 1990; **336**: 201–6.

18 Sherman MP, Goetzman BW, Ahlfors CE & Wennberg RP. Tracheal aspiration and its clinical correlates in the diagnosis of congenital pneumonia. *Pediatrics* 1980; **65**: 258–63.

19 Sherman MP, Chance KH & Goetzman BW. Gram's stains of tracheal secretions predict neonatal bacteremia. *Am J Dis Child* 1984; **138**: 848–50.

20 Rudd PT, Waites KB, Duffy LB *et al. Ureaplasma urealyticum* and its possible role in pneumonia during the neonatal period and infancy. *Pediatr Infect Dis J* 1986; **5**: S288–91.

21 Cassell GH, Waites KB, Crouse DT *et al.* Association of *Ureaplasma urealyticum* infection of the lower respiratory tract with chronic lung disease and death in very low-birth-weight infants. *Lancet* 1988; **ii**: 240–5.

22 Waites KB, Crouse DT, Philips JB *et al.* Ureaplasmal pneumonia and sepsis associated with persistent pulmonary hypertension of the newborn. *Pediatrics* 1989; **83**: 79–85.

23 Harris H, Wirtshaffer D & Cassady G. Endotracheal intubation and its relationship to bacterial colonization and systemic infection of newborn infants. *Pediatrics* 1976; **58**: 816–23.

24 Sprunt K, Leidy G & Redman W. Abnormal colonization of

neonates in an intensive care unit: means of identifying neonates at risk of infection. *Pediatr Res* 1978; **12**: 998–1002.

25 Isaacs D, Wilkinson AR & Moxon ER. Surveillance of colonisation and late-onset septicaemia in neonates. *J Hosp Infect* 1987; **10**: 114–19.

26 Evans ME, Schaffner W, Federspiel CF *et al.* Sensitivity, specificity and predictive value of body surface cultures in a neonatal intensive care unit. *JAMA* 1988; **259**: 248–52.

27 Slagle TA, Bifano EM, Wolf JW & Gross SJ. Routine endotracheal cultures for the prediction of sepsis in ventilated babies. *Arch Dis Child* 1989; **64**: 34–8.

28 Misra S, Bhakoo ON, Ayyagiri A & Katariya S. Clinical and bacteriological profile of neonatal pneumonia. *Indian J Med Res* 1991; **93**: 366–70.

29 Stagno S, Brasfield DM, Brown MB *et al.* Infant pneumonitis associated with cytomegalovirus, *Chlamydia*, *Pneumocystis* and *Ureaplasma*: a prospective study. *Pediatrics* 1981; **68**: 322–9.

30 Rudd PT & Carrington D. A prospective study of chlamydial, mycoplasmal and viral infections in a neonatal intensive care unit. *Arch Dis Child* 1984; **59**: 120–5.

31 Singhi S & Singhi PD. Clinical signs in neonatal pneumonia. *Lancet* 1990; **336**: 1072–3.

32 Tipple M, Beem MO & Saxon E. Clinical characteristics of the afebrile pneumonia associated with *Chlamydia trachomatis* infection in infants less than 6 months of age. *Pediatrics* 1979; **63**: 192–7.

33 Beem MO & Saxon EM. Respiratory tract colonization and a distinct pneumonia syndrome in infants infected with *Chlamydia trachomatis*. *N Engl J Med* 1977; **296**: 306–10.

34 Harrison HR, English MG, Lee CK & Alexander ER. *Chlamydia trachomatis* infant pneumonitis: comparison with matched controls and other infants pneumonitis. *N Engl J Med* 1978; **298**: 702–8.

35 Baker CJ & Edwards MS. Group B streptococcal infections. In: Remington JS & Klein JO (eds) *Infectious Diseases of the Fetus and Newborn Infant*, 3rd edn. Philadelphia: WB Saunders, 1990: 742–811.

36 Yeung CY & Tam ASY. Gastric aspirate findings in neonatal pneumonia. *Arch Dis Child* 1972; **47**: 735–40.

37 Pole JR & McAllister TA. Gastric aspirate analysis in the newborn. *Acta Paediatr Scand* 1975; **64**: 109–12.

38 Harrison HR, Taussig LM & Fulginiti VA. *Chlamydia trachomatis* and chronic respiratory disease in childhood. *Pediatr Infect Dis J* 1982; **1**: 29–33.

39 Brasfield DM, Stagno S, Whitley RJ *et al.* Infant pneumonitis associated with cytomegalovirus, *Chlamydia*, *Pneumocystis* and *Ureaplasma*: follow-up. *Pediatrics* 1987; **79**: 76–83.

10 | Osteomyelitis and septic arthritis

EPIDEMIOLOGY

Before antibiotics were widely available, about 10% of cases of septicaemia resulted in osteomyelitis [1]. Neonatal osteomyelitis is a rare condition with a reported incidence of from one in 5000 live births in the UK [2] to one in 15 000 in the United States [3]. Certain organisms are more likely to cause osteomyelitis: during the epidemics of neonatal *Staphylococcus aureus* infection in the 1950s and 1960s there was a higher incidence of neonatal osteomyelitis. Methicillin-resistant strains of *S. aureus* (MRSA) cause up to 30% of these infections [4]. Boys are affected more commonly than girls (sex ratio 1.6:1).

Preterm babies are at increased risk of developing osteomyelitis. In a study in the late 1970s, 9 of 39 babies (23%) with neonatal osteomyelitis weighed <2000 g at birth [3], compared with 17 of 30 (57%) in the more recent study of Wong *et al.* [5], reflecting the increased survival of very premature babies.

PATHOGENESIS

HAEMATOGENOUS SPREAD

The haematogenous route is the most common mechanism for osteomyelitis; about 70% of blood cultures are positive [5,6] and multifocal osteomyelitis occurs in about 40% of cases [4]. Neonatal septicaemia, however, is commoner than neonatal osteomyelitis, so other factors must come into play. One of these, as discussed in Chapter 1, is the relative propensity of different organisms to seed to the bone.

In about one-half of all cases of neonatal osteomyelitis, there is preceding bacterial infection such as skin sepsis, peri-umbilical sepsis, otitis media, pneumonia, conjunctivitis, or deep abscess, suggesting that the pathogenesis involved haematogenous spread to the bones. Bacterial osteomyelitis is also a rare complication of neonatal virus infections caused by varicella and herpes simplex viruses.

Umbilical catheters are associated with an increased risk of osteomyelitis [7]. This may be due to septic emboli from the catheter tip or direct inoculation of organisms from the umbilicus into the bloodstream at the time of catheter insertion. Cases of osteomyelitis have occurred following brief umbilical catheterization for exchange transfusion. *Staphylococcus aureus* is the commonest organism, but Gram-negative bacilli and fungi can also be responsible. The hips or knees are usually involved, generally on the same side as the catheter tip [7].

Haematogenous infection of the long bones usually starts in the most vascular part of the bone, the metaphysis, where there is sluggish blood flow through the arteriolar loops [8]. From there, infection can spread to the adjacent growth plate (the physis), across the growth plate via transphyseal blood vessels to the epiphysis, or may rupture into the joint space, because in neonates the synovial membrane extends down to the metaphysis (Figure 10.1). The transphyseal vessels which connect the metaphysis with the epiphysis disappear with increasing age and by 1 year of age are absent. In addition, the

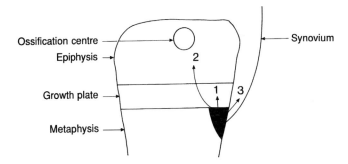

Figure 10.1 Haematogenous osteomyelitis of long bones in neonate, e.g. femur, humerus. Infection originates in vascular area of metaphysis (shaded area); may spread (1) to involve growth plate, (2) to involve epiphysis, (3) into joint space causing septic arthritis

bone is very thin in neonates and the periosteum loosely attached. Infection of neonatal bone almost always decompresses spontaneously with rupture into the joint, causing concomitant septic arthritis. Lifting of the periosteum occurs, often involving much of the length of the bone, and pus may track through the periosteum to form a subcutaneous abscess. It is because of ready decompression of pus in the bone into joint or subcutaneous tissues that neonatal osteomyelitis is relatively painless.

As bone is very vascular, it heals rapidly. Sequestrum rarely forms; when it does, it is often resorbed. However, the rich blood supply also facilitates infection of the cartilaginous growth plate and epiphysis, and the resulting damage to the cartilage is generally irreparable. Neonatal osteomyelitis of the long bones often results in impaired growth of the bone [9,10].

DIRECT INOCULATION

Heel-pricks should always be done in the fleshy side of the heel; the point of the heel overlies the os calcis (Figure 10.2), and calcaneal osteomyelitis or osteochondritis, commonly due to *S. aureus* or *Proteus mirabilis,* can complicate heel-pricks performed too near the midline (Colour plate 10.1).

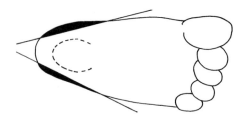

Figure 10.2 Safe area of heel in which to do heel-prick (shaded). Position of os calcis is shown to indicate danger of performing heel-prick on point of heel

Femoral stabs should no longer be necessary in neonatal care. They can cause femoral osteomyelitis, usually due to *S. aureus, S. epidermidis* or *Proteus mirabilis.*

Use of fetal scalp monitors can occasionally lead to osteomyelitis due to *S. aureus, S. epidermidis,* anaerobes or a variety of other organisms.

CONTIGUOUS SPREAD

Scalp abscesses, usually caused by *S. aureus,* can spread to involve the underlying parietal or occipital bone. Cephal-haematomas may become infected, generally with *S. aureus* or Gram-negative bacilli (*Escherichia coli, Pseudomonas*) and extend to involve the parietal bone. Paronychias may occasionally spread to the bone of the underlying finger. Maxillary osteomyelitis may extend from maxillary antral sinusitis, although it can also occur in the absence of sinusitis, presumably due to haematogenous spread.

TRANSPLACENTAL INFECTION

This is the mode of infection in osteitis associated with congenital syphilis. It is an extremely rare cause of bacterial osteomyelitis occurring in association with early-onset sepsis.

TRAUMA

Although in many series of babies with neonatal osteomyelitis, there has been some association with obstetric trauma, such as forceps delivery, the proportion of babies with osteomyelitis experiencing such trauma has not generally exceeded that of normal babies.

MICROBIOLOGY

As with older children, *Staphylococcus aureus* is the commonest cause of neonatal osteomyelitis, accounting for more than 80% of all cases up to the early 1970s, and continuing to be the major cause in most countries. However, in the USA there has been a shift to group B streptococcus (GBS) as an important and sometimes the major organism [11]. When MRSA is prevalent on the neonatal unit, this organism has been found to be an important cause of osteomyelitis. It is particularly likely to colonize and infect very preterm babies [4,12].

Although the organisms causing osteomyelitis might be expected to reflect the organisms causing sepsis, and in particular early-onset septicaemia, certain organisms seem to have a tropism for bone and occur in the absence of overt septicaemia. Most cases of GBS osteomyelitis occur in previously healthy babies who did not have clinical early-onset sepsis. In contrast, certain organisms that are fairly common causes of sepsis, such as Gram-negative bacilli, are relatively rare causes of osteomyelitis, although they were the commonest cause in a series from India [13]. Faecal streptococci, increasingly described as causes of late-onset sepsis, have not been reported to cause neonatal osteomyelitis. *Haemophilus influenzae* is a very rare cause of neonatal and infantile osteomyelitis, although a well-documented cause of infantile septic arthritis. Organisms reported to cause osteomyelitis are given in Table 10.1. In about 5–10% of cases, two or more organisms are isolated from bone (usually *S. aureus* and a β-haemolytic streptococcus).

In summary, it is clear that in many cases the organisms causing osteomyelitis seed bone at the time of acute septicaemia, which may be of early or late onset. Some organisms virtually never cause osteomyelitis despite causing septicaemia; other organisms, such as *S. aureus*, cause osteomyelitis

Staphylococcus aureus (methicillin-sensitive or MRSA)
Group B streptococcus
Gram-negative bacilli
    Escherichia coli
    Pseudomonas sp.
    Serratia sp.
    Enterobacter sp.
    Proteus sp.
    Klebsiella sp.
    Salmonella sp.
    Haemophilus influenzae
Group A streptococcus
Miscellaneous
    Coagulase-negative staphylococci
    Neisseria gonorrhoeae
    Treponema pallidum
    Anaerobes
    Fungi

Table 10.1 Organisms causing neonatal osteomyelitis

disproportionately often. Thus, the tropism for bone of different organisms varies. In the case of some organisms, such as group B streptococcus, osteomyelitis appears often to result from an occult episode of bacteraemia.

CLINICAL PRESENTATION

The onset is either insidious or fulminant. In the insidious form, which is the commoner presentation, the baby is feeding and developing normally and often afebrile. In a recent series of babies with osteomyelitis, two-thirds were afebrile [5]. The initial presentation is with swelling of a limb or joint and reluctance to move the limb. Redness is rarely present and 'point tenderness' is absent or difficult to elicit. There may be irritability on handling, for example when having nappies changed. Sometimes the reluctance to move a limb is so severe as to cause a pseudoparalysis, which can be misdiagnosed as nerve palsy [14]. The classic example is a mistaken diagnosis of Erb's palsy: the main distinction is that Erb's palsy is pain-less, whereas in osteomyelitis of the clavicle or humerus, movement of the arm is painful (Figure 10.3). Involvement of the femur can cause foot drop, and the resulting septic arthritis of the hip may cause the baby to hold the leg flexed, abducted and externally rotated. Pseudoparalysis of a limb may also be caused by the osteitis of congenital syphilis. Oedema may be a prominent feature.

In the newborn period, not only is the presentation often insidious, but multiple bones are involved in about 40% of cases. The infection commonly decompresses into the adjacent joint, and the initial presentation may be with an abscess or an unexplained swelling. In contrast, osteomyelitis in older chil-dren is acute, with fever; a single bone is most commonly involved, and exquisite local tenderness is the rule. It is, there-fore, extremely important to examine assiduously *all* the joints and bones of a baby with possible osteomyelitis.

If the clinical diagnosis of osteomyelitis is not made early, the baby may develop a subcutaneous abscess with more

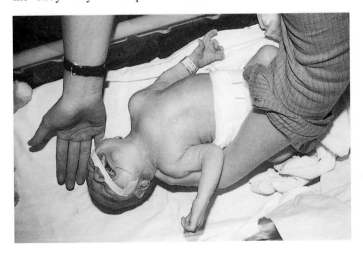

Figure 10.3 Baby with cleft lip and palate who developed *S. aureus* osteomyelitis of clavicle. Absent left Moro response due to pseudoparalysis mimicking Erb's palsy

evident inflammation. Thus, retroperitoneal abscesses should suggest vertebral osteomyelitis, whereas an abscess in the thigh, buttock, groin or iliac fossa suggests femoral or pelvic osteomyelitis.

Maxillary osteomyelitis presents with fever, poor feeding, conjunctivitis, and erythema and oedema of the eyelid. Proptosis and chemosis are common. The cheek often becomes swollen and inflamed and an abscess may form which can drain below the eye. There is often unilateral purulent nasal discharge and swelling of the hard palate, which may become a draining abscess. The commonest error is to misdiagnose maxillary osteomyelitis as peri-orbital cellulitis.

In the 'fulminant' form of osteomyelitis, signs of bone and joint involvement may occur at the time of, or some time after, signs of sepsis. The babies are lethargic, with or without fever, do not tolerate feeds, and have abdominal distension and jaundice. Multiple bones or joints may be involved (see Case history, below). There is often evidence of abscess formation elsewhere, e.g. liver abscesses or pleural empyema, and babies are gravely ill. The commoner sites of neonatal osteomyelitis are shown in Table 10.2.

Site	Frequency (%)
Femur	35
Humerus	17
Tibia	14
Maxilla	6
Radius	5
Clavicle	3
Phalanges	2
Ulna	2
Skull	2
Ribs	2
Miscellaneous (vertebrae, pelvis, mandible, scapula, sternum, etc.)	12

Table 10.2 Commoner sites of neonatal osteomyelitis and approximate frequency

Case History 10.1

A 15-month-old boy was referred for surgery for patent urachus after passing urine through his umbilicus. His umbilicus was not obviously infected, he was afebrile and feeding well. His left thigh was noted to be swollen, but not tender or inflamed and he had left foot drop (Colour plate 10.2). Sciatic nerve palsy secondary to an intramuscular vitamin K injection was diagnosed. The patent urachus was tied off surgically. Two days later, erythematous patches appeared over the right shoulder, wrist and left middle finger (Colour plate 10.3). Blood cultures, urine and pus aspirated from the thigh, shoulder and wrist grew *S. aureus*. The initial radiograph of his left hip showed evidence of osteomyelitis with periosteal elevation and bite-like erosions of the metaphysis and epiphysis. At surgery there was septic arthritis of the left hip and extensive destruction of the femoral head.

Infection was eventually controlled with antibiotics and repeated surgical drainage of affected joints. At follow-up, the boy has shortening of his left femur with loss of the left femoral head and dislocation of the hip (Figure 10.4), a flexion contracture of the left proximal interphalangeal joint and limited dorsiflexion of the right wrist.

DIAGNOSIS

CLINICAL

The most important diagnostic test is clinical acumen. The possibility of neonatal osteomyelitis should be considered in any baby with soft tissue or joint swelling, subcutaneous abscess, cellulitis or immobility of a limb. Groin abscesses secondary to septic arthritis of the hip may be misdiagnosed as hernias or lymphadenopathy. Cellulitic lesions may be erroneously treated with 5–7 days of antibiotics without considering possible underlying osteomyelitis. Limb immobility may be misdiagnosed as due to nerve palsy.

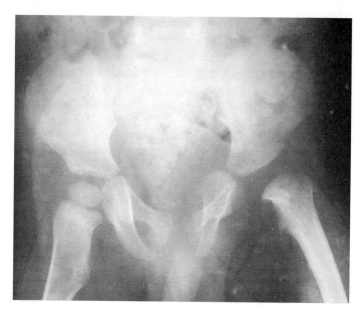

Figure 10.4 Case history: staphylococcal septic arthritis. Follow-up showing loss of left femoral head and dislocation of left hip

Staphylococcus aureus septicaemia

In a study by Wong and colleagues, 27 babies with *S. aureus* septicaemia but no clinical signs of osteomyelitis or septic arthritis were investigated by bone scan [5]. Four (15%) had positive bone scans, suggesting *S. aureus* septicaemia alone may be an indication for bone scan.

RADIOGRAPHS

Unlike older children, radiographic changes appear early in neonatal osteomyelitis. The thin periosteum ruptures easily, and osteolytic lesions (Figures 10.5 and 10.6), soft tissue swelling (Colour plate 10.2 and Figure 10.6) and periosteal elevation (Figure 10.7) are often seen within 7 days of onset of infection.

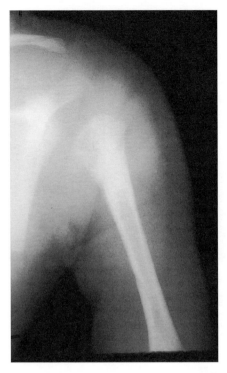

Figure 10.5 Group B streptococcal osteomyelitis of humerus. Punched-out lesion of head of humerus

Radiographs should be obtained in all newborns with suspected osteomyelitis and septic arthritis, and it is helpful to X-ray the opposite limb for comparison.

ULTRASONOGRAPHY

Although septic arthritis is primarily a clinical diagnosis, ultrasonography of the joint space can confirm joint effusion(s) in septic arthritis, and is particularly useful in doubtful cases and in babies with multiple joint involvement.

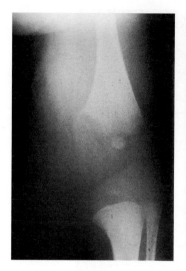
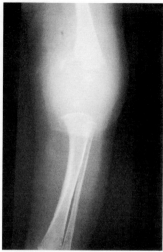

Figure 10.6a   **Figure 10.6b**

Figure 10.6 (a) Plain radiograph of osteomyelitis and septic arthritis of distal femur. Symptoms for 5 days. Soft tissue swelling, widening of joint space, and bony erosion. (b) Plain radiograph of distal femur. Same patient, 14 days after onset. Extensive joint swelling, new bone formation

BONE SCAN

It used to be thought that technetium-99m methylene diphosphonate (^{99m}TC) bone scan was insensitive in neonatal osteomyelitis [15]. With improved resolution of scanners, bone scan is now both sensitive and specific: the sensitivity in a recent study was 84%, specificity 89%, positive predictive value 79% and negative predictive value 92% [5].

Technetium is taken up by active osteoblasts, so is of no value in septic arthritis unless there is concomitant osteomyelitis. In osteomyelitis, enhanced uptake of ^{99m}TC is usual (Figure 10.8), but occasionally vascular compromise results in 'cold spots' of reduced uptake (Figure 10.9).

Bone scans are often abnormal within 2–3 days of onset of symptoms, whereas radiographs are often not abnormal until symptoms have been present for 6–7 days (Figure 10.10).

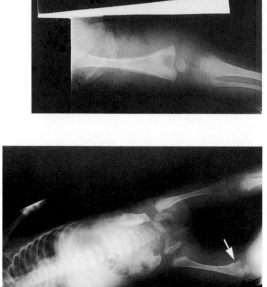

Figure 10.7a

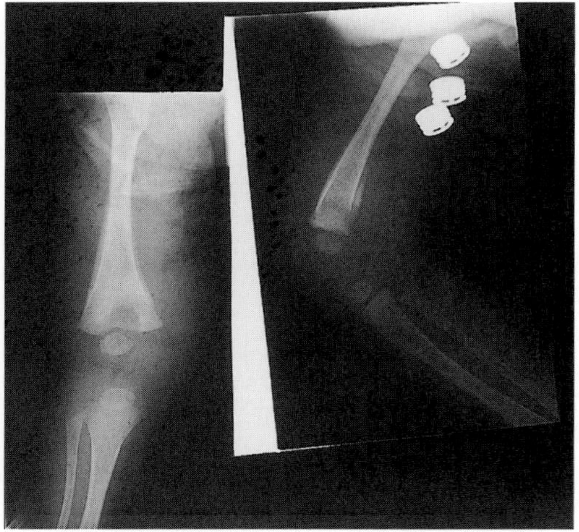

Figure 10.7b

Figure 10.7 Pathological metaphyseal fracture in right distal femur of a 4-month-old girl born at 30 weeks' gestation. Originally misdiagnosed as non-accidental injury. *Proteus* osteomyelitis secondary to necrotizing enterocolitis 2 months earlier. Arrow shows fracture. Periosteal reaction seen in lateral.

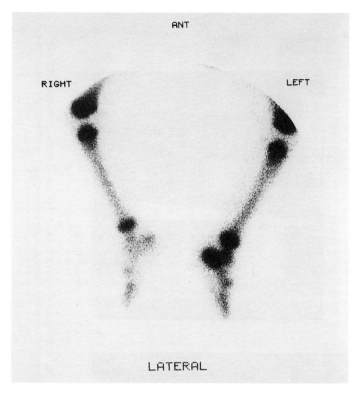

Figure 10.8 Technetium-99m bone scan in osteomyelitis of the foot. Increased uptake in left os calcis and left ankle.

GALLIUM SCAN

Gallium-67- labelled citrate is taken up by iron-metabolizing cells, including neutrophils. It delivers five to six times the radiation dose of bone scan and is slower to be absorbed (48 hours), so is very much a second-line investigation. However, gallium scanning can be useful when bone scan is equivocal, or when osteomyelitis or septic arthritis is strongly suspected, but radiographs and bone scans are normal or inconclusive. In Wong's study, the use of gallium scans in addition to bone scans in selected patients gave improved sensitivity

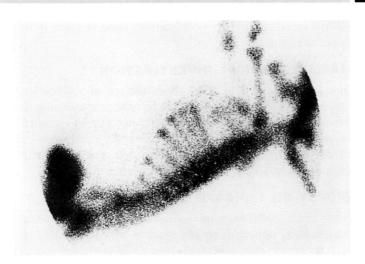

Figure 10.9 Technetium-99m bone scan of spine. Vascular compromise secondary to osteomyelitis of left second to fifth ribs appearing as 'cold spot'

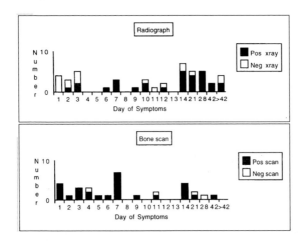

Figure 10.10 Timing of radiograph and bone scan results in relation to onset of symptoms in babies with proven osteomyelitis [5]. Bone scans are more likely to be positive than radiographs in the first 3 days

(90%), specificity (97%), positive (93%) and negative (95%) predictive values [5].

HAEMATOLOGICAL INVESTIGATIONS

The ESR is raised in only about half of all babies with osteomyelitis [5,16] and should not be used as a screening test for osteomyelitis. Other acute-phase reactants such as serum C-reactive protein (CRP) are similarly unreliable, and white cell counts, neutrophil ratios, platelet counts, etc. give non-specific information and may be normal in osteomyelitis [4].

BIOPSY OR ASPIRATE

A tissue diagnosis, by bone biopsy or joint aspirate, improves the reliability of identifying an organism only marginally from 70% for blood culture alone, to about 80% [4]. An orthopaedic opinion should be sought on every baby with probable osteomyelitis or septic arthritis.

SEPTIC ARTHRITIS

Septic arthritis complicates about 50% of cases of neonatal osteomyelitis, particularly osteomyelitis of the long bones. Occasionally, septic arthritis occurs in the absence of demonstrable osteomyelitis, in which case the pathogenesis is either direct haematogenous seeding of the joint (primary septic arthritis) or secondary to occult osteomyelitis. *Staphylococcus aureus* is the commonest single cause of all cases of primary septic arthritis (about 45%) but Gram-negative bacilli (25%) cause proportionately more cases than of osteomyelitis. Other organisms that cause septic arthritis are those described as causing osteomyelitis (Table 10.1). Neonatal gonococcal infection is very rare in the UK, but not in parts of the world where the prevalence of gonorrhoea is high.

Clinically, septic arthritis usually presents with obvious swelling of one or more joints. The overlying skin is often not red, fever is absent more often than not, and, although the presence of pain on moving the joint and paucity of movement of a limb will differentiate septic arthritis from most other diagnoses, there may be surprisingly little discomfort or impairment of function.

The commonest joints involved are the hip and the shoulder, followed by the knee, elbow and ankle [4].

Septic arthritis, if untreated, will cause growth plate disturbances and subsequent shortening of an affected limb. Hence the need for urgent diagnosis and treatment.

MANAGEMENT

In view of the wide range of organisms that can cause neonatal osteomyelitis and septic arthritis, and the long duration of antibiotic treatment, it is particularly important to identify the organism responsible. Pus should, therefore, be aspirated by needle or open drainage from bone, joint or soft tissue abscesses. Blood should always be cultured, because up to 20% of joint aspirates are sterile in septic arthritis, possibly because joint fluid is bacteriostatic or because organisms are limited to the synovium. Urine and CSF should also be cultured, as the likelihood of metastatic spread through bacteraemia is high.

Surgical drainage is necessary for large soft-tissue abscesses, and open surgical drainage of the relevant joint is essential to prevent necrosis of the head of the femur or humerus. Smaller joints can usually be effectively treated by regular aspiration and rarely need open surgical drainage. Because there is spontaneous decompression of infection of the shaft, it is not usually necessary to drill the cortex of the long bones [3] but pus in the bone under pressure should be drained surgically.

Antimicrobial therapy is guided by Gram stain on the aspirated pus. If no organisms are seen, or no pus is obtained, empirical therapy might comprise a penicillinase-resistant penicillin (flucloxacillin, oxacillin) to cover staphylococci and streptococci and an aminoglycoside or third-generation cephalosporin for Gram-negative bacilli.

Anaerobic infection will normally respond to this regimen, but, if this seems a likely cause, either the addition of metronidazole (favoured in the UK) or the use of clindamycin (favoured in the USA) is advisable. Clindamycin is excellent treatment for Gram positive cocci (except MRSA).

Data concerning older children are accumulating to the effect that treatment can be given orally after a few days. As oral absorption is uncertain in neonates, oral therapy is not advised. Oral therapy can only ever be countenanced if the baby is observed in hospital to monitor clinical progress and measure weekly serum bactericidal titres (titration of the patient's serum against the patient's organism or a laboratory strain of *S. aureus* [17]). Treatment of osteomyelitis for a period of 3 weeks or less results in at least a 15% failure rate, whereas treatment for a period of 4 weeks or more has a 5% or lower failure rate [18]; therefore treatment should be for at least 4 weeks.

Early immobilization of the limb and joint is usually necessary, but as soon as there is no further pain physiotherapy should be started to mobilize affected joints.

SILENT OSTEOMYELITIS

The management of 'silent lesions' is controversial. If these are found by bone scan in addition to a clinically evident focus, the baby will obviously be treated for at least 4 weeks with antibiotics. More of a problem is the baby with *S. aureus* septicaemia, who is found to have a positive bone scan, but no clinical signs, i.e. 'silent osteomyelitis'. Should this baby be treated for 7–10 days as for septicaemia, or for 4 weeks? The improved reliability argues for a full 4 weeks, but presumably, in pre-bone scan days, these babies rarely developed later overt osteomyelitis, so 7–10 days of treatment sufficed. There does not seem to be a clear-cut answer to which regimen is 'correct'.

PROGNOSIS

The prognosis of neonatal osteomyelitis and/or septic arthritis is much worse than for older children. Shortening of an affected limb is a common outcome, particularly in preterm babies, occurring in 30–50% of babies [10,16]. Early diagnosis and treatment is vital to limit long-term sequelae.

PREVENTION

Heel-pricks should never be done on the point of the heel. If staff see a baby with a sticking plaster overlying the os calcis, careful enquiry should be made to find who performed the heel-prick; – for educational, not punitive, reasons.

Invasive procedures should, of course, be kept to a minimum, and particular care should be taken when needles are introduced near bone or joint space.

SUMMARY

- The neonatal periosteum is thin and the joint space large, so osteomyelitis and septic arthritis often coexist as pus ruptures from the bone into the joint.
- The presentation may be insidious or with fulminant sepsis.
- In the insidious form there may be no fever, normal feeding and few signs.
- The possibility of osteomyelitis should be considered in any baby with soft tissue or joint swelling, subcutaneous abscess, cellulitis or immobility of a limb.
- Radiographic changes appear early in neonatal osteomyelitis, usually within 1 week of symptoms, and radiographs should always be obtained of the affected area and the opposite side for comparison.
- Ultrasonography is useful in suspected septic arthritis.
- Bone scan is quick, has a low radiation dose and is sensitive and specific in neonatal osteomyelitis.
- Gallium scan is slow, has a high radiation dose, but is useful if bone scan is inconclusive.
- Clinical suspicion needs to be high, as early diagnosis and treatment improve the outcome of osteomyelitis.

- The prognosis of neonatal osteomyelitis is poor, with limb shortening a common complication in 30–50%.

References

1 Dunham EC. Septicemia in newborn. *Am J Dis Child* 1933; **45**: 229–53.

2 Craig WS. *Care of the Newly Born Infant*. Baltimore: Williams & Wilkins, 1962.

3 Fox L & Sprunt K. Neonatal osteomyelitis. *Pediatrics* 1978; **62**: 535–42.

4 Wong M. Osteomyelitis and septic arthritis. *Semin Neonatal* 1996; **1**: 761–8.

5 Wong M, Isaacs D, Howman-Giles R & Uren R. Clinical and diagnostic features of osteomyelitis occurring in the first three months of life. *Pediatr Infect Dis J* 1995; **14**: 1047–53.

6 Mok PM, Reilly BJ & Ash J. Osteomyelitis in the neonate. *Radiology* 1982; **145**: 677–82.

7 Lim MO, Gresham EL, Franken EA & Leake RD. Osteomyelitis as a complication of umbilical artery catheterization. *Am J Dis Child* 1977; **131**: 142–4.

8 Ogden JA & Lister G. The pathology of neonatal osteomyelitis. *Pediatrics* 1975; **55**: 474–8.

9 Trueta J. The three types of acute haematogenous osteomyelitis: a clinical and vascular study. *J Bone Joint Surg* 1959; **41**: 671–80.

10 Williamson JB, Galasko CSB & Robinson MJ. Outcome after acute osteomyelitis in preterm infants. *Arch Dis Child* 1990; **65**: 1060–2.

11 Edwards MS, Baker CJ, Wagner ML *et al.* An etiologic shift in infantile osteomyelitis: the emergence of the group B streptococcus. *J Pediatr* 1978; **93**: 578–83.

12 Ish-Horowicz MR, McIntyre P & Nade S. Bone and joint infections caused by multiply resistant *Staphylococcus aureus* in a neonatal intensive care unit. *Pediatr Infect Dis J* 1992; **11**: 82–7.

13 Kumari S, Bhargava SK, Baijal VN & Ghosh S. Neonatal osteomyelitis: a clinical and follow-up study. *Indian Pediatr* 1978; **15**: 393–7.

14 Isaacs D, Bower BD & Moxon ER. Neonatal osteomyelitis presenting as nerve palsy. *BMJ* 1986; **292**: 1071.

15 Ash JM & Gilday DL. The futility of bone scanning in neonatal osteomyelitis: concise communication. *J Nucl Med* 1980; **21**: 417–20.

16 Fredericksen B, Christiansen P & Knudsen FU. Acute osteomyelitis and septic arthritis in the neonate, risk factors and outcome. *Eur J Pediatr* 1993; **152**: 577–80.

17 Prober CG & Yeager AS. Use of the serum bactericidal titer to assess the adequacy of oral antibiotic therapy in the treatment of acute haematogenous osteomyelitis. *J Pediatr* 1979; **95**: 131–5.

18 Syriopoulou VP & Smith AL. Osteomyelitis and septic arthritis. In: Feigin RD & Cherry JD (eds) *Textbook of Pediatric Infectious Diseases*, 2nd edn. Philadelphia: WB Saunders, 1987: 759–79.

11 | Urinary tract infection

DEFINITION

A urinary tract infection (UTI) may involve any or all parts of the renal tract, from the kidneys to the bladder. It is diagnosed by culturing voided urine or urine obtained by catheterization or by needle aspiration of the bladder. Voided urine is often contaminated with bacteria; as the doubling time of coliform bacteria is only about 20 minutes, delays in transit result in significant increases in the number of organisms cultured.

Conventionally, UTI is defined as the culture of $\geq 10^5$ colonies of a single organism from each millilitre of urine. However, this definition is based on Kass's studies of midstream urine specimens cultured from adult women who were about to undergo bladder catheterization [1]. The applicability of such diagnostic criteria to neonatal UTI has never been assessed. Nevertheless, it is generally accepted that a diagnosis of neonatal UTI should be made only on a suprapubic aspirate, where any growth is significant, or on growth of $\geq 10^3$ organisms per ml from a catheter sample of urine [2,3].

EPIDEMIOLOGY

Given the difficulties of making a secure diagnosis, it is not surprising that the reported incidence of neonatal UTI has varied: estimates have ranged from 0.1 to 1% of all infants. This incidence has been found in the USA, UK, New Zealand, Sweden [2] and Nigeria [4]. The incidence is higher in preterm babies, with figures of 3–10% reported for babies <2500 g birthweight [2]. In the newborn period, boys experience between three and eight times as many urinary tract infections as girls [5–9]. Circumcision may reduce the incidence of UTI in boys, although a small number of babies will develop UTI as a complication of the operation (see below). Breastfeeding is probably protective against UTI.

PATHOGENESIS

Neonatal UTI is often stated to occur secondary to bacteraemia. In contrast, UTI in older children usually results from ascending infection. In the neonate, blood cultures are more often positive and symptoms of systemic sepsis often precede the appearance of urinary abnormalities. However, there is little evidence to support the contention that UTI in neonates is secondary to bacteraemia, and it is equally likely that in neonatal UTI the urinary tract is the primary site of infection and bacteraemia occurs secondarily.

Obstructive abnormalities of the urinary tract such as posterior urethral valves, vesico-ureteric or pelvi-ureteric junction stenosis are responsible for only about 5–10% of infections in boys [7,8], and this proportion may be even lower since the use of antenatal ultrasonography. Vesico-ureteric reflux (VUR) is found in 30–50% of newborn babies of either sex with UTI [8,10]. VUR is considered by many, but not all, authorities to be an important factor in the pathogenesis of UTI.

The increased susceptibility to neonatal UTI of boys, who have a 3- to 8-fold higher incidence than girls, compared with the 1.5- to 2-fold increase for other forms of sepsis, suggests that other factors may be important. Underlying structural renal tract anomalies are equally common in girls. The male prepuce becomes heavily colonized with *Escherichia coli* during the first few days after birth [11] and uropathogenic P-fimbriated *E. coli* are particularly likely to bind to the foreskin [12]. Wiswell and colleagues have provided evidence, based on retrospective studies, that circumcision reduces the incidence of UTI in boys [13–15]. Circumcision reduces urethral as well as peri-urethral colonization with *E. coli* [16] and *Proteus* [17].

A host factor correlating with susceptibility to UTI is the P-1 blood group antigen, a glycolipid that is a receptor for the adherence of P-fimbriae. In a study of girls, 97% with recurrent UTI had the P-1 phenotype compared with 75% of controls [18]. Antigens in the P blood group system can also act as epithelial cell receptors that can bind *E. coli*.

Host factors are clearly important in determining susceptibility to UTI, but there are also organism factors which affect virulence (see Microbiology below). Tullus and colleagues examined host risk factors for sepsis and virulence-associated bacterial characteristics in neonates with *E. coli* bacteraemia, including UTI or meningitis [19]. Just over half the babies (59%) were considered at risk for sepsis and just under half (45%) of the clones were considered virulent. However, the association between *E. coli* and P-fimbriae (see below) was one of the stronger associations.

MICROBIOLOGY

Escherichia coli causes about 75% of cases of neonatal UTI and *Klebsiella* about 13% [2]. The remainder are caused by miscellaneous Gram-negative organisms (*Proteus, Pseudomonas, Serratia, Enterobacter*) and Gram-positive cocci (enterococci, *Staphylococcus aureus, Staphylococcus epidermidis*). Multiple organisms were found in almost 10% of cases in one series [8].

E. coli causing UTI are faecal strains, but those that cause UTI and pyelonephritis differ in a number of ways from other faecal strains, suggesting that certain virulence factors are important in causing infection. The restricted serotypes of *E. coli* causing pyelonephritis stick to uroepithelial cells more avidly, resist serum bactericidal activity, and produce haemolysins [20]. *E. coli* adheres to uroepithelial cells using fimbriae, and there is much interest in the role of different fimbriae, particularly P-fimbriae, in the pathogenesis of UTI [21], and the way their expression is subject to phase variation (being switched on and off). Certain clones seem to be particularly virulent or uropathogenic [22,23]. These P-fimbriae or P-pili are thin, flexible polymers and the adhesin responsible for attachment is a component of distinct fibrillar structures at the tips of the pili [24].

The urinary tract may be involved by metastatic spread as part of a pattern of disseminated sepsis with *Staphylococcus aureus* or group B streptococcus. *S. aureus* UTI occasionally occurs in isolation, i.e. without evidence of dissemination. Infection with *Proteus or Pseudomonas* is more likely to occur in babies with underlying renal tract pathology.

The pattern of organisms causing nosocomial UTI has changed markedly in the USA since the 1970s, when 75% of episodes were due to *E. coli*. In the early 1990s, about 30% of cases were due to coagulase-negative staphylococci, with 10–15% each caused by *E. coli*, *Klebsiella* species, *Enterobacter* species, enterococci and *Candida* [2].

CIRCUMCISION

There is good evidence that male circumcision reduces the incidence of UTI in boys under 1 year of age [2,25]. The mechanism seems to be increased per-urethral colonization of the uncircumcised prepuce by uropathogenic organisms. Adherence of these organisms to non-keratinized mucosa such as the prepuce is enhanced [12].

Craig points out that, before advocating routine male neonatal circumcision to prevent UTI, the risks and benefits should be examined [25]. The surgical complication rate of circumcision is from 0.2% to 4%, mainly due to local infection and haemorrhage, but with some far more serious complications. If the odds ratio for non-circumcision compared to circumcision being associated with UTI is 10:1, and the incidence of UTI is 1% in the first year of life, 1000 circumcisions would be needed to prevent nine cases of UTI, with 2–40 children developing complications of surgery.

At present the evidence would support circumcision only for boys at high risk of UTI in the first year of life, and for whom UTI might significantly impair already compromised renal function.

CLINICAL MANIFESTATIONS

UTI may manifest early as part of generalized early-onset sepsis, or may appear late, usually more insidiously. Sometimes UTI may be diagnosed in completely asymptomatic babies who, none the less, have significant bacteriuria.

In early-onset sepsis the signs or symptoms of UTI are non-specific. Over a 12-month period Visser and Hall cultured urine and blood from 188 babies with suspected early-onset sepsis [26]. Nine babies had bacteraemia but only one of these, with group B streptococcal (GBS) infection, had a positive urine culture. Two babies had bacteriuria with negative blood cultures: one had *Staphylococcus epidermidis* grown from a suprapubic aspirate but recovered without antibiotics (i.e. the organism was probably a contaminant) and the other grew *Escherichia coli*. Over 5 years in Oxford we have seen positive urines in suspected early-onset sepsis only in association with generalized GBS sepsis (three cases) or as probable contaminants, and we no longer perform suprapubic aspirates as part of the routine cultures for suspected early-onset sepsis.

In infants presenting with late-onset UTI, the main clinical features are failure to thrive (50%), fever (40%), vomiting and/or diarrhoea (40%), jaundice (20%) and irritability or lethargy (20%) [2]. Intolerance of feeds and abdominal distension may be prominent. Although the sudden onset of, or increase in, jaundice is well recognized as suggesting UTI, particularly *E. coli* UTI with septicaemia, jaundice is recorded in less than one-quarter of all cases of UTI. If jaundice does occur it may be conjugated, unconjugated or mixed. Hepatosplenomegaly may be present. Obstructive uropathy can result in severe hyponatraemia sufficient to cause convulsions. Hypertension is rare.

Renal tract abnormalities may be diagnosed antenatally by ultrasonography scan. They are also associated with other congenital anomalies, as for example in the CHARGE (Coloboma, Atresia choanae, Retardation of growth and development, Genital hypoplasia and Ear defects of external ear and hearing) and VATER (Vertebral, Anorectal, Tracheo-oEsophageal and Radial anomalies) groups of anomalies. A single umbilical artery is often, although not always, associated with renal tract anomalies, as are abnormalities of the ears. Thus, a full examination is important: the kidneys should be palpated bimanually for abnormalities in size and position, the external genitalia should be examined and the urinary stream observed.

Occasionally, there may be signs of localized sepsis. Suppurative orchitis has been described, caused by various organisms (*Staphylococcus aureus*, *E. coli*, *Pseudomonas*), and prostatitis and epididymitis occur very occasionally. One outbreak of *Serratia* UTI, attributable to contaminated umbilical wash solution, was associated with balanitis.

DIAGNOSIS

The growth of organisms from a suprapubic aspirate (SPA) of urine is the generally accepted 'gold standard' for diagnosing UTI, and it is usually stated that any growth of bacteria is significant. However, even SPA urines can be contaminated with skin bacteria from the baby, or occasionally the bowel can be punctured, although this is less likely if ultrasonography is used first to confirm a full bladder. Suprapubic aspiration causes significant haematuria in 0.6% of cases [27] and is a traumatic procedure for babies, parents and staff. As discussed in Chapter 5, our policy is to reserve SPA for babies in whom UTI seems highly probable and for whom antibiotics need to be started immediately. SPA should also be used to confirm UTI after one or more positive bag urine specimens.

Bag urines are highly likely to be contaminated by the baby's faeces. Cleancatch urines, in which the pot is held poised over the penis or the vagina until the baby urinates, are a decided improvement, although they may require considerable patience. Catheter specimens, particularly from girls, may be less invasive than repeated failed attempts at SPA and should perhaps be used more often. If antibiotics are to be started, and an SPA is unsuccessful, catheterization is indicated to obtain a sample. The doubling time of *E. coli* at room temperature is about 20 minutes. Urine for culture should be taken to the laboratory immediately or refrigerated overnight.

MANAGEMENT

INVESTIGATION

Babies with proven UTI should have cultures of blood and CSF taken before starting treatment, since UTI is often septicaemic. Microscopic examination of the urine sediment can be helpful. However, normal babies without UTI may have up to 50 white blood cells per mm^3 [28] while about a quarter of babies with proven UTI do not have pyuria [9].

ANTIBIOTICS

The decision whether to initiate immediate antibiotic treatment of UTI while awaiting culture results depends on the level of clinical suspicion of systemic sepsis and whether organisms are seen on Gram staining of the urine. Although the relative distribution of the different organisms causing UTI differs from that of late-onset septicaemia (more Gram-negative bacilli, fewer staphylococci, rarely enterococci), the range of organisms does not differ substantially. Therefore, if a baby is systemically unwell, and whether or not there is evidence from urine microscopy of a UTI, our policy has been to treat with flucloxacillin and an aminoglycoside, the same antibiotics as for late-onset sepsis. This provides good cover against staphylococci as well as against Gram-negative bacilli.

If a baby is known to have renal tract anomalies, is systemically unwell and urine microscopy shows Gram-negative bacilli, we use cefotaxime and an aminoglycoside. On the other hand, if the baby has a positive culture from a bag urine, obtained because of relatively minor symptoms, and is not systemically unwell, we reassess the baby clinically. If the baby is well, we repeat the bag urine microscopy and culture but do not start antibiotics. If the baby is moderately unwell, we perform an SPA and full septic screen including CSF, and start antibiotics based on the antibiotic susceptibility of the organism from the previous bag urine culture. We repeat urine cultures after 48 hours' treatment to determine whether the urine is sterile, and if UTI is confirmed continue treatment for at least 7 days. Abscesses or complicated infections may require surgical exploration and extended antibiotic treatment.

Babies absorb oral antibiotics relatively poorly, particularly when sick. UTI is often a septicaemic illness and should not be treated with oral antibiotics: intravenous therapy should be used for the full treatment course. Oral antibiotics are suitable for prophylaxis.

SUPPORTIVE TREATMENT

Urinary tract infection, particularly when there is obstructive uropathy, can result in severe hyponatraemia sufficient to mimic salt-losing congenital adrenal hyperplasia. Hypertension is rare but shock may result from systemic sepsis; the blood pressure should always be measured. Haemolytic anaemia can be associated with the jaundice of UTI. The usual supportive measures for sepsis should be employed where appropriate, as outlined in Chapter 7, and a full blood count, serum creatinine and urea and electrolyte levels should be obtained.

INVESTIGATION OF URINARY TRACT

It is important to detect obstructive lesions early, so, once UTI is diagnosed, immediate investigations of the structure of the urinary tract should be performed (Figure 11.1). The commonest abnormality that can be detected is vesico-ureteric reflux (VUR), present in about one-half of all newborns with UTI [10]. The combination of both intrarenal reflux and urinary infection predisposes to renal damage with scarring, although it is controversial whether either alone causes scarring.

In the past, intravenous pyelography (IVP) was used to diagnose structural abnormalities, but this has largely been superseded by the use of real-time ultrasound. The reliability of ultrasound depends on the experience of the examiner. Ultrasound-based investigation of the urinary tract should be performed only when the appropriate expertise is available. It will detect obstructed systems, showing one or both kidneys dilated with or without dilatation of one or both ureters. Gross VUR

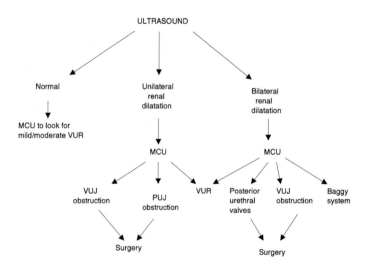

Figure 11.1 Management of neonate with confirmed urinary tract infection. MCU, micturating cysto-urethrography; VUJ, vesico-ureteric junction; PUJ, pelvi-ureteric junction

will also be detected by ultrasonography, but not milder degrees of reflux, and most neonatologists would perform micturating cysto-urethrography (MCU) as well as ultrasonography in the initial examination. (NB: Babies should be given oral or i.v. chemoprophylaxis before MCU to reduce the risk of UTI from the procedure.)

PREVENTION

The whole issue of prevention of further renal damage by preventing UTIs or treating them early is unresolved. Nevertheless, most authorities consider that at least some cases of chronic pyelonephritis might be prevented by preventing recurrences of UTI.

Thus babies with correctable lesions should have early surgery. Babies with proven UTI are usually treated with prophylactic oral antibiotics, trimethoprim or cotrimoxazole, at least until investigations are complete. Some would continue antibiotic prophylaxis for 12 months, because of the risk of recurrence, but others would stop prophylaxis if the urinary tract was normal. Surgical correction of moderate to severe ureteric reflux is considered for babies with breakthrough UTI. Babies undergoing MCU should be given oral or i.v. prophylaxis so that the MCU does not cause UTI.

SCREENING TO PREVENT UTI

Antenatal screening of fetuses for urinary tract abnormalities, notably hydronephrosis, is controversial. Gunn and colleagues found no renal ultrasonographic abnormalities before 28 weeks' gestation in over 3000 screened fetuses, while later examination of 761 fetuses yielded 8% with renal pelvis dilatation, of whom 16% had serious renal abnormalities [29]. Others have described false-positive fetal renal ultrasonographic scans, which cause great anxiety and waste resources; false positives may be less common with experience. Evidence does not support the use of routine fetal renal ultrasonography.

Ultrasonographic screening of newborn babies for abnormalities, and particularly for dilatation due to ureteric reflux, may be indicated under certain circumstances. Routine screening of all newborns by renal ultrasonography is not cost-effective. Hiraoka and colleagues scanned 300 unselected newborns [30]. They identified 53 with a dilated renal pelvis or other minor abnormality, 9 of whom were investigated by MCU and 3 of whom had VUR of grade III or above. Ultrasonography is indicated where fetal abnormalities have been detected by antenatal ultrasonography; in this case ultrasonography should be delayed for at least 48 hours after birth to avoid false-negative scans due to a low glomerular filtration rate (GFR). There is strong evidence that ureteric reflux is familial, and screening of the siblings and offspring of patients with known reflux, by ultrasonography and/or MCU, has been advocated.

SUMMARY

- Neonatal UTI is usually a septicaemic illness, so:
  (a) meningitis should be excluded by lumbar puncture;
  (b) treatment should be intravenous for the full course.
- UTI is 3–8 times more common in male than in female newborns.
- Host risk factors and organism virulence factors both contribute to the pathogenesis of UTI.
- It would require 100 circumcisions to prevent one UTI: routine male neonatal circumcision is probably not indicated, but circumcision might be recommended for babies at high risk of UTI.
- Oral antibiotic chemoprophylaxis (trimethoprim or cotrimoxazole) should be given to babies with proven UTI and babies due to have an MCU examination.

References

1 Kass EH. Asymptomatic infections of the urinary tract. *Trans Assoc Am Physicians* 1956; **69**: 56–64.

2 Klein JO & Long SS. Bacterial infections of the urinary tract. In: Remington JS & Klein JO (eds) *Infections of the Fetus and Newborn Infant*, 3rd edn. Philadelphia: WB Saunders, 1995: 925–34.

3 Pryles CV, Lüders D & Alkan MKA. A comparative study of bacterial cultures and colony counts in paired specimens of urine obtained by catheter versus voiding from normal infants and infants with urinary tract infection. *Pediatrics* 1961; **27**: 17.

4 Airede AI. Neonatal bacterial meningitis in the middle belt of Nigeria. *Dev Med Child Neurol* 1993; **35**: 424–30.

5 Lincoln K & Winberg J. Studies of urinary tract infections in infancy and childhood. II. Quantitative estimation of bacteriuria in unselected neonates with special reference to the occurrence of asymptomatic infections. *Acta Paediatr Scand* 1964; **53**: 307–16.

6 Littlewood JM, Kite P & Kite BA. Incidence of neonatal urinary tract infection. *Arch Dis Child* 1969; **44**: 617–20.

7 Bergstrom T, Larson H, Lincoln K & Winberg J. Neonatal urinary tract infections. *J Pediatr* 1972; **80**: 859–66.

8 Maherzi M, Guignard J-P & Torrado A. Urinary tract infection in high-risk newborn infants. *Pediatrics* 1978; **62**: 521–3.

9 Ginsburg CM & McCracken GH. Urinary tract infections in young infants. *Pediatrics* 1982; **69**: 409–12.

10 Rolleston GL, Shannon FT & Utley WLF. Relationship of infantile vesicoureteric reflux to renal damage. *BMJ* 1970; **1**: 460–3.

11 Bollgren I & Winberg J. The periurethral aerobic bacterial flora in healthy boys and girls. *Acta Paediatr Scand* 1976; **65**: 74–80.

12 Fussel EN, Kaack B, Cherry R & Roberts JA. Adherence of bacteria to human foreskins. *J Urol* 1988; **140**: 997–1001.

13 Wiswell TE, Smith FR & Bass JW. Decreased incidence of urinary tract infections in circumcised male infants. *Pediatrics* 1985; **75**: 901–3.

14 Wiswell TE, Enzenauer RW, Holton ME *et al.* Declining frequency of circumcision: implications for changes in the absolute incidence and male to female sex ratio of urinary tract infections in early infancy. *Pediatrics* 1987; **79**: 338–42.

15 Wiswell TE & Roscelli JD. Corroborative evidence for the decreased incidence of urinary tract infections in circumcised male infants. *Pediatrics* 1986; **78**: 96–9.

16 Wiswell TE, Miller GM, Gelston HM *et al.* Effect of circumcision status on periuretheral bacterial flora during the first year of life. *J Pediatr* 1988; **113**: 442–6.

17 Glennon J, Ryan PJ, Keane CT & Rees JPR. Circumcision and periurethral carriage of *Proteus mirabilis* in boys. *Arch Dis Child* 1988; **63**: 556–7.

18 Lomberg H, Hanson LA, Jacobsson B *et al.* Correlation of P blood group, vesicoureteral reflux, and bacterial attachment in patients with recurrent pyelonephritis. *N Engl J Med* 1983; **308**: 1189–92.

19 Tullus K, Brauner A, Fryklund B *et al.* Host factors versus virulence-associated bacterial characteristics in neonatal and infantile bacteraemia and meningitis caused by *Escherichia coli*. *J Med Microbiol* 1992; **36**: 203.

20 Svanborg C, Hausson S, Jodal U *et al.* Host–parasite interaction in the urinary tract. *J Infect Dis* 1988; **157**: 421.

21 de Man P, Claeson I, Johanson IM *et al.* Bacterial attachment as a predictor of renal abnormalities in boys with urinary tract infection. *J Pediatr* 1989; **115**: 915–22.

22 Vaisanen-Rhen V, Elo J, Vaisanen E *et al.* P-fimbriated clones among uropathogenic *Escherichia coli* strains. *Infect Immun* 1984; **43**: 149–55.

23 Marild S, Jodal U, Orskov I *et al.* Special virulence of the *Escherichia coli* O1:K1:H7 clone in acute pyelonephritis. *J Pediatr* 1989; **115**: 40–5.

24 Kuehn MJ, Heuser J, Normark S & Hultgren SJ. P pili in uropathogenic *E. coli* are composite fibres with distinct fibrillar adhesive tips. *Nature* 1992; **356**: 252–5.

25 Craig J. Urinary tract infection. In: Isaacs D & Moxon ER (eds) *A Practical Approach to Pediatric Infections*. London: Churchill Livingstone, 1996: 235–7.

26 Visser VE & Hall RT. Urine culture in the evaluation of suspected neonatal sepsis. *J Pediatr* 1979; **94**: 635–8.

27 Saccharow L & Pryles CV. Further experience with the use of percutaneous suprapubic aspiration of the urinary bladder. Bacteriologic studies in 654 infants and children. *Pediatrics* 1969; **43**: 1018–24.

28 Lincoln K & Winberg J. Studies of urinary tract infections in infancy and childhood. III. Quantitative estimation of cellular excretion in unselected neonates. *Acta Paediatr Scand* 1964; **53**: 447–53.

29 Gunn TR, Mora JD & Pease P. Outcome after antenatal diagnosis of upper urinary tract dilatation by ultrasonography. *Arch Dis Child* 1988; **63**: 1240.

30 Hiraoka M, Kasuga K, Hori C & Sudo M. Ultrasonic indicators of ureteric reflux in the newborn. *Lancet* 1994; **343**: 519–20.

12 | Infections of the eye

DEFINITION

It might be thought that the definition of conjunctivitis would cause little problem, because inflammation of the conjunctiva should be readily identifiable. In practice, however, it has been difficult to compare different studies of neonatal conjunctivitis because of variation in definitions or even complete failure to define what is meant by conjunctivitis.

Many babies present with 'sticky eyes' caused by purulent discharge, and this can be associated with a varying degree of conjunctival reddening and oedema. Conjunctivitis has been defined as purulent ocular discharge or inflammation of the conjunctivae. The term 'ophthalmia neonatorum' has been used to mean all neonatal eye infections or, alternatively, as synonymous with gonococcal ophthalmitis, the first-described and most serious cause of neonatal conjunctivitis.

Significant inflammation of the nasolacrimal duct is termed 'dacryocystitis', a condition diagnosed by finding a purple swelling lateral to the bridge of the nose from which purulent discharge can be expressed through the lacrimal punctum.

In conjunctivitis there may also be significant involvement of the eyelids and surrounding orbital tissues amounting to cellulitis. Periorbital cellulitis can be subdivided into preseptal cellulitis, with mild inflammation confined to the orbital margins, and orbital cellulitis, with severe inflammation beyond the margins of the orbit and often proptosis.

Most eye infections are confined to the conjunctivae, but there may be involvement of the cornea, of the inner eye (perforating keratitis and endophthalmitis) or of the whole eye (panophthalmitis).

EPIDEMIOLOGY

Conjunctivitis is the commonest neonatal infection. The incidence in industrialized countries, as judged by prospective studies, has been reported as 2–12% [1–4]. In one study from Belgium, 11% of babies had conjunctivitis by the time of discharge at 7–10 days, and a further 13% developed red or sticky eyes at home before 1 month of age [5]. Since many babies develop conjunctivitis after leaving hospital, retrospective hospital-based studies will greatly underestimate the incidence.

The incidence of neonatal conjunctivitis depends to a large extent on that of the sexually transmitted organisms *Neisseria gonorrhoeae* and *Chlamydia trachomatis* in the adult population. It also depends on ocular hygiene and access to clean water. In developing countries, a much higher incidence of neonatal conjunctivitis (15–34%) has been reported, of which gonococcal and chlamydial infection together contribute approximately one-half [6–10].

A complicating factor is the use of ocular prophylaxis against infection (see below), because the solutions used, particularly silver nitrate, are irritant and cause a chemical conjunctivitis in about 90% of babies. Conjunctivitis is common in babies receiving phototherapy, possibly because of the protective eyepads or even the lights.

Staphylococcus aureus is an important cause of conjunctivitis, and when there is much spread of staphylococci, as for example when umbilical cord care is not given, epidemics of staphylococcal conjunctivitis may occur.

Eyewash solutions may become contaminated with water-loving Gram-negative bacilli, such as *Pseudomonas* and *Serratia*, and outbreaks of Gram-negative conjunctivitis in neonatal units have been traced to contaminated eyewash solutions.

Disposable single-use saline sachets have largely prevented this problem.

MICROBIOLOGY

The three major causes of neonatal eye infections are *Neisseria gonorrhoeae*, *Chlamydia trachomatis* and *Staphylococcus aureus*.

Gonococcal ophthalmitis used to be the commonest cause of blindness, even in industrialized countries. Three British studies, in which ocular prophylaxis was not given, found no cases of gonococcal ophthalmitis [2,3,11], although 11 of 103 babies with therapy-resistant conjunctivitis in Liverpool had gonococcal infection [12]. In Britain and the Netherlands, eye prophylaxis has been discontinued and the rare cases of gonococcal ophthalmitis are used as a signal for treating baby and parents. A study from Australia, where a similar approach is used, found that eight (1.4%) of 571 babies with conjunctivitis had gonococcal infection, 0.4 per 1000 live births [13]. In the United States, where ocular prophylaxis is almost universal, the incidence of gonococcal ophthalmitis is about 0.1 per 1000 live births [14].

In contrast, *N. gonorrhoeae* has been responsible for between 15% and 44% of all eye infections in studies from Africa. When these figures are combined with the incidence data, they suggest that 2–18% of babies from the African populations studied can be expected to develop gonococcal ophthalmitis [15].

The incidence of *C. trachomatis* conjunctivitis in industrialized countries has generally been reported as approximately 2–4 per 1000 live births [2,4,14]. As the incidence is higher in lower socio-economic groups, the reported incidence will vary according to the socio-economic status of the local population. If milder cases of conjunctivitis and those occurring after leaving the maternity hospital are included, a higher incidence of chlamydial conjunctivitis is found. In the United States, such studies have reported an incidence of chlamydial conjunctivitis of 10–63 per 1000 live births [16]. This represents up to 43% of all cases of neonatal conjunctivitis [17]. About 60–70% of babies born to mothers with chlamydial infection of the cervix become colonized. Chlamydial conjunctivitis develops in 25–50% of exposed infants and, if untreated, pneumonitis develops in 10–20%.

In Africa a greater proportion of cases of conjunctivitis is probably caused by *C. trachomatis*, with reports suggesting that 13–35% of babies with conjunctivitis, and 2–10% of all babies, have chlamydial conjunctivitis [8–10].

Staphylococcus aureus is the commonest organism other than *N. gonorrhoeae* and *C. trachomatis* to cause conjunctivitis. Other bacteria have been isolated from the eyes of babies with conjunctivitis but can also colonize eyes without causing infections. Studies in which appropriate controls have been included have shown that conjunctivitis may be caused by *Pseudomonas aeruginosa*, group A and B streptococci, pneumococci, *Haemophilus influenzae*, meningococci, *Moraxella* (originally *Branhamella) catarrhalis*, coliforms, enterococci and *Streptococcus viridans*. Occasional cases due to *Corynebacterium diphtheriae*, *Pasteurella multocida* and *Clostridia* have been reported. Herpes simplex virus, echoviruses, adenoviruses, *Candida* and *Mycoplasma hominis* are all rare causes. Dacryocystitis and dacryostenosis are more likely with infections due to *Haemophilus* and pneumococci [18].

Pseudomonas aeruginosa may cause a mild conjunctivitis or a fulminant panophthalmitis. Other organisms such as group B streptococci, pneumococci, *S. aureus* (particularly in the older literature), *H. influenzae* type b, meningococci and *Salmonella enteritidis* may very occasionally cause severe endophthalmitis, probably due to metastatic foci following septicaemia. In a German study, 13 of 16 cases of bacterial endophthalmitis were caused by *P. aeruginosa,* two by group B streptococci and one by *Streptococcus pneumoniae* [19].

PATHOLOGY AND PATHOGENESIS

Neisseria gonorrhoeae replicates rapidly and induces a vigorous host leukocyte response. There is eyelid oedema and profuse purulent exudate which may be under pressure and may damage the cornea, causing ulceration. If treatment is delayed, corneal perforation and endophthalmitis may ensue. In pre-antibiotic days, gonococcal ophthalmia caused about a quarter of all cases of blindness in the USA.

Chlamydia trachomatis infection is associated with purulent eye discharge, oedema and pseudomembrane, but corneal ulceration is extremely rare. Resolution is slow, even with treatment, and babies often develop micropannus and conjunctival scarring, although conjunctival follicles are less common than in older children and adults with trachoma.

Herpes simplex virus causes a keratoconjunctivitis which can progress to corneal ulceration classically with a branching pattern (dendritic ulcer).

Other forms of conjunctivitis, bacterial, viral or chemical, are usually less severe, although *Pseudomonas* may sometimes progress rapidly from conjunctivitis to a life-threatening panophthalmitis.

CLINICAL FEATURES

Gonococcal infection usually presents as an acute severe purulent conjunctivitis, 2–5 days after birth. It may, however, present earlier, be indolent, present later or occasionally be asymptomatic. Typically, the baby develops eyelid oedema, chemosis and a profuse purulent discharge (Colour plate 12.1). If untreated, corneal involvement with ulceration, perforation and, very occasionally, panophthalmitis occurs, and corneal scarring can lead to blindness.

Gonococcal infection is particularly likely to result in severe conjunctivitis. However, chlamydial infection can also be severe, and gonococcal infection may be modified by prior topical or systemic antibiotic therapy.

Infection with *Chlamydia trachomatis* usually presents between 5 and 14 days after birth, as it is acquired predominantly by passage through an infected birth canal. However, early cases occur and there have been occasional reports of babies developing infection despite caesarean delivery with intact membranes. *Chlamydia* causes a more severe conjunctivitis than other organisms except gonococcus [4]. A watery discharge rapidly becomes purulent and the eyes are red with oedematous lids (Colour plate 12.2a). There is marked conjunctival inflammation, sometimes with formation of a pseudomembrane of inflammatory material (Colour plate 12.2b). Infection may be suppressed, but not cured, by topical antibiotics and will then recur or become chronic. Most untreated cases eventually resolve spontaneously, but chronic infection may lead to conjunctival follicles and even corneal neovascularization (pannus) with 'sheet scarring' or linear scarring as in trachoma.

It may be impossible to distinguish gonococcal and chlamydial infection clinically. The Gram stain is a sensitive test of gonococcal infection (see Diagnosis below), provided that no antibiotics have been given.

Pseudomonas conjunctivitis usually appears at between 4 and 18 days of age. There may be mild infection limited to the conjunctiva, or lid oedema and erythema. In the fulminant form, there is corneal involvement with pannus formation and sometimes perforation, exudate in the anterior chamber and adherence of the iris to the cornea. Although the initial conjunctivitis is usually bilateral, the endophthalmitis is usually (although not always) unilateral [19].

There are no distinctive clinical features to distinguish the other bacterial causes of conjunctivitis [18]. Herpes simplex causes dendritic or geographical corneal ulcers. *Candida* can cause fluffy infiltrates in the retina or aqueous humour. Maxillary osteomyelitis often presents with purulent conjunctivitis and eyelid oedema before swelling of the cheek develops (Chapter 10).

DIAGNOSIS

The degree of assiduity with which the cause of conjunctivitis is pursued depends on the availability of tests, the severity of the conjunctivitis and the epidemiology. In industrialized countries, for example, chlamydial conjunctivitis is rare except in very poor populations. We look for *Chlamydia* only in severe or refractory cases.

Gram stain for gonococcus is over 90% sensitive in untreated cases [20] so an immediate Gram stain is mandatory. Conjunctival swabs for gonococcal culture need to be charcoal impregnated, calcium alginate or Dacron swabs, since others are toxic to the organism. Gonococci need a high CO_2 concentration for optimal growth (5%) and are quite fastidious, needing incubation on enriched media, e.g. chocolate agar. Specimens that need to be transported any distance for which laboratory delay is anticipated should be inoculated into isolation media or transport media and transported or incubated in 5% CO_2. Swabs should be processed as soon as possible, certainly within 48 hours.

Various techniques have been used to detect chlamydial infection. A conjunctival smear, taken by rubbing the lower lid conjunctiva with a glass rod, can be stained with Giemsa for inclusion bodies, but is fairly insensitive. Rapid tests employed in different laboratories include immunofluorescent staining, ELISA and polymerase chain reaction (PCR) testing; all these are highly sensitive and specific. Specific immunoglobulin A (IgA) levels in tears rise too late to be useful. Serum IgM concentration only rises in up to two-thirds of babies and is unreliable. Culture for *Chlamydia* on McCoy cells is time consuming, but still used for definitive diagnosis by some laboratories.

HSV infection can be diagnosed rapidly by immunofluorescence on a conjunctival smear, taken simply by streaking a swab on a glass slide (see Figure 16.3).

TREATMENT

Mild conjunctivitis often responds to saline washes alone. Topical antibiotics such as chloramphenicol or trimethoprim–polymyxin will be sufficient to treat most cases of neonatal conjunctivitis.

Gonococcal ophthalmia requires systemic penicillin G; the dose for sensitive organisms is 25 000 units/kg per dose 12-hourly, given intravenously. Babies infected with resistant penicillinase-producing *Neisseria gonorrhoeae* should be treated with ceftriaxone (50–100 mg/kg) or cefotaxime (100 mg/kg), which is sometimes recommended as a single intramuscular or intravenous injection [15,21] although many authorities would treat for 7 days with the same antibiotics. Frequent eye irrigation is important, but topical antibiotics are unnecessary. The baby should be isolated for 24 hours as the organism is highly contagious, and both parents and any sexual contacts should be screened for gonorrhoea and treated.

Chlamydial conjunctivitis should be treated with topical tetracycline, erythromycin or sulphonamides. Because recurrences are frequent and there is some evidence of a consequent reduction in the incidence of pneumonitis, it is usual to give oral erythromycin 10 mg/kg per dose, 6-hourly for 14 days. Both parents should be screened and treated for *Chlamydia* infection.

PREVENTION

It was in 1881 that Credé first introduced the practice of cleaning the newborn's eyelids and instilling a drop of 1% silver nitrate solution as prophylaxis against ophthalmia neonatorum. This greatly reduced the incidence of blindness, and is still used in many countries.

However, silver nitrate frequently (up to 90% of babies) causes a chemical conjunctivitis, and its disadvantages for non-industrialized countries, which usually have the highest incidence of ophthalmia neonatorum, are its expense and evaporation from the heat with resultant concentration.

In a study in Kenya, silver nitrate was 83% effective in preventing gonococcal ophthalmia, but only 68% effective for *Chlamydia,* whereas 1% tetracycline ointment prophylaxis prevented 93% of gonococcal and 77% of chlamydial conjunctivitis [22]. Tetracycline ointment is about one-twentieth the price of silver nitrate solution.

Cheaper still is 2.5% povidone–iodine. This costs about one-third of the price of tetracycline and in a large trial, also in Kenya, was far more effective than silver nitrate or erythromycin ointment against *Chlamydia*, although slightly less effective than silver nitrate against gonococcal ophthalmia [23]. Povidone–iodine 2.5% solution is a cheap, effective and non-toxic measure which should be routinely introduced in non-industrialized countries.

In some industrialized countries, such as the Netherlands and the UK, the incidence of gonococcal and chlamydial conjunctivitis is low. Prophylaxis is not used; each case is diagnosed and treated, and is used as a marker of maternal disease.

The incidence of neonatal ophthalmia can be reduced by preventing sexually transmitted diseases and/or by screening pregnant women for genital infection.

Babies born to mothers with gonococcal infection can be protected with a single i.v. or i.m. dose of 50 000 units penicillin (20 000 units for babies of low birthweight). Such a regimen has been used as routine prophylaxis for all babies in some North American hospitals. Siegel and colleagues randomly allocated babies to receive a single dose of penicillin G i.m. at birth, or tetracycline eye ointment [24]. The penicillin group had a lower incidence of group B streptococcus (GBS) infections, but a higher incidence of penicillin-resistant enterococcal infections and a mortality rate 2.4 times higher; thus, prophylactic penicillin is not without risks.

Case history 12.1

A baby girl, the first child of an 18-year-old mother and 20-year-old father, was born vaginally at term, weighing 3440 g. Mother said she had had some vaginal discharge throughout pregnancy, but thought it was normal. The baby developed conjunctivitis at 2 days of age. She went home at 3 days, breastfeeding well. She was given chloramphenicol eyedrops, with no improvement. An eye swab taken at 12 days of age showed multiple pus cells, but no organisms were seen and none grew. She was changed to tobramycin drops, but purulent discharge continued, and the eyes became increasingly haemorrhagic over the next 2 days.

At 14 days of age, when she was referred, she was well, afebrile and still feeding well. Both eyes were gummed shut with thick, sticky, brownish-red pus oozing out. The eyes were cleaned with normal saline, after prior administration of amethocaine drops, and fluorescein staining showed that there were no corneal ulcers and no keratitis. The remainder of the examination was normal, and in particular the joints showed no abnormality. Gram stain of an eye swab showed copious pus cells, but no organisms.

The mother's vaginal swab also had a negative Gram stain for organisms, making gonococcal ophthalmitis unlikely. It was decided to treat the baby both for gonorrhoea with i.v. cefotaxime and for *Chlamydia* infection with oral erythromycin, pending further results.

Bacterial cultures from the baby's eye and the mother's vagina were negative. The baby's serum immunoglobulins showed a raised serum level IgG of 9.2 g/L (normal 2.4–8.6), but normal IgA and IgM levels. PCR for *Chlamydia* was performed and was positive on the baby's eye swab and the mother's vaginal swab. The baby's cefotaxime was stopped, and oral erythromycin was continued for 14 days, while both parents were treated with erythromycin. The baby's eyes improved slowly for the first week, but eventually recovered completely.

Gonococcal ophthalmitis typically presents at 2–5 days, although, because the initial course may be indolent, babies may not present until later in the first month. *Chlamydia* conjunctivitis tends to present somewhat later, at 5–14 days of age. The organism cannot usually be demonstrated in the conjunctiva within 24 hours of birth and, as the organism's growth cycle is about 48 hours, it is somewhat surprising that this baby's conjunctivitis was already present at 48 hours.

There are no clinically distinguishing features between gonococcal and chlamydial conjunctivitis. In this case, the onset at 2 days seemed to favour gonococcus, while the prolonged failure to respond to topical antibiotics was more suggestive of chlamydial infection. It seemed sensible to treat empirically for both organisms until results were back. In the past, it took a number of days before chlamydial cultures became positive. Nowadays, however, culture has been largely superseded by antigen detection and more recently by PCR techniques. Serum levels of immunoglobulins G, A and/or M are raised in over 90% of babies with *Chlamydia* pneumonitis, but in a smaller proportion of babies with *Chlamydia* ophthalmitis. There are no controlled treatment trials, but epidemiological studies have suggested that 50% of babies with untreated *Chlamydia* ophthalmitis develop pneumonitis, which itself has a high risk of leading to recurrent small airways disease.

For babies with *Chlamydia* ophthalmitis, oral erythromycin therapy virtually abolishes the risk of subsequent pneumonitis, whereas topical therapy alone will not reduce the risk at all.

SUMMARY

- Gonococcal and chlamydial ophthalmia present early and may be clinically indistinguishable.
- Gram stain for gonococcus is sensitive and specific.
- *Chlamydia* can be detected rapidly by immunofluorescence, ELISA or PCR.
- Gonococcal conjunctivitis should be treated with parenteral penicillin, ceftriaxone or cefotaxime.
- Chlamydial conjunctivitis should be treated with 14 days' oral erythromycin to prevent chlamydial pneumonitis.
- Parents of babies with gonococcus or *Chlamydia* must be screened and treated.

References

1 Johnson D & McKenna H. Bacteria in ophthalmia neonatorum. *Pathology* 1975; **7**: 199–201.

2 Prentice MJ, Hutchinson CR & Taylor-Robinson D. A microbiological study of neonatal conjunctivae and conjunctivitis. *Br J Ophthalmol* 1977; **61**: 601–7.

3 Pierce JM, Ward ME & Seal DV. Ophthalmia neonatorum in the 1980's: incidence, aetiology and treatment. *Br J Ophthalmol* 1982; **66**: 728–31.

4 Sandstrom I. Etiology and diagnosis of neonatal conjunctivitis. *Acta Paediatr Scand* 1987; **76**: 221–7.

5 Fransen L, van den Berghe P, Mertens A *et al.* Incidence and bacterial aetiology of neonatal conjunctivitis. *Eur J Pediatr* 1987; **146**: 152–5.

6 Sowa S, Sowa J & Collier LH. Investigation of neonatal conjunctivitis in the Gambia. *Lancet* 1968; **ii**: 243–7.

7 Otiti JML. Ophthalmia neonatorum in Mbale Hospital, Uganda. *East Afr Med J* 1975; **52**: 644–7.

8 Maybe DCW & Whittle HC. Genital and neonatal chlamydial infection in a trachoma endemic area, Gambia. *Lancet* 1982; **ii**: 300–1.

9 Meheus A, Delgadillo R, Widy-Wirsky R & Piot P. Chlamydial ophthalmia neonatorum in Central Africa. *Lancet* 1982; **ii**: 882.

10 Fransen L, Nsawze H, Klauss V *et al.* Ophthalmia neonatorum in Nairobi, Kenya: the roles of *Neisseria gonorrhoeae* and *Chlamydia trachomatis*. *J Infect Dis* 1986; **153**: 862–9.

11 McGill RET. Neonatal eye infections. *Communicable Diseases Scotland; Weekly Rep.* 1979; **22**: 12.

12 Rees E, Tait IA, Hobson D *et al.* Neonatal conjunctivitis caused by *Neisseria gonorrhoeae* and *Chlamydia trachomatis*. *Br J Vener Dis* 1977; **53**: 173–9.

13 Johnson D & McKenna H. Bacteria in ophthalmia neonatorum. *Pathology* 1975; **7**: 199–201.

14 Armstrong JH, Zacarias F & Rein MF. Ophthalmia neonatorum: a chart review. *Pediatrics* 1976; **57**: 84–92.

15 Foster A & Klaus V. Ophthalmia neonatorum in developing countries. *N Engl J Med* 1995; **332**: 33–61.

16 Schachter J & Grossman M. Chlamydial infections. *Annu Rev Med* 1981; **32**: 45–61.

17 Rapoza PA, Quinn TC, Kiessling LA & Taylor HR. Epidemiology of neonatal conjunctivitis. *Ophthalmology* 1986; **93**: 456–61.

18 Sandstrom I, Bell TA, Chandler JW *et al.* Microbial causes of neonatal conjunctivitis. *J Pediatr* 1984; **105**: 706–11.

19 Lohrer R & Belohradsky BH. Bacterial endophthalmitis in neonates. *Eur J Pediatr* 1987; **146**: 354–9.

20 Gilbert GL. *Infectious Disease in Pregnancy and the Newborn Infant*. Harwood: Chur, 1991.

21 World Health Organization. *Conjunctivitis of the Newborn: Prevention and Treatment at the Primary Health Care Level*. Geneva: WHO, 1986.

22 Laga M, Plummer FA, Piot P *et al*. Prophylaxis of gonococcal and chlamydial ophthalmia neonatorum: a comparison of silver intrate and tetracycline. *N Engl J Med* 1988; **318**, 653–7.

23 Isenberg SJ, Apt L, Wood MA. A controlled trial of povidone–iodine as prophylaxis against ophthalmia neonatorum. *N Engl J Med* 1995; **332**: 562–6.

24 Siegel JD, McCracken GH, Threlkeld N *et al*. Single-dose penicillin prophylaxis against neonatal group B streptococcal infections. A controlled trial in 18,738 newborn infants. *N Engl J Med* 1980; **303**: 769–75.

13 | Intestinal infections

GASTROENTERITIS

Gastroenteritis is relatively uncommon in neonatal units in industralized countries, but life-threatening outbreaks continue to occur in many non-industrialized countries [1].

As with all infections, the most important determinants can be divided into host factors, organism factors and the environment.

THE HOST

The newborn baby has poor secretory antibody production and is, therefore, relatively susceptible to gastrointestinal infection. Breast milk, which contains secretory immunoglobulin A (IgA) and lymphocytes, is protective against gastroenteritis. Other factors that protect against infection are gastric acid, gastric motility, normal intestinal flora and intestinal mucus.

THE ORGANISM

Pathogens can be ingested at the time of birth from the birth canal or perineum (vertical transmission), e.g. enteropathogenic *Escherichia coli* and enteroviruses, or can be acquired later by horizontal transmission from other babies. Infections may be sporadic or part of a nursery outbreak.

A wide range of organisms has been associated with neonatal enteric infections (Table 13.1). In general, bacteria cause diarrhoea either by direct invasion of intestinal mucosa (enteroinvasive) or by colonization and toxin production (enterotoxic). Some strains of *E. coli* are enteroinvasive, while others are enterotoxic, and yet others act through less well-characterized mechanisms, such as enteropathogenic and enterohaemorrhagic *E. coli*.

E. coli is a normal commensal of the neonatal intestine, and, although the association of diarrhoea in calves (scours) with certain strains of *E. coli* was recognized in the nineteenth century, it was not until the 1930s that strains of *E. coli* responsible for human neonatal and infantile diarrhoea were distinguished serologically. Enteropathogenic forms of *E. coli* (EPECs), such as strain 0111, were described in association

---

Bacteria
   Escherichia coli
      Enterotoxigenic (ETEC)
      Enteropathogenic (EPEC)
      Enterohaemorrhagic
      Enteroinvasive
   Salmonella species
   Shigella species
   Campylobacter species
   Yersinia species
   Clostridium difficile
Viruses
   Rotavirus
   Echovirus
   Coxsackieviruses
   Adenoviruses (enteric)
   Small round viruses, e.g. Norwalk
   Astroviruses
   Coronaviruses

Table 13.1 Organisms causing neonatal enteric infection

with nursery epidemics and infantile diarrhoea in the 1950s onwards to the mid-1970s in the UK, the USA and Uganda. They do not produce toxins, nor do they invade the mucosa, and the mechanism by which they produce diarrhoea is ill understood. Infection is by the faecal–oral route. EPECs are now a rare cause of neonatal diarrhoea in developed countries, although they are still important when there is overcrowding and poor sanitation.

Enterotoxigenic forms of *E. coli* (ETECs) produce enterotoxins that are classified as heat-labile (LT) or heat-stable (ST). Although there were reports of outbreaks of ETEC infection in neonatal units in the USA and Scotland in the 1970s, ETEC was a less common cause of neonatal gastroenteritis than EPEC.

Although EPEC and ETEC are more commonly associated with diarrhoea in infants, older children and adults in developing countries, neonatal diarrhoea attributable to these organisms is relatively rarely reported. This may be because of difficulty with culture techniques, but also because home delivery is common and breastfeeding, which is protective, is virtually universal. The decline in incidence of neonatal diarrhoea due to these organisms in developed countries may be attributable to improved hygiene, increased use of human breast milk for feeding preterm babies or to a decline in virulence.

In areas of the world where *Salmonella* infection (excluding typhoid, which is extremely rare in neonates) is common or endemic, this can be an important cause of neonatal gastroenteritis, albeit accounting for a small proportion of all cases of gastroenteritis. Salmonellae invade the intestinal mucosa, replicate in the lamina propria and invade mesenteric lymph nodes. They may then spread via lymphatics or blood to distant sites. Infection is primarily acquired at the time of birth from ingesting infected faeces or cervical secretions. Outbreaks in neonatal units may occur, with organisms transmitted on the hands of staff, who may themselves develop intestinal colonization. Infection rates in neonatal units have varied from 10% to 85% of exposed babies. Up to one-half may be asymptomatic and the remainder generally have a non-specific gastroenteritis with foul-smelling green 'pea-soup' stools containing mucus and often flecks of blood.

About 5% of neonates with non-typhoid *Salmonella* infection have an associated septicaemia, although in some outbreaks the incidence of septicaemia is higher. More neonates than older children develop septicaemia. Septicaemic babies may have rose spots or purpura, but fever may be absent and the symptoms and signs are generally non-specific. Metastatic spread can cause meningitis, osteomyelitis, septic arthritis, pericarditis, pneumonia, empyema, pyelonephritis, cholecystitis, endophthalmitis and skin sepsis. Very occasionally, the metastatic manifestations may be the presenting symptom. Many infected neonates will develop a carrier state for many months, which is generally asymptomatic, although chronic *Salmonella* enteritis with intractable diarrhoea has been described. Oral antibiotics prolong the carrier state and increase the risk of relapse, yet neonatal salmonellosis may be associated with septicaemia and the risk of metastatic spread. Blood, urine and CSF cultures should be taken from newborns with *Salmonella* gastroenteritis, and intravenous ampicillin (100–200 mg/kg per day in four divided doses) started if there is fever, toxicity or severe diarrhoea.

Shigella is an uncommon cause of neonatal diarrhoea, even in endemic countries. *Shigella*, like enteroinvasive *E. coli*, attaches to the colonic enterocyte and penetrates by pinocytosis, spreading to neighbouring cells by bacteria-induced pseudopodia. This results in a colitis with shallow ulcers and exudate. Clinical manifestations include blood and mucous stools, with fever and abdominal pain. If disease occurs in neonates, they may perforate and develop peritonitis. *Shigella dysenteriae* 1 is toxigenic, elaborating an exotoxin called shiga toxin which is cytotoxic. Neonatal *Shigella* infection may be complicated by *Shigella* septicaemia, and even occasionally meningitis. In addition, bowel necrosis caused by *Shigella* may result in secondary septicaemia due to other bowel organisms.

Campylobacter jejuni and *Campylobacter fetus* have both been associated with nursery outbreaks of diarrhoea in which the index case acquired the infection from the mother at delivery. Outbreaks have also been associated with the use of unpasteurized milk. The index case in an outbreak is generally born preterm and presents within 12–24 hours of birth with fever, respiratory distress, vomiting, diarrhoea, cyanosis and convulsions. Septicaemia progresses rapidly to meningitis. Secondary cases have diarrhoea, often with mucus, pus and blood, but rarely fever unless they develop septicaemia with or without meningitis. Oral erythromycin is the treatment of choice for enteritis, but intravenous chloramphenicol and an aminoglycoside is probably the regimen of choice for meningitis. However, in a report of a nosocomial outbreak when 11 babies developed *Campylobacter jejuni* meningitis, Goossens and colleagues successfully treated them with ampicillin and gentamicin, although a β-lactamase-producing strain was isolated [2]. One baby had mild hydrocephalus, but the rest recovered uneventfully.

Yersinia enterocolitica is a rare cause of neonatal gastroenteritis. It invades and replicates in the Peyer's patches. It can cause bloody diarrhoea with mucus, but also severe abdominal pain mimicking appendicitis.

Enterotoxins can cause profuse watery diarrhoea by stimulation of intracellular adenylate cyclase, leading to altered chloride secretion from villi; examples are the heat-labile toxin of enterotoxigenic *E. coli* (ETEC) and the closely related cholera toxin. The heat-stable toxins produced by other strains of ETEC activate guanylate cyclase, leading to cyclic GMP accumulation and secretory diarrhoea. Neonatal disease due to ETEC and cholera is fortunately rare.

Staphylococcus aureus occasionally proliferates in the intestine, producing a clinical picture identical to necrotizing enterocolitis, with bloody diarrhoea, abdominal distension and tenderness (see staphylococcal enterocolitis below).

Clostridium difficile is a frequent commensal of the neonatal gut. Although *C. difficile* can elaborate an enterotoxin (toxin

A) and a potent cytotoxin (toxin B), there is little evidence for *C. difficile* causing neonatal disease. Colonization with toxin-producing *C. difficile* is common in the neonatal period, and almost always asymptomatic [3,4].

A number of different viruses has been associated with neonatal gastroenteritis. The most commonly identified virus is rotavirus. Asymptomatic shedding of rotaviruses is common in the neonatal period, unlike later in life, but rotaviruses can also cause severe neonatal disease [5]. Rotavirus infection can result in watery diarrhoea, or bloody diarrhoea with a clinical picture mimicking necrotizing enterocolitis [6]. Rotaviruses mainly cause lytic infection of mature enterocytes at the tips of small intestinal villi.

Enteric adenoviruses (types 40 and 41) cannot be cultured in conventional tissue culture, but can be seen by electron microscopy of stools. They infect enterocytes causing villus atrophy and crypt hypertrophy. Astroviruses cause similar pathology in experimental animals.

Enteroviruses may be horizontally or vertically acquired. Gastroenteritis is more likely following horizontal acquisition, for example in nursery outbreaks, but vertical acquisition may result in fulminant and often fatal disease characterized by hepatitis and/or myocarditis and/or meningitis (see Chapter 16).

CLINICAL FEATURES

Bloody diarrhoea with mucus, i.e. colitis, is likely to be due to *Salmonella*, *Shigella*, *Campylobacter* or, rarely, *Yersinia* species. Profuse watery diarrhoea may be caused by enterotoxin-producing organisms, such as ETEC or *Vibrio cholerae*, although non-toxin-producing organisms, like EPEC and viruses, also cause watery diarrhoea. In general, the clinical features in neonatal gastroenteritis are rarely diagnostic of any particular pathogen and the organism needs to be identified in the laboratory.

Bacteraemic dissemination may occur with *Salmonella* (bone, joint, meninges), *Shigella* (meninges) and less commonly with other bacteria. Signs of bone, joint or meningeal involvement should, therefore, be sought in each baby with gastroenteritis.

DIAGNOSIS

Bloody diarrhoea with mucus suggests colitis and hence bacterial gastroenteritis, but otherwise there are few clinical features to suggest the aetiology in gastroenteritis. In most cases we are dependent on the laboratory to identify the cause. Stool microscopy can reveal white cells, suggesting colitis, and Gram stain will show profuse Gram-positive cocci in staphylococcal enterocolitis (see below). Routine bacterial cultures will identify *Salmonella*, *Shigella*, *Campylobacter* and *S. aureus*, but not *Yersinia* or *Vibrio* species, which require special media, nor the various strains of *E. coli*, which also require selective media.

If viruses are suspected, a separate stool specimen needs to be sent, asking specifically for viruses. Rotaviruses, enteric adenoviruses, small round viruses, astroviruses and coronaviruses cannot be cultured, and are usually identified by electron microscopy (EM), either direct negative-staining EM or immune EM. EM has the advantage that it detects small numbers of viruses, and will identify any of the above viruses. It is expensive and requires specialist expertise. ELISA tests are available for rotavirus; these are cheap and more freely available, but there are problems with false-positive tests, particularly when rotavirus ELISA is used to screen asymptomatic babies [1,6]. Latex agglutination assays for rotavirus are available, but are not preferred to ELISA generally. ELISAs for enteric adenoviruses are also available. PCR for different viruses is being developed.

Enteroviruses (echo, coxsackie, polio) are not identifiable by EM, and stool culture on appropriate cell monolayers is the diagnostic method of choice. If enteroviruses are suspected from the maternal or neonatal history, viral cultures of stool (and throat swab) should be specifically requested.

TREATMENT

Fluid and electrolyte balance are the mainstay of treatment. If the baby is shocked or significantly volume-depleted, rapid volume replacement with colloid is indicated.

Parenteral antibiotics are indicated in babies with *Shigella* diarrhoea, and in babies with *Salmonella* or *Campylobacter* who have high swinging fever and probable bacteraemia. Staphylococcal enterocolitis is treated with parenteral antibiotics and oral vancomycin. It should not be forgotten that systemic sepsis may present with gastrointestinal symptoms (diarrhoea, vomiting, abdominal distension).

Babies with suspected gastroenteritis who are severely unwell warrant treatment with antibiotics that will cover staphylococci, faecal streptococci and enteric Gram-negative bacilli until blood culture results are available.

PREVENTION

Gastrointestinal pathogens are either acquired at the time of delivery or via the faecal–oral route postnatally. Outbreaks of gastroenteritis in neonatal nurseries are almost always the result of poor infection control practices. Organisms are carried on the hands of staff and outbreaks can be prevented by handwashing. If they do occur, outbreaks can often be terminated rapidly by strict attention to handwashing [7]. For further discussion of management of outbreaks, see Chapter 18.

Rotavirus vaccines, based on bovine rotaviruses or rhesus and human reassortants, are being developed and evaluated. They are not yet in routine use.

NECROTIZING ENTEROCOLITIS

DEFINITION

Necrotizing enterocolitis (NEC) is a disease, mainly of preterm infants, that was barely recognized until the 1960s. Although there is no evidence that NEC is a primary infection, it is covered in this book because there is circumstantial evidence that microbes are implicated, at least in part, in its pathophysiology. NEC is currently the commonest cause of neonatal peritonitis and a major cause of mortality and morbidity.

NEC is essentially a pathological diagnosis. Classical cases have unique clinical features, such as intramural gas, which are diagnostic. Because of the serious implications, clinicians are often obliged to make a presumptive diagnosis of NEC without firm evidence. Bell and colleagues suggested a three-step staging system that takes into account the weight of evidence in favour of a diagnosis of NEC [8]. In Oxford, a five-step system is used (Table 13.2): grades I and II indicate a low probability of NEC, but identify occasional cases which progress later to a more advanced grade; grade III is 'probable NEC', whereas grades IV and V represent 'definite NEC'. The Oxford gradings correspond closely to Bell's definitions, but allow a more precise clinical description for purposes of comparison.

EPIDEMIOLOGY

The incidence of NEC is greatest in infants of very low birthweight and lowest in term infants. As the number of cases varies considerably over time within any hospital, it should not be assumed that temporal clustering of cases within a hospital

Grade	Clinical description
I	Bloody stools, no clotting abnormality. No abdominal distension. Tolerate early reintroduction of enteral feeds (within 48 hours)
II	Abdominal distension. Suspicious abdominal radiograph without intramural gas. No blood in stools. Tolerate early reintroduction of enteral feeds
III	Bloody stools, abdominal distension, ileus with dilated small bowel loops on abdominal radiograph, no intramural gas
IV	Bloody stools, abdominal distension, intramural gas, with or without gas in biliary tree or intestinal perforation
V	Operative or autopsy diagnosis, histologically confirmed

Table 13.2 Clinical grading of nectrotizing enterocolitis (Oxford)

represents an outbreak. Outbreaks of colitis attributable to a number of different microorganisms may be indistinguishable clinically and histopathologically from NEC. Clustering of cases should therefore be interpreted with caution: in small clusters many of the babies have risk factors for NEC and their simultaneous occurrence is usually due to chance. In larger clusters, a search should be made for an infectious cause of colitis.

The reported incidence of NEC ranges from 0.5 to 15 per 1000 live births [9] and develops in about 2% (range 1–5%) of babies admitted to neonatal intensive care units [10]. The incidence is inversely related to gestational age and birthweight: Stoll and colleagues reported NEC in 6.5% of babies with birthweight <1500 g, 1% of babies 1500–2000 g, 0.27% of 2000–2500 < g and 0.04% of >2500 g [11]. Nevertheless, about 10% of all cases of NEC occur in full-term infants; 90–95% of cases occur in babies who have received enteral feeds [10]. The mortality rate is 10–50%, while survivors may suffer from short bowel syndrome [12].

PATHOGENESIS

One theory is that NEC results from an initial episode of intestinal ischaemia, subsequently compounded by bacterial invasion of the disrupted intestinal mucosa. The multiplication of anaerobic (e.g. *Clostridium*) and aerobic (e.g. *E. coli*) gas-forming organisms within the bowel wall is thought to result in the formation of intramural gas [13]. Bacterial invasion of the intestinal wall and local cytokine release may result in an inflammatory cascade, in which interferon γ and nitric oxide are implicated, which may contribute to further damage [14].

Early reports of associations with NEC were uncontrolled and so did not prove causality. In controlled studies, birth asphyxia, placental abruption, early enteral feeding, patent ductus arteriosus, polycythaemia, exchange transfusion, umbilical vein or artery catheterization, and hypothermia have been implicated by some (but not all) workers as significant risk factors [10,11,15–18]. All these risk factors for NEC could result in intestinal ischaemia and hence local hypoxia. It is interesting that none of them is consistently found to predispose to NEC. It has been suggested that neonates may exhibit the mammalian 'diving reflex' in which cerebral perfusion is protected during hypoxia at the expense of the splanchnic circulation.

NEC almost always develops in association with enteral feeding and it has been suggested that delaying enteral feeding might decrease the risk of NEC. However, La Gamma and co-workers found in a controlled trial that four of 18 (22%) babies given early enteral feeds developed NEC compared with 12 of 20 (60%) in whom enteral feeds were delayed for 2 weeks, a significant increase in incidence of NEC in the delayed feed group [19]. Their observations contrast with the sequential but uncontrolled observations of Brown and Sweet who 'abolished' an outbreak of NEC by delaying enteral feeding [20].

Lake and Walker suggested that NEC might result from a breakdown in the intestinal mucosal barrier which would allow absorption of macromolecules [21]. Gray and colleagues showed an immune complex vasculitis in the damaged intestinal wall of two of four babies with NEC and speculated whether the antigens might be macromolecules [22]. Such an immune complex vasculitis would further contribute to bowel wall ischaemia. The macromolecules might be from milk or alternatively from intestinal microorganisms. Breast milk appears to be relatively protective compared with feeds based on cow's milk [10]. Human breast milk contains immunological factors such as secretory IgA that may be important in protecting against direct bacterial invasion or the action of bacterial exotoxins, whereas cow's milk contains many macromolecules that might contribute to disease.

Is NEC an infectious disease?

There have been clusters of cases in association with a number of different pathogens, including Gram-negative enteric bacilli (e.g. *Klebsiella*) and anaerobes (e.g. *Clostridia*), and viruses such as rotavirus, coronavirus and enteroviruses [10]. No single organism has been consistently isolated in NEC. *Clostridia* and clostridial toxins are found as commonly in control babies as in those with NEC [23]. Some workers have emphasized that *Klebsiella* species are cultured more frequently and in higher numbers from the faeces of babies with NEC. Kosloske presents a theory in which bacteria, particularly Gram-negative enteric bacteria, are central in the pathogenesis of NEC [24,25]. Lawrence and colleagues showed that germ-free rats that became colonized with one of a number of single organisms developed NEC; these organisms were *Staphylococcus aureus*, *S. epidermidis*, *Pseudomonas aeruginosa*, *Clostridium perfringens*, *C. butyricum* and *Bacillus cereus*, all of which produce exotoxins [26]. *E. coli* and *Klebsiella* outnumbered *S. aureus* by 10 000 to 1. Lawrence *et al.* suggested, therefore, that bacterial cultures at the time of symptoms may not reveal the causative organism, and they postulated that NEC in the human neonate may be similar to the model infection in the germ-free rat [26]. Exotoxin-producing bacteria could contribute to mucosal damage and this would explain the propensity of NEC to affect the lower ileum where bacterial counts are highest and where macromolecular uptake of bacterial toxins might occur. Such a sequence seems particularly likely in the neonatal unit when normal colonization of the intestine is delayed by relatively sterile conditions, by lack of enteral feeding and by antibiotics. Scheifele and co-workers found an exotoxin produced by coagulase-negative staphylococci in the faeces of 56% of babies with NEC, but in only 6% of controls [27].

It seems highly likely that NEC is multifactorial. The increased susceptibility of very preterm infants might be due to immaturity of local host defences such as IgA against microorganisms, to an increased risk of ischaemic injury to the intestine, or to differences in regulation of circulation. Ischaemic injuries have generally been found to be a risk factor for NEC. The enteral flora seems to be an important factor, and it is possible that bacterial exotoxins contribute to NEC (Figure 13.1). Finally, in some cases, particularly those associated with

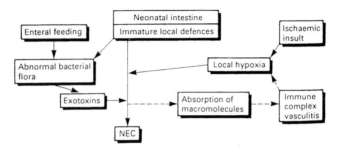

Figure 13.1 Some possible mechanisms in the pathogenesis of necrotizing enterocolitis (NEC)

exchange transfusion and the sporadic cases that occur shortly after a blood transfusion has been given to an apparently well infant, NEC is probably caused by emboli.

PATHOLOGY

In the early stages, there is mucosal oedema, haemorrhage and superficial ulceration, but little or no inflammation or necrosis. With advancing disease there is transmural necrosis and an acute inflammatory cellular infiltrate affecting primarily the terminal ileum and ascending colon. In severe cases the entire bowel may be involved; a pseudomembrane of exudate and cell debris may cover necrotic ulcerated mucosa, large vessels may be thrombosed, and perforation of the terminal ileum or colon occurs in up to one-third of cases.

CLINICAL FEATURES

The usual onset of symptoms is at 3–10 days of age, although babies may present on the first day after birth or as late as 2–3 months old. Presentation may be insidious, with apnoea, brady-cardia, temperature instability, intolerance of feeds, bilious vomiting and abdominal distension; alternatively, it may be fulminant, with shock, bloody diarrhoea and gross distension of the abdomen, which is red, tense and shiny. Very occasion-ally, abdominal crepitus may be felt. In the early stages, the

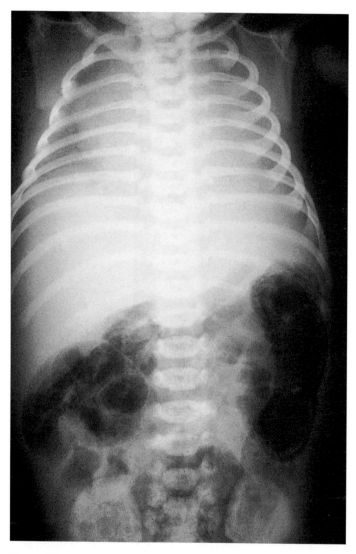

Figure 13.2a

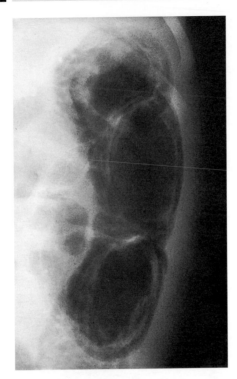

Figure 13.2b

Figure 13.2 Plain abdominal radiograph in necrotizing enterocolitis: (a) film showing pneumatosis intestinalis; (b) detail of (a) showing double shadow of wall of descending colon

diagnosis may be difficult to differentiate from sepsis or non-infectious causes of ileus.

The abdominal radiograph may show only distended, centrally placed loops of small bowel or a single, persistently dilated loop. Oedema of the bowel wall leads to separation of small bowel loops. In classical NEC, there is pneumatosis intestinalis with a generalized bubbly appearance in the bowel lumen and air visible in the bowel wall (Figure 13.2). Air may be seen in the liver outlining the biliary tree, a sign once thought to be a terminal finding, and one which may appear and disappear over minutes (Figure 13.3). Pneumoperitoneum may be apparent on the plain radiograph, but is best seen on a lateral decubitus film with the right side up, when air appears above the liver (Figure 13.4).

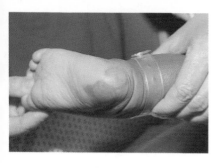

plate 10.1 Osteomyelitis of the calcaneus (*os calcis*) caused by heel-prick into bone.

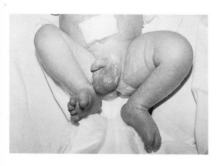

plate 10.2 Case history: patent urachus. Left thigh swollen, leg externally rotated.

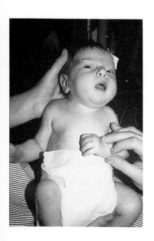

plate 10.3 Case history: disseminated joint involvement (hip, shoulder, finger, elbow) due to *Staphylococcus aureus*.

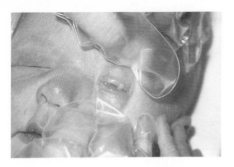

plate 12.1 Gonococcal opthalmitis.

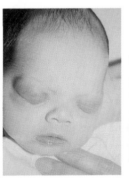 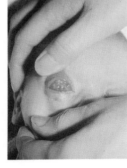

plate 12.2 Chlamydia conjunctivitis: (a) red, swollen lids; (b) exuber inflammation with pseudomembrane formation.

(a) (b)

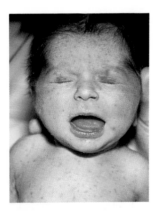

plate 14.1 Granulomatous rash of congenita listeriosis.

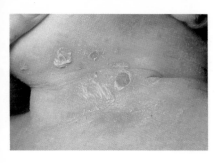

plate 14.2 Bullous impetigo.

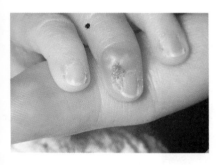

plate 14.3 Paronychia.

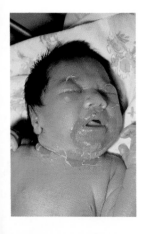

plate 14.4 Staphylococcal scalded-skin syndrome.

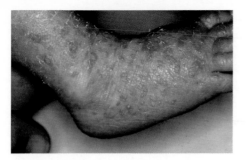

plate 15.1 Congenital candidiasis. Vesicular lesions of foot.

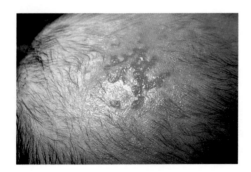

(a)

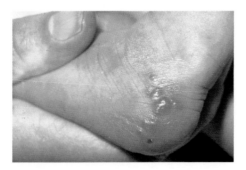

(b)

plate 16.1 Herpes simplex virus infection. Blistering lesions (a) on scalp and (b) heel.

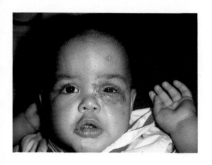

plate 16.2 Herpes simplex virus infection. Lesions around eyes.

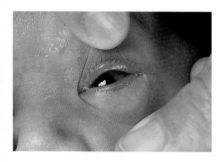

plate 16.3 Herpes simplex virus conjunctivitis.

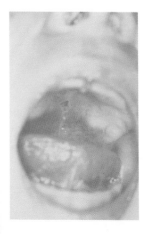

plate 16.4 Herpes simplex virus infection. Lesion on palate.

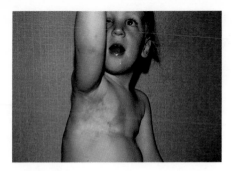

plate 16.5 Congenital varicella syndrome. Skin scarring in a dermatomal distribution.

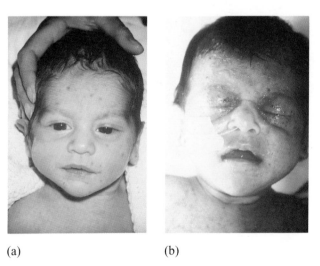

(a)   (b)

plate 16.6 Perinatal chickenpox: (a) baby born with maternal antibody and rash, but well; maternal chickenpox 10 days before delivery; (b) baby born well, developed rash on day 5 with fatal pneumonitis, despite ZIG and acyclovir; maternal chickenpox 3 days before delivery; (c) chest radiograph of (b) showing varicella pneumonitis.

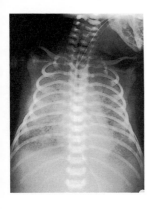

plate 16.6 (c)

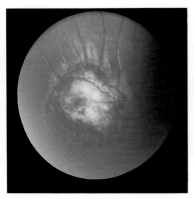

plate 17.1 Congenital toxoplasmosis: optic fundus; area of chorioretinitis with surrounding pigmentation.

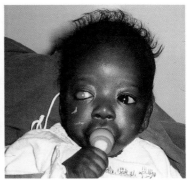

plate 17.2 Congenital rubella syndrome: microcephaly and cloudy cornea.

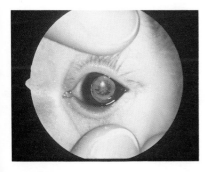

plate 17.3 Congenital rubella: cataract.

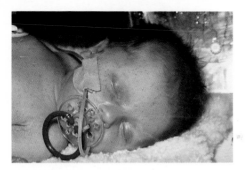

plate 17.4 Congenital CMV infection: thrombocytopenia.

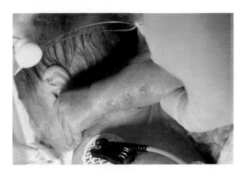

(a)

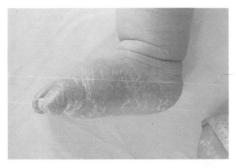

(b)

plate 17.5 Congenital syphilis: (a) bullous lesions on arm, (b) red, indurated, peeling sole.

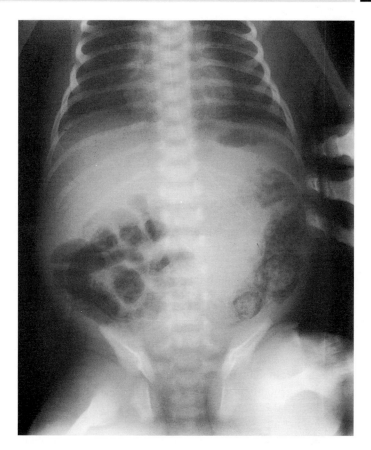

Figure 13.3 Necrotizing enterocolitis. Air in biliary tree

Blood cultures are positive at the time of diagnosis in about one-third of patients, mainly with *E. coli*, *Klebsiella* species, *Pseudomonas* species or *S. aureus*. There may be anaemia, neutropenia and thrombocytopenia with disseminated intravascular coagulation. The serum level of C-reactive protein (CRP) is raised at the time of diagnosis in >80% of cases [28].

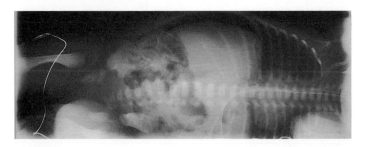

Figure 13.4 Lateral decubitus radiograph showing free air above the liver

TREATMENT

The most important aspect of treatment is early diagnosis. At the first suspicion of NEC, enteral feeds should be stopped, a nasogastric tube passed to aspirate the stomach contents, and intravenous fluids and antibiotics started after taking blood cultures. The antibiotics used should provide cover against Gram-negative bacilli, *S. aureus* and anaerobes. We use flucloxacillin, an aminoglycoside and metronidazole, but reasonable alternatives would be clindamycin and an aminoglycoside or a third-generation cephalosporin with metronidazole. Faix and colleagues compared ampicillin and gentamicin therapy with ampicillin, gentamicin and clindamycin in the only randomized controlled trial of antibiotic therapy in NEC [29]. They found no difference in mortality, but an increase in late strictures in the latter group. However, the association between clindamycin and strictures is unconfirmed and seems biologically implausible. We have not found stool cultures very useful, although we always send stools for bacteriology and virology to exclude staphylococcal enterocolitis (see below) and in case other babies develop NEC. Umbilical catheters are removed.

The next priority is vigorous resuscitation, because hypovolaemia is an almost invariable sequel of NEC. Even if the blood pressure is normal there is often a core–peripheral temperature difference of >3°C, indicating poor perfusion. We almost always resuscitate babies immediately with 10 ml/kg fresh frozen plasma i.v. (or fresh whole blood if there is significant blood loss), as this will support the circulation and replace consumed clotting factors. Close monitoring, as for sepsis, then helps to determine the need for further volume replacement. Ventilatory support is always considered and is often necessary in severe cases.

The necessity for immediate surgical intervention is debatable. Many neonatologists would consider perforation to be an absolute indication for surgery and would often operate when there were signs of peritonism. On the other hand, others, including those at the John Radcliffe Hospital, Oxford, have recently taken a much more conservative approach to surgical intervention. Virtually all babies are initially managed medically. Babies with perforations are resuscitated vigorously and operation is delayed until their clinical condition has improved, although almost all later require surgery to remove necrotic bowel and abscess. Babies with gross ascites that is impairing respiration are often managed by inserting an indwelling catheter to drain the ascites. Early diagnosis and a more conservative approach to surgery has kept the mortality rate from NEC in Oxford to under 10% [28].

Continual monitoring of progress is necessary. We have found serum CRP measurements to be a useful adjunct to clinical assessment, as these levels return to normal in uncomplicated NEC, but remain raised when complications such as stricture or abscess develop [28]. Babies with probable or definite NEC continue without enteral feeds and with antibiotics for 10 days; earlier reintroduction of feeds has led to relapse. The duration of antibiotics is empirical, and others have stopped these sooner if blood cultures are negative. For more dubious cases of NEC (grades I and II in Table 13.2), we reassess the babies with repeat abdominal radiographs after 48 hours. If there has been rapid resolution of any radiographic signs of ileus and NEC seems unlikely, enteral feeds are cautiously reintroduced. Most babies tolerate this, although occasional babies again develop abdominal distension and large aspirates, and are then treated as for probable NEC.

PROGNOSIS

The commonly reported mortality rate of NEC is 20–40%, largely attributable to septicaemia, disseminated intravascular coagulation, massive intestinal necrosis and extreme prematurity [10,12].

Strictures develop in up to 10% of patients, sometimes many days after apparent recovery. Barium studies are necessary, therefore, if intestinal obstruction develops and some centres perform such studies routinely. Many perforations are undiagnosed clinically and abscesses may develop at the site of such perforations. Short-bowel syndrome due to massive resection of necrotic bowel is rare. Recurrences of NEC occur in 3–7% of patients [10].

PREVENTION

In a randomized controlled trial, Eibl and co-workers reported a significant reduction in NEC in babies given an enteral immunoglobulin preparation containing IgG and IgA [30]. This was used only for babies for whom breast milk was not available. The use of breast milk is a cheaper and more physiological alternative to oral immunoglobulins, and significantly decreased the incidence of NEC in preterm babies in a large multicentre study [31].

Oral aminoglycosides have been used as prophylaxis against NEC, but their efficacy is, at best, anecdotal and, because of their toxicity, dubious effectiveness and great propensity to select for resistant strains [12], they are rarely used. Standard infection control measures (handwashing, use of gowns and gloves, cohorting of babies) have been reported to be effective in limiting apparent outbreaks of NEC. Neu points out that babies of mothers treated with antenatal glucocorticoids have a significantly lower incidence of NEC [12].

STAPHYLOCOCCAL ENTEROCOLITIS

Very occasionally, a disease similar to NEC may develop in association with *Staphylococcus aureus* infection. Staphylococcal enterocolitis is characterized by acute onset of bloody or non-bloody diarrhoea with abdominal distension and ileus. In its most severe form, there is marked mucosal necrosis and pseudomembrane formation. It is not clear how often this disease is diagnosed as NEC or, indeed, whether it is the same disease. Large numbers of neutrophils and grapelike clusters of Gram-positive cocci are seen on Gram staining of the faeces and a pure, heavy growth of *S. aureus* can be cultured. The role of staphylococcal toxins in this disease has not been elucidated. An outbreak of four cases in a neonatal unit was described by Gutman and colleagues [32]. We have seen a baby with *S. aureus* septicaemia, diarrhoea and abdominal distension whose abdominal symptoms did not settle with 48 hours of appropriate parenteral antibiotics. The baby responded rapidly to oral vancomycin (40 mg/kg per day for 3 days), which is the treatment of choice for staphylococcal enterocolitis.

HIRSCHSPRUNG'S ENTEROCOLITIS

Babies with Hirschsprung's disease may develop a fulminant enterocolitis with abdominal distension, profuse diarrhoea which is watery, but rarely bloody, and shock. Vigorous resuscitation is required before surgery. Babies with Hirschsprung's disease also have an increased incidence of acute appendicitis with perforation [33].

ACUTE APPENDICITIS

This condition is extremely rare in the neonatal period, and only about 50 cases have been reported worldwide. The diagnosis is often made late. Most cases occur within 2 weeks of birth and babies present with abdominal distension, bilious vomiting and pain. Fever is variable. The clinical features are generally indistinguishable from NEC or other causes of peritonitis, although the radiograph may show a mass in the right iliac fossa. If peritonitis develops, Gram-negative organisms (*E. coli*, *Klebsiella* and *Enterobacter* species) predominate but streptococci, *S. aureus* and anerobes may also be cultured from peritoneal fluid.

PERITONITIS

Peritonitis may occur in association with NEC, appendicitis, perforation of the intestine secondary to structural abnormalities, infected omphaloceles or gastroschisis and as a sequel to abdominal surgery. In such cases, the infecting organisms are those to be expected from the gut flora. The infected peritoneal fluid often grows multiple isolates of Gram-negative bacilli, *S. aureus* and anaerobes. Boys are more commonly affected. The mortality rate from gastrointestinal perforation and peritonitis is 25–50% [34].

In contrast, primary peritonitis may occasionally develop in the absence of apparent underlying gastrointestinal pathology. In such cases, as in older children, girls predominate and the organisms responsible are predominantly streptococci (pneumococci and β-haemolytic streptococci). It is possible that an important route of infection in primary peritonitis is ascending infection from the neonatal vagina.

References

1 Kinney JS & Eiden JJ. Enteric infectious disease in neonates. *Clin Perinatol* 1994; **21**: 317–33.
2 Goossens H, Henocque G, Kremp L *et al.* Nosocomial outbreak of *Campylobacter jejuni* meningitis in newborn infants. *Lancet* 1986; **ii**: 146–9.
3 Donta ST & Myers MG. *Clostridium difficile* toxin in asymptomatic neonates. *J Pediatr* 1982; **100**: 431.
4 Kotloff KL, Wade JC, Morris J *et al.* Lack of association between *Clostridium difficile* toxin and diarrhea in infants. *Pediatr Infect Dis J* 1988; **7**: 662.
5 Haffeejee IE. Neonatal rotavirus infectious. *Rev Infect Dis* 1991; **13**: 957–62.

6 Rotbart HA, Levin MJ, Volken RH *et al.* An outbreak of rotavirus-associated neonatal necrotizing enterocolitis. *J Pediatr* 1983; **103**: 454.

7 Isaacs D, Dobson SRM, Wilkinson AR *et al.* Conservative management of an echovirus 11 outbreak in a neonatal unit. *Lancet* 1989; **i**: 543–5.

8 Bell MJ, Ternberg JL & Feigin RD. Neonatal necrotising enterocolitis: therapeutic decisions based upon clinical staging. *Ann Surg* 1978; **187**: 1–7.

9 Wilson R, Kanto WP, McCarthy BJ *et al.* Epidemiological characteristics of necrotising enterocolitis: a population based study. *Am J Epidemiol* 1981; **114**: 880–7.

10 Kliegman RM & Fanaroff AA. Necrotising enterocolitis. *N Engl J Med* 1984; **310**: 1093–103.

11 Stoll BJ, Kanto WP, Glassri RI *et al.* Epidemiology of neonatal necrotising enterocolitis: a case control study. *J Pediatr* 1980; **96**: 447–51.

12 Neu J. Necrotizing enterocolitis: the search for a unifying pathogenic theory leading to prevention. *Pediatr Clin North Am* 1996; **43**: 409–32.

13 Gall LS. The role of intestinal flora in gas formation. *Ann NY Acad Sci* 1968; **150**: 27–30.

14 Ford HR, Sorrells DL & Knisely AS. Inflammatory cytokines, nitric oxide, and necrotizing enterocolitis. *Semin Pediatr Surg* 1996; **5**: 155–9.

15 Ryder RW, Shelton JD & Guinan ME. Committee on necrotising enterocolitis. Necrotising enterocolitis: a prospective multicenter study. *Am J Epidemiol* 1980; **112**: 113–23.

16 Kliegman RM & Fanaroff AA. Neonatal necrotising enterocolitis: a nine-year experience. I. Epidemiology and uncommon observations. *Am J Dis Child* 1981; **135**: 603–7.

17 Yu VH, Joseph R, Bajuk B *et al.* Perinatal risk factors for necrotising enterocolitis. *Arch Dis Child* 1984; **59**: 430–4.

18 Barnard JA, Cotton RB & Lutin W. Necrotizing enterocolitis. Variables associated with the severity of disease. *Am J Dis Child* 1985; **139**: 375–7.

19 La Gamma EF, Ostertag SG & Birenbaum H. Failure of delayed oral feedings to prevent necrotizing enterocolitis. *Am J Dis Child* 1985; **139**: 385–9.

20 Brown EG & Sweet AY. Preventing necrotizing enterocolitis in neonates. *JAMA* 1978; **240**: 2452–4.

21 Lake AM & Walker AA. Neonatal necrotizing enterocolitis: a disease of altered host defense. *Clin Gastroenterol* 1977; **6**: 463–80.

22 Gray ES, Lloyd DJ, Miller SS *et al.* Evidence for an immune complex vasculitis in neonatal necrotising enterocolitis. *J Clin Pathol* 1981; **34**: 759–63.

23 Thomas DFM, Fernie DS, Bayston R & Spitz L. Clostridial toxins in neonatal necrotising enterocolitis. *Arch Dis Child* 1984; **59**: 270–2.

24 Kosloske AM. Pathogenesis and prevention of necrotizing enterocolitis. *Pediatrics* 1984; **74**: 1086–92.

25 Kosloske AM. A unifying hypothesis for pathogenesis and prevention of necrotizing enterocolitis. *J Pediatr* 1990; **117** (Suppl): 68–74.

26 Lawrence G, Bates J & Gaul A. Pathogenesis of neonatal necrotising enterocolitis. *Lancet* 1982; **i**: 137–9.

27 Scheifele DW, Bjornson GL, Dyer RA & Dimmick JE. Delta-like toxin produced by coagulase-negative staphylococci is associated with neonatal necrotizing enterocolitis. *Infect Immun* 1987; **55**: 2268–73.

28 Isaacs D, North J, Lindsell D & Wilkinson AR. Serum acute phase reactants in necrotizing enterocolitis. *Acta Paediatr Scand* 1987; **76**: 923–7.

29 Faix RG, Polley TZ & Grasela TH. A randomized, controlled trial of parenteral clindamycin in neonatal necrotizing enterocolitis. *J Pediatr* 1988; **112**: 271–7.

30 Eibl MM, Welf HM, Furnkranz H & Rosenkranz A. Prevention of necrotizing enterocolitis in low-birth-weight infants by IgA–IgG feeding. *N Engl J Med* 1988; **319**: 1–7.

31 Lucas A & Cole TJ. Breast milk and neonatal necrotizing enterocolitis. *Lancet* 1990; **336**: 1519.

32 Gutman LT, Idriss ZH, Gehlbach S & Blackmon L. Neonatal staphylococcal enterocolitis: association with indwelling feeding catheters and *S. aureus* colonization. *J Pediatr* 1976; **88**: 836–9.

33 Srouji MN & Buck BE. Neonatal appendicitis: ischemic infarction in incarcerated inguinal hernia. *J Pediatr Surg* 1978; **13**: 177–9.

34 Grosfeld JL, Molinari F, Chaet M *et al.* Gastrointestinal perforation and peritonitis in infants and children: experience with 179 cases over ten years. *Surgery* 1996; **120**: 650–5.

14 Infections with specific bacteria

GROUP B STREPTOCOCCUS

Group B streptococci are the most important cause of early-onset sepsis in industrialized countries, are an important cause of late-onset sepsis with meningitis, and are beginning to be described as an important cause of sepsis in some non-industrialized countries [1]. The first reported case of neonatal group B streptococcal (GBS) sepsis was in 1939, but it was not until after 1970 that the increasing incidence became apparent in the United States and Europe.

It is estimated that in 1990 in the USA there were 7600 episodes of early-onset neonatal GBS sepsis, at a rate of 1.8 cases per 1000 live births, and 310 deaths [2].

The main route of neonatal infection is undoubtedly from a mother who is colonized rectally or vaginally. About 15–20% of women are colonized at the time of delivery, although reported colonization rates have varied from 5 to 30%. The yield of positive GBS cultures from women is increased by taking cultures from the anorectal area as well as from the vaginal introitus, and by using selective media (broths with antimicrobials to suppress growth of competing organisms). Colonization rates are higher in sexually experienced women, during the first half of the menstrual cycle, in women with an intrauterine device, in women less than 21 years of age and in women with lower parity [3]. GBS colonization is *not* a sexually transmitted disease, an important point in talking to parents of infected babies: colonization does not increase with the number of sexual partners, with oral contraceptive use, with vaginal discharge or with gonococcal infection [3]. If colonized women are treated with antibiotics during pregnancy, the organism may be temporarily suppressed, but organisms can usually be cultured again once therapy is discontinued. Maternal colonization is associated with an increased risk of preterm delivery and of premature rupture of membranes. Colonized preterm babies have a greater risk of systemic GBS sepsis with a poorer outcome than full-term babies. Thus, although it has been shown that treatment of colonized mothers with oral penicillin for the last 2 weeks of pregnancy can reduce colonization, failures do occur and such a strategy presupposes that most colonized mothers will deliver at term.

Without intervention, 40–70% of babies of colonized mothers become colonized, and of these about 1% become infected (Figure 14.1). Early-onset disease, associated with ascending infection and in most cases with the maternal risk factors outlined in Chapter 1, is responsible for about 70% of the cases of sepsis. The incidence of early-onset GBS sepsis is about 0.3 per 1000 live births in the UK, but up to 3 per 1000 in the USA, despite similar rates of maternal colonization.

This suggests that the American strain or strains of GBS are more virulent than the British equivalent, and indeed highly virulent strains have been described in the USA. Socio-economic and possibly racial factors are important: the rate of early neonatal GBS sepsis is two to three times higher in black than white Americans [2,4] and more than three times higher in Aboriginal than non-Aboriginal Australians [5]. Using a definition of early-onset disease as sepsis occurring in the first 5 days after birth, Anthony and Okada found that 60% of early-onset cases presented before 24 hours of age [6], and many babies with early-

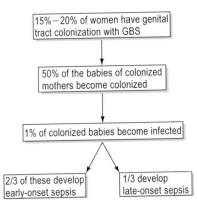

Figure 14.1 Approximate rates of colonization and infection of mothers and babies with group B streptococci

onset GBS sepsis are bacteraemic at birth [7]. About one half of early-onset cases present with pneumonia and septicaemia, one-third with septicaemia alone and up to 20% with meningitis. Although about 75% of cases of early-onset disease are associated with maternal risk factors, this still means that one-quarter of cases occur in term infants in the absence of maternal fever or prolonged rupture of the membranes [8]. The mortality rate is highest in preterm babies, but morbidity rate from meningitis remains high at all gestational ages.

Pregnant women are colonized approximately equally commonly with serotypes I, II or III. In early-onset sepsis without meningitis, the same frequency distribution of serotypes is seen. In contrast, >90% of cases of late-onset sepsis and 85% of cases of early-onset meningitis are caused by serotype III group B streptococci. This supports the concept that different pathogenetic mechanisms are involved in early and late sepsis and in meningitis. In early sepsis, group B streptococci infect the amniotic fluid and have direct access to lung tissue, so that the relative virulence of the different serotypes is less important. In late sepsis, the organism has not only to survive in the baby's nasopharynx, but to invade the mucosa, to survive and multiply in the bloodstream and to invade the meninges. Thus, serotype III appears to have increased virulence compared with the other serotypes, and is more likely to cause meningitis.

The main determinant of this increased virulence appears to be the group III capsule: antibodies to the capsular polysaccharide are protective, while babies born to a mother lacking such antibody are at greater risk of sepsis [3].

Late-onset GBS sepsis primarily occurs in the second, third and fourth week with approximately equal frequency, and thereafter with decreasing frequency to 12 weeks of age. Infection after this time is rare, although it may occur up to 3–5 months of age [6].

Most cases of late-onset infection probably result from GBS colonization of the nasopharynx at birth, secondary to maternal colonization, with later invasion of the bloodstream. Transmission via breast milk has been postulated as another mechanism of transmission [9]. Nosocomial colonization has been well described and, although subsequent infection is rare, sporadic cases and even neonatal unit outbreaks [10] of nosocomial GBS sepsis have been described. The great majority of cases of late-onset meningitis occur in full-term babies.

Meningitis is the commonest manifestation of late-onset GBS sepsis, occurring in up to 85% of cases, although recent data suggest that the proportion of GBS cases with meningitis has fallen to about 50%, perhaps due to early recognition and treatment of septicaemia before meningitis develops [3,6].

Other manifestations are bacteraemia without an established source of infection, osteomyelitis and septic arthritis. Rarer presentations include facial cellulitis, which causes unilateral swelling and erythema of the cheek, submandibular or preauricular region; pleural empyema; endophthalmitis; breast abscess; endocarditis and suppurative pericarditis.

The mortality rate from early-onset GBS sepsis is up to 20% and generally has remained high despite early recognition of symptoms and prompt treatment, often from birth. However, a large population-based US study found a mortality rate from early-onset GBS disease of only 6%, perhaps due to increasing use of maternal intrapartum antibiotics. The mortality rate from late-onset sepsis is about 10%, but about one-half of the survivors of GBS meningitis have neurological sequelae, mostly severe [11].

CLINICAL FEATURES

About half of all babies with early-onset GBS sepsis have pneumonia, somewhat under half have septicaemia without focus and up to 20% have meningitis. Over 80% of babies with early-onset GBS infection have non-specific respiratory signs such as apnoea or tachypnoea, grunting or cyanosis [3]. GBS may cause antepartum infection and babies can be born shocked and acidotic. Other non-specific signs of lethargy, hypothermia, poor feeding, etc., as described in Chapter 3, are no different to those due to sepsis from other organisms.

Babies with early-onset GBS pneumonia may have a ground glass radiographic appearance mimicking hyaline membrane disease or idiopathic respiratory distress syndrome, consolidation, increased vascular markings, a small pleural effusion, or the initial chest radiograph may occasionally be normal.

About 40% of all babies with late-onset GBS sepsis have septicaemia without focus, 50% have meningitis and 10% have osteomyelitis or septic arthritis. There is nothing specific about the presentation of the first two of these entities. GBS osteomyelitis often affects only one bone and/or its adjoining joint and is characteristically indolent (see Chapter 10).

Facial cellulitis due to GBS, which may be buccal, preauricular or submandibular, with or without adenitis, is increasingly described. Almost all of the babies are bacteraemic [3].

Rare manifestations of GBS include cardiac (endocarditis, pericarditis and myocarditis), neurological (brain abscess), gastrointestinal (peritonitis, hepatitis), ocular (conjunctivitis, endophthalmitis), respiratory (supraglottitis) and dermatological (abscesses, omphalitis, necrotizing fasciitis) presentations. All are extremely uncommon.

Relapses of infection during treatment or recurrences after treatment has been stopped, occasionally more than one recurrence, have been described in a small number of babies. Often no cause is found, although sometimes the dose of penicillin is too low, it is stopped too early, or the organism is found to be penicillin-tolerant. Rifampicin may be used to stop further recurrences (see Treatment section below).

PREVENTION

Many babies with early-onset GBS sepsis are septicaemic at birth, and it seems unlikely that further advances in antibiotic or supportive treatment will greatly affect the mortality or morbidity. What then of prevention? The possible strategies are to attempt to reduce maternal colonization during pregnancy, to treat all babies from birth, to attempt passive protection of the baby by giving antibodies to the mother or by actively immunizing her, and to attempt to reduce maternal–fetal transmission during labour. Screening all women for GBS carriage during pregnancy and treating carriers with oral antibiotics during the third trimester has proved impractical because women usually become recolonized once antibiotics are stopped and because the highest mortality is in preterm babies. Siegel and colleagues apparently reduced the incidence of early-onset GBS sepsis in preterm and full-term babies by giving a single intramuscular dose of penicillin G at birth [12]. However, no cultures were obtained before treatment, so the results are difficult to interpret. There was an increase in infections with penicillin-resistant enteric bacilli and the mortality rate was two to four times higher in the treated than in the control group. Subsequently Siegel and Cushion have reconsidered the data and found that rates of early-onset GBS sepsis were significantly lower in babies given intramuscular penicillin at birth, both in a controlled study and in sequential observations [13] (Table 14.1). They also found no increase in disease due to resistant organisms. However, there was no improvement in mortality from early-onset GBS infection and no reduction in incidence of late-onset GBS infection. Pyati and colleagues found that intramuscular penicillin at birth did not reduce the incidence or mortality of early-onset GBS sepsis in babies <2000 g [7].

Years	Intervention	Incidence per 1000 live births	
		No penicillin	Penicillin
1972–77	None treated	1.59	–
1977–81	Controlled trial	1.19	0.25
1981–86	All treated		0.63
1986–94	None treated	1.95	
Adapted from ref. [13].			

Table 14.1 The effect of penicillin at birth on incidence of early-onset GBS infection in Texas

Whether they develop early- or late-onset sepsis, it has been found that babies who become infected with serotypes II and III group B streptococci have absent or very low levels of maternally acquired opsonic immunoglobulin G (IgG) antibody against the type II or III capsular polysaccharide, compared with babies who do not become infected.

Baker and colleagues immunized 40 pregnant women with the type III capsular polysaccharide to try to produce protective antibody levels [14]. Only 20 (57%) of the 35 with low levels responded to the vaccine, although, if they did respond, IgG crossed the placenta.

Those women who fail to produce antibodies in response to natural colonization with group B streptococci *may* respond to the vaccine [15], but polysaccharide vaccines are unsatisfactory because of the low proportion of women who respond. Conjugate vaccines, using tetanus toxoid or other proteins conjugated to different GBS capsular polysaccharides, have proved immunogenic in laboratory animals and early human studies are in progress [16]. Suitable vaccines will need to incorporate conjugates using all important serotype capsular polysaccharides. Maternal immunization with GBS conjugate vaccines appears the most promising approach to effective prevention of neonatal (and maternal) GBS sepsis.

Hyperimmune immunoglobulin, plasma with high titre IgG antibody, could be prepared by immunizing adult volunteers.

Such a preparation might be used for passive immunization of mothers or of high-risk neonates [17].

The approach to prevention of early-onset GBS sepsis that has proved most successful is the use of intrapartum antibiotics, usually ampicillin or penicillin (see chapter 19) G. Boyer and S. Gotoff screened women for GBS carriage at 26–28 weeks' gestation [18]. They randomized 160 women who had fever (>37.5°C), premature onset of labour (<37 weeks) and/or prolonged rupture of membranes (>12 hours) to intrapartum ampicillin 2 g i.v. at once, then 1 g i.v. 4-hourly until delivery, or no treatment. Maternal fever was reduced by ampicillin from 21 to 8%, colonization of babies was reduced from 51 to 9% and there were five cases of early-onset GBS sepsis in the control group, but none in the treatment group, a significant reduction. Selective intrapartum chemoprophylaxis of carriers at high risk will not protect the 26% of cases of early-onset GBS sepsis with no risk factors, although in Chicago these accounted for only 6% of all fatal cases [8]. It also relies on a single screening culture for carriage, which will fail to identify approximately 8% of women who become colonized by delivery [8]. Early recommendations on prevention of neonatal GBS sepsis by the use of intrapartum antibiotics emphasized the use of screening cultures on pregnant women to identify GBS carriers. This reduces the number of women being given antibiotics in labour and thus the risk of anaphylaxis due to antibiotics, but screening is expensive. Cost-benefit analyses have suggested that a rate of GBS of 2 per 1000 live births is necessary before maternal screening is justified.

Alternative approaches have been discussed by various groups [2,19], and include the empirical use of intrapartum antibiotics for high-risk pregnancies without antenatal screening.

If antenatal screening for GBS carriage is used, this can be at any gestation from 26 weeks to 37–38 weeks. Some authorities have advocated the use of intrapartum antibiotics for all colonized women [20], whereas the US approach has been selective intrapartum chemoprophylaxis for carriers with risk factors.

The CDC has recommended a double strategy [2]:

1. intrapartum antibiotic prophylaxis for *all* women identified as carriers by routine antenatal screening cultures at 35–37 weeks' gestation; and/or
2. empirical antibiotic prophylaxis intrapartum for any women with risk factors: spontaneous preterm onset of labour or rupture of membranes (<37 weeks), prolonged rupture of membranes (>18 hours), maternal fever, and a previous child with GBS infection [2].

Where strategy (1) is used, women with risk factors for neonatal sepsis who deliver prior to screening should also be given intrapartum antibiotics.

The CDC estimates that combining the two strategies would result in 27% of US women being eligible for chemo-prophylaxis and would prevent 86% of early-onset GBS infections, while the respective figures for the second strategy alone are 18% and 70%.

Where screening is not possible, the latter approach alone might be considered to be a cheap, effective way of preventing most cases of early-onset GBS sepsis and of early sepsis with other penicillin-sensitive organisms (e.g. pneumococcus, *Listeria*) at minimal risk and expense.

In the UK, screening of pregnant women for GBS carriage has been done for research purposes only and because of the low incidence is not considered cost-effective. Screening may also be important, however, in preventing some cases of preterm labour. Maternal GBS colonization is associated with an increased risk of preterm labour [21,22]. In Denmark, GBS screening has been performed by culturing urine, as opposed to cervical secretions. Thomsen and colleagues cultured urine from 4122 women at 27–31 weeks' gestation, and randomly allocated the 69 colonized women to oral penicillin (10 units 8-hourly for 3 days) or placebo, repeated if colonization recurred [23]. Penicillin reduced the incidence of preterm delivery from 12 of 32 (38%) to 2 of 37 (5%) and increased the mean gestational age from 36.2 to 39.6 weeks. If oral penicillin can really avoid 10 preterm deliveries a year in 4000 deliveries, this strengthens the argument for routine urine screening of pregnant women. However, only 1.7% of Thomsen's study population had GBS-uria, so screening for GBS-uria identifies far fewer women than screening for vaginal carriage.

Is it possible to prevent late-onset GBS sepsis by treating asymptomatic babies who are colonized with GBS? Paredes and co-workers showed that even i.v. penicillin treatment did not eliminate nasopharyngeal carriage in babies with GBS sepsis [24]. Although it is possible that this selected group of babies was unrepresentative, it is generally acknowledged that penicillin does not eradicate colonization nor prevent late sepsis. Indeed, Pyati *et al.* found that intramuscular penicillin prophylaxis was associated with an increase in the incidence of late-onset GBS sepsis from 0.5 to 1.5 per 1000 live births [7].

Penicillin treatment will alter normal flora and may cause moniliasis. There is no evidence that penicillin treatment can prevent late-onset GBS infection in asymptomatic, colonized babies, and it may be disadvantageous.

There is modest *in vivo* evidence that rifampicin eradicates GBS colonization in babies. It eradicates colonization in infant rats [25] and was used to eradicate colonization in a baby with recurrent GBS infections [26]. In Sydney we have successfully used rifampicin (10–15 mg/kg once daily, orally) to eradicate GBS carriage after a baby relapsed from GBS meningitis, and when one of twins and one of triplets developed late GBS sepsis, to eradicate colonization in the other siblings, because of the high risk of concordance for sepsis (unpublished).

Nosocomial transmission of group B streptococci is most likely when there is overcrowding, and can be prevented by handwashing [3]. We do not isolate babies with GBS sepsis or colonization in Oxford or Sydney, but do re-emphasize the importance of handwashing.

TREATMENT

Penicillin G or ampicillin are the antibiotics of choice for GBS sepsis. An aminoglycoside is often given initially because of synergy *in vitro* rather than any proven clinical efficacy. The recommended dose of penicillin G is high because of the high minimum inhibitory concentration (MIC) of the organism and poor CSF penetration [27]. The dose of penicillin G for bacteraemia without meningitis is 200 000 units/kg per day for 7–10 days (150–200 mg/kg per day of ampicillin) and for meningitis is 400 000 units/kg per day (300–400 mg/kg per day of ampicillin) for at least 14 days. Endocarditis is treated with 300 000 units/kg per day for at least 4 weeks. Relapses or recurrences of meningitis occasionally occur; these may be caused by ventriculitis or arguably occasionally by tolerant organisms with a much higher minimum bactericidal concentration (MBC) than MIC, suggesting that they might be suppressed, but not killed, by antibiotics. However, tolerance can also be demonstrated in populations of group B streptococci that respond rapidly to antibiotic treatment. The outcome from early-onset GBS sepsis is worse in babies of low birthweight with neutropenia, acidosis, apnoea or pleural effusion [28].

LISTERIA MONOCYTOGENES

Listeria monocytogenes is a Gram-positive rod that causes serious infections especially in fetuses and newborns, pregnant women, elderly and immunocompromised individuals. It is an intracellular organism; cellular immunity is probably critical in recovery, therefore, although the incidence and severity of infection is not greatly increased in HIV infection. It causes monocytosis in rabbits (hence the name), although not usually in humans, and the CSF pleocytosis in *Listeria* meningitis is usually predominantly neutrophilic. Listeriosis was originally thought to be primarily a zoonosis because 50 species of animals can be infected and there is little person-to-person spread, but there is increasing evidence of food-borne spread. *Listeria* can exist in soil and can contaminate crops. Most cases are sporadic, but outbreaks of listeriosis have occurred.

One outbreak in Canada occurred when people ate coleslaw made with cabbage that had been fertilized with sheep manure [29]. Listeria readily contaminates both fresh and frozen poultry carcasses, and will survive the 'cook–chill' process [30].

In an investigation of 154 sporadic cases of listeriosis, Schwartz and colleagues found that about 20% of the cases could be attributed to eating uncooked hot dogs or undercooked chicken [31]. Both cow's and goat's milk may contain *Listeria*; not only is unpasteurized milk a vehicle of infection, but one outbreak implicated pasteurized milk [32]. Milk products such as cheese, and particularly soft cheeses from endemic areas such as France and Switzerland, may contain high concentrations of *Listeria* and have caused outbreaks. Belgian pâté has been implicated in an outbreak in Britain, and possibly shellfish in New Zealand. The organism can be isolated from salami and continental sausage [33]. It might seem that there is little that is safe for the pregnant woman to eat, but prudent dietary advice might include the avoidance of unpasteurized milk, soft cheeses, prepacked salads, pâtés and undercooked meat, particularly 'cook–chill' poultry. The organism grows well at refrigerator temperatures (4–8°C), but is killed by thorough cooking.

The incidence of congenital listeriosis is highest in Germany, Holland, Switzerland and France, but is rising in America [34] and Britain [35]. The reported UK incidence of perinatal listeriosis is 1 in 20 000 (5 in 100 000) live births [35]. Perinatal listeriosis, although more common in France, remains a sporadic infection: at the Hôpital Robert Debré there were 12 cases in 6 years, equivalent to an incidence of 0.4 per 1000, live births or 7% of all early-onset infections [36] (40 per 100 000) compared with 2% at Yale [37].

Early-onset neonatal infection probably results primarily from bacteraemic infection of the mother, with infection of the placenta and transplacental spread. The placenta is often covered with miliary granulomata such as are seen in the baby (granulomatosis infantiseptica). On the other hand, some babies present with pneumonia without granulomata, a picture more suggestive of ascending infection.

Most cases of early-onset neonatal listeriosis are associated with symptomatic maternal illness [35,38], often bacteraemic, suggesting that maternal bacteraemia is probably an important predisposing factor.

Extensive maceration of the fetus may be found soon after maternal symptoms, and in some instances the infected fetus may serve as a reservoir of infection and infect the mother.

Pregnant women present with a febrile illness in which sore throat, headache and chills are prominent. Diarrhoea, pyelitis and backache have all been reported. Blood and urine cultures are usually positive, as well as vaginal swabs. Symptoms generally resolve even without treatment, although *Listeria* meningitis develops in a small number of women. Infections before 24 weeks' gestation generally result in spontaneous abortion, whereas later infections may cause stillbirth even at term, or spontaneous preterm onset of labour.

Meconium staining of the liquor (which is thin and may in fact be a pigment rather than true meconium) during preterm labour is highly suggestive of *Listeria* infection: Becroft *et al.* reported it in 9 of 13 cases of congenital listeriosis [38]. However, other organisms such as *Escherichia coli* may also cause meconium staining of the liquor during preterm labour, so this occurrence should not be assumed to be pathognomonic of listeriosis.

Neonatal infection, as for group B streptococcus, may be of early or late onset. Most early-onset cases present at, or soon after, birth [38,39]. Respiratory distress is the most consistent finding, with a radiographic appearance that may mimic hyaline membrane disease or be more suggestive of pneumonia (Figure 9.3). Other presenting features include hepatosplenomegaly, apnoea, convulsions, hypotonia or hypertonia, vomiting, and mucous stools sometimes with blood. The classical rash is rarely present, but consists of tiny white or pink pinpoint granulomata on the face, trunk and notably the posterior pharyngeal wall (Colour plate 14.1). This rash is frequently misinterpreted as petechial. Meningitis occurs in about 30% of early-onset cases; neutrophils usually predominate in the CSF, but sometimes there may be a preponderance of mononuclear cells (mainly monocytes and macrophages). Very occasionally, all the cells are mononuclear, but the associated clinical features and a raised CSF protein and low CSF glucose level should distinguish it from viral meningitis. When organisms are seen on Gram staining, they are not infrequently misinterpreted as Gram-negative rods (*Haemophilus influenzae*) or Gram-positive cocci (group B streptococci).

Late-onset infection presents at 1–4 weeks of age, almost exclusively with non-specific features of meningitis. In over 90% of cases there is no history of maternal illness [35] and it is thought that late-onset infection results from nasopharyngeal colonization at birth, acquired from a mother with asymptomatic perineal carriage, and from later invasion of the bloodstream. McLaughlin reported that 12 of 50 cases of late-onset infection were probably due to cross-infection [35].

An outbreak in a newborn unit has been reported in which the mode of transmission may have been a communal rectal thermometer, while cross-contamination has occurred in a delivery suite, and an infected mother, whose baby with known congenital listeriosis was on the neonatal unit, infected a term baby on the maternity ward. Thus, it is wise to isolate both mother and baby in cases of proven or suspected congenital listeriosis.

The accepted treatment of choice is ampicillin and an aminoglycoside, because this regimen has been most widely employed and gives the best survival rates in animal models. There is, however, little evidence in human neonates that ampicillin and an aminoglycoside is superior to penicillin G and an aminoglycoside, although high-dose penicillin must be used because of the higher MIC. The addition of an aminoglycoside has a synergistic effect both *in vitro* and in animal models of *Listeria* meningitis, where ampicillin therapy alone is associated with a high relapse rate. *Listeria* is resistant to all cephalosporins. Because of the intracellular nature of *Listeria*, we treat septicaemia for 14 days and meningitis for 21 days, although we stop the aminoglycoside after 7 days.

Most US practitioners use 10 days of i.v. therapy for *Listeria* sepsis and 14 days for meningitis (C. Baker, personal communication). These regimens are purely empirical. In our experience, about one-third of babies with clinical congenital listeriosis are colonized with *Listeria*, but have negative blood and CSF cultures and normal CSF microscopy; we treat them as for *Listeria* septicaemia.

The mortality rate from early-onset *Listeria* sepsis is up to 50%, although considerably lower for late-onset meningitis. Survivors of meningitis may develop hydrocephalus, ptosis, strabismus and other neurological sequelae. There are no large studies of the outcome of neonatal *Listeria* infection. A recent French study of 12 babies with early-onset *Listeria* sepsis had no deaths and eight babies had a favourable outcome [36].

STREPTOCOCCUS PNEUMONIAE

Early-onset infection with pneumococcus, acquired by ascending infection from the maternal genital tract, is relatively uncommon. The clinical features are identical to those of early-onset GBS infection. Babies often have the same risk factors as for GBS infection, and present early with respiratory distress, a chest radiograph showing pneumonia or mimicking hyaline membrane disease, and with hypotension and leucopenia [40]. The infection is often fulminant with a poor outcome. Meningitis can be present in early-onset sepsis, but babies may also present at 2–4 weeks of age with pneumococcal meningitis. Although pneumococcal meningitis is generally considered to be rare in the neonatal period, the neonatal incidence in the USA is 3 per 100 000 population, which is greater than that at any age after 1 year [41].

HAEMOPHILUS INFLUENZAE

Early-onset *Haemophilus influenzae* infection is rare, but apparently increasing in incidence in both the USA [42] and the UK [43]. In both countries the incidence of septicaemia is from 0.1 to 0.23 per 1000 live births. The clinical picture may resemble that of hyaline membrane disease, or early conjunctivitis may be the presenting feature with or without septicaemia [43]. Most cases are associated with maternal chorioamnionitis and preterm labour. The great majority of cases are due to non-typable *H. influenzae* and ampicillin resistance is currently rare. Only approximately 1% of women have vaginal carriage of *H. influenzae* [41]. *H. influenzae* is a rare cause of late-onset meningitis, which then occurs mainly in term babies and is attributable to *H. influenzae* type b.

STAPHYLOCOCCUS AUREUS

Staphylococcus aureus is a rare cause of early-onset sepsis, but an extremely important cause of late sepsis. *S. aureus* can be a vaginal commensal, and in an Australasian study 2 of 100 cases of early-onset sepsis were caused by *S. aureus* [44]. Outbreaks of staphylococcal infection in neonatal units have been described since 1889, with epidemics in the 1920s, 1950s and early 1970s.

Although outbreaks are now rare in industrialized countries, they are still a major problem in developing countries. When routine umbilical cord care (topical chlorhexidine) was inadvertently stopped in Oxfordshire, a small outbreak of omphalitis and bullous impetigo was a potent reminder that *S. aureus* is still ubiquitous and no less virulent.

S. aureus may be carried on the hands of staff, and overcrowding of neonatal units has been shown to be a major factor in spread to babies [45]. *S. aureus* can also be carried in the nose or rectum of members of staff, which may sometimes be an important mode of transmission. Nevertheless, handwashing as opposed to elimination of nasal and rectal carriage has consistently been shown to be a better way of limiting outbreaks. The application of topical bacitracin antiseptics, in liquid or powder form, such as hexachlorophene, chlorhexidine, gentian violet or triple dye to the umbilical stump is important in preventing infection [46,47]. Bathing of babies in hexachlorophene has been abandoned because of severe neurological toxicity from absorption through the skin, described in babies in France, when baby powder was accidentally contaminated with hexachlorophene. Eichenwald and colleagues identified four babies with asymptomatic echovirus 20 infection who showered *S. aureus* into the surrounding air [48]. Such 'cloud babies' may occasionally contribute to spread of staphylococcal infection.

Colonization of the umbilicus, nose and skin occurs early, with up to 40–90% of babies colonized by 5 days of age. The commonest manifestation of *S. aureus* infection is probably conjunctivitis. Skin infections of various sorts are, however, common. Bullous impetigo presents with yellow blistering lesions (Colour plate 14.2) round the umbilicus, nappy area, neck or axilla. The bullae contain clear yellow fluid that can easily be aspirated and shown by Gram staining to contain numerous neutrophils and Gram-positive cocci. Strains of phage type II are particularly associated with bullous impetigo. Other skin manifestations include skin abscesses, often at the site of cannulas, paronychia (Colour plate 14.3), cellulitis (often periumbilical), and staphylococcal scalded-skin syndrome (Colour plate 14.4). The last of these, sometimes called Ritter's disease or (erroneously) toxic epidermal necrolysis, is the result of an exotoxin produced by *S. aureus*. A scarlatiniform rash progresses to wrinkling of skin and widespread desquamation, which can be produced by rubbing the skin gently (Nikolsky's sign). Staphylococcal scalded skin syndrome can occur as an outbreak, with the toxin-producing strain passed from baby to baby [49]. Loughead described a baby whose rash developed at 8 hours of age, the first reported case of congenital staphylococcal skin syndrome [50]. Toxic shock syndrome is exceedingly rare in newborns. Babies with microabscesses (septic spots) can sometimes be managed by rubbing the heads off the spots with an alcohol-based swab. All the other skin manifestations described above require a systemic antistaphylococcal antibiotic such as flucloxacillin. Although bullous impetigo is a superficial infection, it may be associated with septicaemia, as may any of the above infections.

S. aureus may cause a wide range of systemic manifestations. Septicaemia may be primary without an obvious focus, or secondary to a focus of infection. Infection may be localized to the skin, lungs (pneumonia often with pneumatoceles and/or empyema), bone, joint, kidneys, heart (endocarditis) or gut (enterocolitis). Meningitis is rare in the absence of an intraventricular shunt, although it may occasionally arise following an intraventricular haemorrhage or by metastatic spread in disseminated disease. Staphylococcal endocarditis is extremely rare, except in association with intravascular catheter-associated thrombus.

The other diseases are described in the relevant chapters. Disseminated staphylococcal infection with metastatic spread to bone, joint, skin, kidneys, liver, spleen, lung and (very occasionally) CNS has a grave prognosis, the mortality rate being approximately 50%.

Methicillin-resistant *S. aureus* (MRSA) has become an increasing problem in adult and neonatal intensive care units worldwide. The resistance genes code for a penicillin-binding protein that prevents the action of β-lactam antibiotics on cell wall synthesis. They are usually chromosomally mediated, rather than plasmid-mediated. The gene alters the bacterial cell wall and appears to render the organisms more stable [51]. *S. aureus*, and particularly MRSA, appears to have a particular predilection for bones and joints; *S. aureus* is the commonest cause of neonatal osteoarticular infections, and up to 30% of strains of *S. aureus* are methicillin resistant [52,53]. The spread of MRSA within units occurs mainly via the hands of staff and can be controlled by improved handwashing and cohorting of colonized babies [54,55].

Nasal mupirocin (pseudomonic acid) may eradicate nasal and skin carriage, but recurrence is common [54]. Haley and co-workers attributed eradication of MRSA colonization from their unit to the use of triple dye on babies' umbilical cords, but they improved their chronic understaffing and employed an infection control nurse to reinforce infection control practices, such as handwashing and cohorting [56]. All these measures were probably important in successful MRSA eradication.

STAPHYLOCOCCUS EPIDERMIDIS

Staphylococcus epidermidis, or more precisely coagulase-negative staphylococcus, is increasingly being recognized as a cause of late-onset neonatal sepsis, particularly in preterm babies. In almost all neonatal units in industrialized countries worldwide *S. epidermidis* is now the leading cause of late-onset sepsis. The organism has a particular predilection for synthetic plastics in cannulas and shunts, eroding into the plastic and possibly thereby obtaining nourishment. Some of the colonies thus formed secrete a glycocalyx or 'slime' layer around them, which may protect them against host defences and antibiotics. Septicaemia may be associated with indwelling umbilical catheters or Silastic central lines, although half the babies with *S. epidermidis* septicaemia in Oxford had never had such a line.

In a study of seven babies with longstanding umbilical catheterization who developed *S. epidermidis* sepsis, the isolates from the blood were the same as those from the catheter site in only four of the babies [57].

Coagulase-negative staphylococci virtually never cause early-onset infection, and blood cultures taken in the first day of life which grow this organism are assumed to be contaminated. Stoll *et al.* reported 11 newborn babies with blood cultures positive for coagulase-negative staphylococci on day 1 of life, which they considered to represent true sepsis [58]. The diagnosis of sepsis was based on clinical symptoms and most babies had abnormal blood counts. Whether they truly had early-onset coagulase-negative staphylococcal sepsis is doubtful.

S. epidermidis is a frequent contaminant of blood and CSF cultures, contamination occurring from the skin of the baby or the person taking the cultures, or alternatively in the laboratory. There is always a problem, therefore, in distinguishing contamination from true septicaemia. Clinical features of infection and the presence of an umbilical catheter or a central line may be highly suggestive. Serum C-reactive protein (CRP) level may be raised in *S. epidermidis* septicaemia, although usually not to such a level as that in septicaemia caused by other bacteria, and the immature to total white cell ratio may be increased. The platelet count is low in about 50% of cases. Quantitative or semi-quantitative blood cultures show low colony counts in presumed contaminated cultures and high colony counts in presumed sepsis. Such cultures are time consuming, however, and rarely available as a routine service. In septicaemia, organisms tend to grow more quickly (within 24–48 hours) and often in both aerobic and anaerobic blood culture bottles, although neither of these can be taken as an absolute indicator of true sepsis.

The features of sepsis with *S. epidermidis* are non-specific, and often more insidious and less fulminant than with other organisms. In one study, 14 of 29 babies with *S. epidermidis* sepsis had pneumonia [59]. Thrombocytopenia is found in about one-half of infected babies, and we have found the trend in platelet counts to be a useful way of monitoring the response to antibiotic treatment in those babies with sepsis and a central line in whom we have attempted to leave the central line in place (Chapter 6). In general, it can be expected that *S. epidermidis* septicaemia in the presence of a central line will often resolve with antibiotics and without removing the line [60], but shunt infections virtually never resolve without removing the entire shunt tubing.

Endocarditis is a rare complication of *S. epidermidis* septicaemia, almost always in a structurally abnormal heart. Meningitis virtually never occurs, except in association with an intraventricular shunt, or rarely an intraventricular haemorrhage. Shunt infections can present insidiously or as fulminant meningitis.

Infections of ventriculoperitoneal shunts may cause peritonitis, whereas infections of ventriculoatrial shunts can cause a chronic nephritis ('shunt nephritis') with microscopic haematuria, anaemia, failure to thrive and hypertension. *S. epidermidis* is one of the organisms described as causing persistent bacteraemia, which may be symptomatic [61] or asymptomatic [62].

Multiple antibiotic resistance of *S. epidermidis*, including resistance to methicillin/flucloxacillin, is increasing, and some hospitals use vancomycin as empirical therapy for late-onset sepsis. On the other hand, the emergence of vancomycin-resistant enterococci has caused many hospitals to develop policies restricting vancomycin use [63].

In many neonatal units, vancomycin is still used, with an aminoglycoside or cephalosporin, as initial empirical treatment for suspected late-onset sepsis. Our policy has been to treat suspected late-onset sepsis with flucloxacillin and an aminoglycoside and to consider removing any umbilical catheter or central line, although increasingly we are attempting to preserve these. Blood cultures are taken from the catheter or central line and from a peripheral vessel. In our experience, babies infected with *S. epidermidis* that is reported as flucloxacillin resistant have often responded to flucloxacillin and an aminoglycoside and/or removal of the catheter by the time that sensitivity results are available. If the baby is not improving, and especially if the platelet count is falling, we would start vancomycin and again consider removing the catheter. We have had no deaths and no long-term complications from *S. epidermidis* sepsis. On the other hand, *S. epidermidis* can be fatal, particularly in very preterm babies – it prolongs hospitalization in survivors by an average of 14 days [64], and many authorities would advise a more aggressive approach to *S. epidermidis* sepsis.

It should be remembered that *S. epidermidis* is a relatively benign organism, and the mortality rate from coagulase-negative staphylococcal sepsis is less than 5%, in contrast to a rate of over 10% for Gram-negative bacilli [65].

In very low birthweight babies the mortality rate from coagulase-negative staphylococcal infection was 10%, compared with 40% from Gram-negative bacilli [66]. It is likely that high-risk preterm babies will develop infection with whatever is the prevalent colonizing organism (see Chapter 1). Thus, extraordinary measures to prevent coagulase-negative staphylococcal sepsis are not justified and are probably counter-productive.

Teicoplanin, a glycopeptide antibiotic related to vancomycin, has been used to treat staphylocccal infections in Europe [67]. It has not been compared with vancomycin in clinical trials, and there is some evidence that teicoplanin resistance is already emerging. In one study, only 70% of coagulase-negative staphylococci were sensitive to teicoplanin [68].

GRAM-NEGATIVE BACILLI

Escherichia coli, and to a lesser extent other enteric bacilli, has always been an important early-onset neonatal pathogen. However, in the 1970s, widespread colonization of babies in neonatal units with Gram-negative enteric organisms was described. Organisms such as *E. coli*, *Klebsiella*, *Enterobacter* and *Serratia* became responsible for an increasing proportion of episodes of late-onset sepsis such as bacteraemia, meningitis, pneumonia and skin sepsis [69]. In the UK, but not the USA, *Pseudomonas* became an important late-onset pathogen [70]. A similar increased incidence in cases of Gram-negative sepsis occurred simultaneously in adult intensive care units. Initially, most organisms were sensitive to ampicillin, but plasmid-mediated β-lactamase resistance rapidly emerged. In addition, several outbreaks of infection due to organisms resistant to aminoglycosides and other antibiotics, such as the third-generation cephalosporins, have now been described [71].

Outbreaks of infection with less well-known Gram-negative bacilli such as *Acinetobacter* have also occurred [72]. Extended-spectrum β-lactamase-producing Gram-negative bacillary infections are increasingly being described.

Most of these organisms are water-loving and, therefore, readily colonize humidified endotracheal tubes and incubators, indicating the need for frequent changes of sterile water in ventilators, incubators and resuscitation equipment. Although *Pseudomonas* may be found on taps and in sinks, careful typing of isolates suggests that these are an infrequent source of colonizing organisms and that most babies become colonized from their mothers or from other babies through poor handwashing by staff [70,73,74]. Gastrointestinal colonization of neonates may be an important reservoir of organisms that can be carried to other babies on the hands of staff. Nasojejunal tube feeding rapidly leads to abnormal colonization of the jejunum with coliform bacilli [75]. The use of antibiotics for more than 3 days is also associated with increased nasopharyngeal colonization with Gram-negative bacteria and bowel colonization with *Klebsiella*, *Enterobacter* and *Citrobacter* [76].

The emergence of extended-spectrum β-lactamase-producing Gram-negative bacilli has been associated with increased use of third-generation cephalosporins.

Gram-negative bacillary septicaemia may accompany necrotizing enterocolitis and urinary tract infections. Like *S. epidermidis*, Gram-negative bacillary septicaemia may occasionally persist. Affected babies may be asymptomatic: Albers and colleagues described two babies, one with *Klebsiella* and one with *Proteus* bacteraemia which persisted for 3–5 days in the absence of symptoms [62]. Babies may have persistent symptomatic Gram-negative bacteraemia despite apparently appropriate antibiotic therapy, and in the absence of a demonstrable focus of infection. We have seen two extremely preterm babies with NEC and *Klebsiella* bacteraemia whose bacteraemia persisted after successful resection of necrotic gut. Both babies remained bacteraemic and unwell for over 7 days, despite appropriate antibiotic therapy, had a laparotomy which showed no gut ischaemia, and multiple investigations which failed to locate a focus; the infections eventually resolved.

There are no specific features of infections with Gram-negative bacilli. Although the skin lesions of ecthyma gangraenosum have been associated with *Pseudomonas* infection, they may also be seen with other organisms, including fungi. All the Gram-negative bacilli have the potential to cause meningitis. They may also cause ascending cholangitis and, very occasionally, pneumonia. Osteomyelitis attributable to Gram-negative enteric bacilli is rare, but, if it does occur, it is often insidious in onset and presentation.

ENTEROCOCCI (FAECAL STREPTOCOCCI)

The enterococci or faecal streptococci, such as *Streptococcus faecalis*, *Streptococcus faecium* and *Streptococcus bovis*, are usually, but not always, Lancefield group D streptococci. Their importance as neonatal pathogens, particularly as a cause of late-onset sepsis, is being recognized increasingly. Coudron and co-workers reported an outbreak of *S. faecium* in which the mode of transmission was thought to be via the hands of the staff [77]. Luginbuhl *et al.*, describing an enterococcal outbreak, found that bowel resection and the presence and duration of central venous catheters were risk factors for enterococcal sepsis [78]. Enterococcal colonization may be selected by the use of cephalosporins, but Dobson and Baker reported increasing numbers of sporadic cases of enterococcal sepsis despite rarely using cephalosporins [79]. In North America, enterococci were found to cause 5% of late-onset infections in very low birthweight babies [66].

Dobson and Baker reported 56 cases of enterococcal sepsis over 10 years in Houston (1977–86), and noted an increased incidence from 1983 to 1986 [79]. Before 1983, the incidence was 0.1–0.4 per 1000 births, but from 1983 it was 0.6–0.8 per 1000. Thirty-six of the babies developed infection after 7 days of age (defined as late-onset) and 20 before this. Twelve of the episodes were associated with necrotizing enterocolitis (10 late, 2 early). The babies with early-onset sepsis tended to be older (mean gestational age 36.9 weeks); two-thirds of them had recognized perinatal risk factors for sepsis, such as prolonged rupture of membranes, maternal fever or spontaneous preterm labour. There were no cases of maternal chorioamnionitis. Eight of the babies developed enterococcal sepsis on the first day of life. Late-onset enterococcal sepsis occurred mainly in babies of very low birthweight (mean gestational age 29.5 weeks) who had undergone multiple invasive procedures. Focal infections were common: 15% had meningitis, 15% pneumonia and 23% scalp abscess, while 23% of infections were catheter-related. Early-onset sepsis caused mild respiratory distress with apnoea and oxygen requirement, but not usually requiring intubation, and not usually with chest radiographic changes. Four of 18 (22%) had diarrhoea. Late-onset sepsis caused severe apnoea and bradycardia, circulatory collapse and increased ventilatory requirements.

Enterococci are relatively resistant to penicillin and the cephalosporins, but are usually sensitive to ampicillin and vancomycin, although neither is bactericidal. The addition of an aminoglycoside to ampicillin or vancomycin gives synergy *in vitro*. Infected catheters must be removed to clear catheter-related enterococcal bacteraemia [79]. The prognosis of enterococcal sepsis is generally good, with most babies responding rapidly to therapy. In the series of Dobson and Baker the mortality rate was 6% for early sepsis, 8% for late sepsis and 17% for sepsis associated with NEC [79]. The emergence of vancomycin-resistant enterococci, which are usually also resistant to ampicillin and other antibiotics, is an increasing problem in industrialized countries and of enormous concern.

TETANUS

Neonatal tetanus is probably the single most important cause of neonatal mortality in developing countries, causing 30–60% of all neonatal deaths, an estimated 800 000 deaths a year [80, 81].

It is called 'eight-day disease', both in the Punjab and on the Hebridean island of St Kilda, because babies die at this age, and 'no suck' disease in Nepal because trismus prevents sucking. The disease is caused by contamination of the umbilical stump with *Clostridium tetani* spores, which are found in animal faeces and survive in the soil. Most cases in Africa have been ascribed to the ceremonial use of mud on the umbilicus. A study from Pakistan showed a significant association between neonatal tetanus and repeated applications of ghee, clarified butter made from the milk of cows or water buffalo [82]. On St Kilda, the disease was caused by anointing the cut umbilical cord with ruby-red oil from a seabird, the fulmar, which was stored in the dried stomach of a solan goose [83]; when this practice was stopped, neonatal tetanus promptly disappeared.

Neonatal tetanus presents at 3–14 days, with muscle rigidity mainly involving the masseter (causing trismus or lockjaw), the facial muscles (risus sardonicus), and the abdominal and spinal muscles (causing opisthotonos).

There are characteristic intermittent muscle spasms which increase in frequency and severity and may be precipitated by loud noises or painful stimuli. Respiratory muscle involvement leads to respiratory failure. The mortality rate can be as high as 60–90% [84,85] although, if artificial ventilation and muscle relaxants are available, it can be reduced to 10% [86]. Conventional treatment is with penicillin G, tetanus antitoxin which can neutralize only unbound toxin, and supportive treatment. Survivors are non-immune and still need to be actively immunized.

The main hope lies in prevention. Education about birth practices and umbilical cord hygiene is obviously important. Women who have been fully immunized against tetanus virtually never have an affected baby. Thus, the main strategy of the World Health Organization has been to eradicate neonatal tetanus by ensuring that all women of childbearing age are fully immunized with three doses of tetanus toxoid [80].

WHOOPING COUGH

There is some controversy whether maternal antibodies against *Bordetella pertussis* are able to cross the placenta.

Cohen and Scadron found that babies of women immunized during pregnancy were protected against infection when exposed to *B. pertussis* [87]. It seems likely that babies whose mothers have had natural pertussis infection are more likely to be protected than babies whose mothers were immunized in childhood [88].

A particular problem arises if the mother or a sibling has whooping cough around the time of delivery. About one-half of the babies might be expected to develop pertussis [87], which can be life-threatening in infancy. Granstrom and co-workers treated 32 of 35 mothers who had peripartum pertussis infection with oral erythromycin (25–500 mg, 8-hourly for 10 days) and 28 of their babies with oral erythromycin ethylsuccinate (40 mg/kg per day, 8-hourly for 10 days) [89]. Other family members with pertussis were also given erythromycin for 10 days. None of the babies developed clinical or laboratory evidence of pertussis infection. These observations, although uncontrolled, suggest that it may be possible to decrease the serious risk of neonatal pertussis infection using erythromycin.

MYCOPLASMAS AND UREAPLASMAS

Mycoplasmas are the smallest free-living microorganisms. They are bacteria which lack cell walls, and as such do not stain well with Gram's iodine and are resistant to antibiotics which inhibit cell wall synthesis. They can be cultured only using special media, and will not grow from routine specimens sent to the laboratory for bacterial culture.

Mycoplasma pneumoniae is not recognized as a neonatal pathogen. The opportunistic genital mycoplasmas, *Mycoplasma hominis* and *Ureaplasma urealyticum*, which can be found in the genital tracts of up to 75% and 20% respectively of healthy women, may cause neonatal disease [90]. However, any proposed association between these low-grade pathogens and disease is bedevilled by the fact that colonization is strongly associated with low socio-economic status, and probably with other unknown risk factors for disease.

MYCOPLASMA HOMINIS

Mycoplasma hominis may be found in women with bacterial vaginosis, endometritis, chorioamnionitis, and postpartum septicaemia [91]. Its association with preterm delivery is less clear-cut than for *U. urealyticum*.

The role of *M. hominis* as a neonatal pathogen is controversial. Babies born to colonized mothers often become colonized. Cassell and colleagues consider *M. hominis* to be an important CNS pathogen [91]; Waites *et al.* isolated *U. urealyticum* from 8 and *M. hominis* from 5 of 100 patients in whom lumbar puncture was performed for suspected or posthaemorrhagic hydrocephalus [92]. In contrast, others have not been able to culture mycoplasmas from CSF from similar babies [93,94].

Even in babies from whom genital mycoplasmas are cultured from CSF, it is unclear that the genital mycoplasmas are pathogenic.

M. hominis can sometimes be isolated from autopsy lung tissue from babies, but is probably merely a commensal, not a pathogen. There are case reports of isolation of *M. hominis* from pericardial effusions, submandibular adenitis and scalp abscesses [91].

UREAPLASMA UREALYTICUM

Ureaplasma urealyticum has been suggested to be a cause of preterm labour and delivery, of congenital pneumonia, of persistent pulmonary hypertension, of chronic lung disease of prematurity, of diseases of the CNS (meningitis, hydrocephalus, intraventricular haemorrhage) and of soft tissue infections [91].

The evidence for all of these assertions is controversial; for example, treatment with erythromycin has not been shown in a controlled trial to be beneficial [95] and there are only occasional anecdotal reports of successful eradication from CSF using erythromycin or doxycycline [96]. These should be counter-balanced against the cardiac toxicity of intravenous erythromycin [97,98].

U. urealyticum has been cultured as the only isolate from some babies with congenital pneumonia and with early bronchopulmonary dysplasia (BPD), particularly babies under 1000 g birthweight [90,96]. There is animal evidence from mice and baboons to support the suggestion that *U. urealyticum* can cause acute pneumonia. There have been fatal cases of neonatal pneumonia when *U. urealyticum* was the only pathogen isolated [99].

However, the radiological, clinical and pathological diagnosis of these conditions is not always clear-cut: very low birthweight babies with peripartum asphyxia have atelectatic lungs and inhale maternal leukocytes. There remains doubt as to how important *U. urealyticum* is as a cause of acute neonatal respiratory disease.

Low birthweight babies colonized with *U. urealyticum* have double the risk of developing chronic lung disease [100] although, because of the possibility of confounding variables, this does not prove causation. Treatment with erythromycin did not alter the clinical course of babies with positive endotracheal cultures in the only reported clinical trial [95].

U. urealyticum has been isolated from the CSF of babies with meningitis and intraventricular haemorrhage, but its significance is uncertain. Soft tissue infections have also been described.

TREATMENT

Erythromycin is the drug of choice for mycoplasma infections [96]. However, oral absorption is erratic and unreliable in the neonatal period, particularly in preterm babies. Intravenous erythromycin is very destructive of veins and usually requires a central venous cannula. There have been anecdotal reports of cardiac arrhythmias in association with i.v. erythromycin lactobionate, and two babies were thought to have died from these [97,98].

Doxycycline has been used to treat babies in whom erythromycin has failed to eradicate mycoplasmas, with occasional success [97].

CHLAMYDIA

Chlamydia species are bacteria but, like viruses, are obligate intracellular pathogens. *C. pneumoniae*, previously called the 'TWAR agent', causes pneumonia in children and young adults, and has not been associated with neonatal disease.

C. trachomatis is an important pathogen which causes adult and neonatal disease. It is of particular importance in non-industrialized countries, where 30% or more of women of child-bearing age may have genital infection, compared with less than 5% in most industrialized countries [90].

In women, *C. trachomatis* can cause urethritis, cervicitis and salpingitis. In babies, the clinical manifestations are conjunctivitis (see Chapter 12) and afebrile pneumonitis (Chapter 9).

References

1 Walsh JA & Hutchins S. Group B streptococcal disease: its importance in the developing world and prospect for prevention with vaccines. *Pediatr Infect Dis J* 1989; **8**: 271–6.

2 CDC (Centers for Disease Control). Prevention of perinatal group B streptococcal disease: a public health perspective. *MMWR* 1996; **45**(RR-7): 1–24.

3 Baker CJ & Edwards MS. Group B streptococcal infections. In: Remington JS & Klein JO (eds) *Infectious Diseases of the Fetus and Newborn Infant*, 4th edn. Philadelphia: WB Saunders, 1995: 980–1054.

4 Schuchat A, Deaver-Robinson K, Plikaytis BD *et al.* Multistate case–control study of maternal risk factors for neonatal group B streptococcal disease. *Pediatr Infect Dis J* 1994; **13**: 623–9.

5 Australasian Study Group for Neonatal Infections. Early-onset group B streptococcal infections in Aboriginal and non-Aboriginal infants. *Med J Aust* 1995; **163**: 302–6.

6 Anthony BF & Okada DM. The emergence of group B streptococci in infections of the newborn. *Annu Rev Med* 1977; **28**: 335–69.

7 Pyati SP, Pildes RS, Jacobs NM *et al.* Penicillin in infants weighing two kilograms or less with early-onset group B streptococcal disease. *N Engl J Med* 1983; **308**: 1383–9.

8 Boyer KM, Gadzala CA, Burd LI *et al.* Selective intrapartum chemoprophylaxis of group B streptococcal early-onset disease. I. Epidemiologic rationale. *J Infect Dis* 1983; **148**: 795–801.

9 Bingen E, Denamur E, Lambert-Zechovsky N *et al*. Analysis of DNA restriction fragment length polymerphisms-extends the evidence for breast milk transmission in *Streptococcus agalactiae* late-onset neonatal infection. *J Infect Dis* 1992; **165**: 569–73.

10 Nota FJD, Rench MA, Metzger TG *et al*. Unusual occurrence of an epidemic of Ib/c group B streptococcal sepsis in a neonatal intensive care unit. *J Infect Dis* 1987; **155**: 1135–44.

11 Edwards MS, Rench MA, Haffar AAM *et al*. Long-term sequelae of group B streptococcal meningitis in infants. *J Pediatr* 1985; **106**: 717–22.

12 Siegel JD, McCracken GH, Threlkeld N *et al*. Single-dose penicillin prophylaxis against neonatal group B streptococcal infections. A controlled trial in 18,738 newborn infants. *N Engl J Med* 1980; **303**: 769–75.

13 Siegel JD & Cushion NB. Prevention of early-onset group B streptococcal disease: another look at single-dose penicillin at birth. *Obstet Gynecol* 1996; **87**: 692–8.

14 Baker CJ, Rench MA, Edwards MS *et al*. Immunisation of pregnant women with a polysaccharide vaccine of group B streptococcus. *N Engl J Med* 1988; **319**: 1180–5.

15 Baker CJ, Rench M & Kasper DL. Response to type III polysaccharide in women whose infants have had invasive group B streptococcal infection. *N Engl J Med* 1990; **322**: 1857–60.

16 Kasper DL. Designer vaccines to prevent infections due to group B streptococcus. *Proc Assoc Am Phys* 1995; **107**: 369–73.

17 Kotloff KL, Fattom A, Basham L, Hawwari A, Harkonen S & Edelman R. Safety and immunogenicity of a tetravalent group B streptococcal polysaccharide vaccine in healthy adults. *Vaccine* 1996; **14**: 446–50.

18 Boyer KM & Gotoff SP. Prevention of early-onset neonatal group B streptococcal disease with selective intrapartum chemoprophylaxis. *N Engl J Med* 1986; **314**: 1665–9.

19 Gilbert GL, Isaacs D, Burgess MA *et al*. Prevention of neonatal group B streptococcal sepsis: is routine antenatal screening appropriate? *Aust NZ J Obstet Gynaecol* 1995; **35**: 120–6.

20 Jeffery HE. Group B streptococcus infections. *Semin Perinatol* 1996; **1**: 77–89.

21 Regan JA, Chao S & James LS. Premature rupture of membranes, preterm delivery and group B streptococcal colonization of mothers. *Am J Obstet Gynecol* 1981; **141**: 184–6.

22 Moller M, Thomsen AC, Borch K, Dinesen K & Zdravkovic M. Rupture of fetal membranes and premature delivery associated with group B streptococci in urine of pregnant women. *Lancet* 1984; **ii**: 69–70.

23 Thomsen AC, Morup L & Hansen KB. Antibiotic elimination of

group-B streptococci in urine in prevention of preterm labour. *Lancet* 1987; **i**: 591–3.

24 Paredes A, Wong P & Yow MD. Failure of penicillin to eradicate the carrier state of group B streptococcus in infants. *J Pediatr* 1976; **89**: 191–3.

25 Millard DD, Shulman ST & Yogev R. Rifampin and penicillin for the elimination of group B streptococci in nasally colonized infant rats. *Pediatr Res* 1985; **19**: 1183–6.

26 Millard DD, Bussey ME, Shulman ST & Yogev R. Multiple group B streptococcal infections in a premature infant: eradication of nasal colonization with rifampin. *Am J Dis Child* 1985; **139**: 964–5.

27 McCracken GH & Feldman WE. Editorial comment. *J Pediatr* 1976; **89**: 203–4.

28 Payne NR, Burke BA, Day DL *et al.* Correlation of clinical and pathologic findings in early onset neonatal group B streptococcal infection with disease severity and prediction of outcome. *Pediatr Infect Dis J* 1988; **7**: 836–47.

29 Schlech WF, Lavigne PM, Bortolussi RA *et al.* Epidemic listeriosis – evidence for transmission by food. *N Engl J Med* 1983; **308**: 203–6.

30 Kerr KG, Dealler SF & Lacey RW. Listeria in cook–chill food. *Lancet* 1988; **ii**: 37–8.

31 Schwartz B, Ciesielski CA, Broome CV *et al.* Association of sporadic listeriosis with consumption of uncooked hot dogs and undercooked chicken. *Lancet* 1988: **ii**: 779–82.

32 Fleming DW, Cochi SL, McDonald KL *et al.* Pasteurised milk as a vehicle of infection in an outbreak of listeriosis. *N Engl J Med* 1985; **312**: 406–7.

33 Hall SM, Crofts N, Gilbert RJ *et al.* Epidemiology of listeriosis in England and Wales. *Lancet* 1988; **ii**: 502–3.

34 Broome CV, Ciesielski CA, Linnan MJ & Hightower AW. Listeriosis in the United States. *J Food Protein* 1986; **49**: 848.

35 McLaughlin J. *Listeria monocytogenes*, recent advances in the taxonomy and epidemiology of listeriosis in humans. *J Appl Bacteriol* 1987; **63**: 1–11.

36 Aujard Y, Bedu A, Mariani-Kurkdjian P, Baumann C & Boissinot C. Infections néonatales à *Listeria monocytogenes* à propos de 12 cas. *Méd Mal Infect* 1995; **25**: 238–43.

37 Gladstone IM, Ehrenkranz RA, Edberg SC & Battimore RS. A ten-year review of neonatal sepsis and comparison with the previous fifty-year experience. *Pediatr Infect Dis J* 1990; **9**: 819–25.

38 Becroft DMO, Farmer K, Seddon RJ *et al.* Epidemic listeriosis in the newborn. *BMJ* 1971; **iii**: 747–51.

39 Teberg AJ, Yonekura ML, Salminen C & Pavlova Z. Clinical man-

ifestations of epidemic neonatal listeriosis. *Pediatr Infect Dis J* 1987; **6**: 817–20.

40 Bortolussi R, Thompson TR & Ferrieri P. Early-onset pneumococcal sepsis in newborn infants. *Pediatrics* 1977; **60**: 352–5.

41 Klein JO & Marcy SM. Bacterial sepsis and meningitis. In: Remington JS & Klein JO (eds) *Infectious Diseases of the Fetus and Newborn Infant*, 4th edn. Philadelphia: WB Saunders, 1995: 835–90.

42 Wallace RJ, Baker CJ, Quinones FJ *et al.* Nontypable *Haemophilus influenzae*. Biotype 4; as a neonatal, maternal and genital pathogen. *Rev Infect Dis* 1983; **5**: 123–36.

43 Milne LM, Isaacs D & Crook PJ. Neonatal infections with *Haemophilus* species. *Arch Dis Child* 1988; **63**: 83–5.

44 Isaacs D, Barfield C, Grimwood K *et al.* Systemic bacterial and fungal infections in infants in Australian neonatal units. *Med J Aust* 1995; **162**: 198–201.

45 Haley RW & Bregman DA. The role of understaffing and overcrowding in recurrent outbreaks of staphylococcal infection in a neonatal intensive care unit. *J Infect Dis* 1982; **145**: 875–85.

46 Johnson JD, Malachowski NC, Vosti KL & Sunshine P. A sequential study of various modes of skin and umbilical care and the incidence of staphylococcal colonization and infection in the neonate. *Pediatrics* 1976; **58**: 354–61.

47 Verber IG & Pagan FS. What cord care – if any? *Arch Dis Child* 1993; **68**: 594–6.

48 Eichenwald HF, Kotsevalov O & Fasso LA. The 'cloud baby': an example of bacterial–viral interaction. *Am J Dis Child* 1960; **100**: 161–73.

49 Dancer SJ, Simmons NA, Poston SM & Ndde WC. Outbreak of staphylococcal scalded skin syndrome among neonates. *J Infect* 1988; **16**: 87–103.

50 Loughead JL. Congenital staphylococcal scalded skin syndrome: report of a case. *Pediatr Infect Dis J* 1992; **11**: 413–14.

51 Editorial. What's to be done about resistant staphylococci? *Lancet* 1985; **ii**: 189–90.

52 Ish-Horowicz MR, McIntyre P & Nade S. Bone and joint infections caused by multiply resistant *Staphylococcus aureus* in a neonatal intensive care unit. *Pediatr Infect Dis J* 1992; **11**: 82–7.

53 Wong M, Isaacs D, Howman-Giles R & Uren R. Clinical and diagnostic features of osteomyelitis occurring in the first three months of life. *Pediatr Infect Dis J* 1995; **14**: 1047–53.

54 Davies EA, Emmerson AM, Hogg GM *et al.* An outbreak of infection with a methicillin-resistant *Staphylococcus aureus* in a special care baby unit. *J Hosp Infect* 1987; **10**: 120–8.

55 Millar MR, Keyworth N, Lincoln C *et al.* 'Methicillin-resistant'

Staphylococcus aureus in a regional neonatology unit. *J Hosp Infect* 1987; **10**: 187–97.

56 Haley RW, Cushion NB, Tenover FC *et al.* Eradication of endemic methicillin-resistant *Staphylococcus areus* infections from a neonatal intensive care unit. *J Infect Dis* 1995; **171**: 614–24.

57 Valvano MA, Hartstein AI, Morthland VH *et al.* Plasmid DNA analysis of *Staphylococcus epidermidis* isolated from blood and colonization cultures in very low birth weight infants. *Pediatr Infect Dis J* 1988; **7**: 116–20.

58 Stoll BJ, Fanaroff A *et al.* Early-onset coagulase-negative staphylococcal sepsis in preterm neonate. *Lancet* 1995; **345**: 1236–7.

59 Hall RT, Hall SL, Barnes WG *et al.* Characteristics of coagulase-negative staphylococci from infants with bacteremia. *Pediatr Infect Dis J* 1987; **6**: 377–83.

60 Sadiq HF, Devaskar S, Keenan WJ & Weber TR. Broviac catheterisation in low birth weight infants: incidence and treatment of associated complications. *Crit Care Med* 1987; **15**: 47–50.

61 Patrick CC, Kaplan SL, Baker CJ *et al.* Persistent bacteraemia due to coagulase-negative staphylococci in low birth weight neonates. *Pediatrics* 1989; **84**: 977–85.

62 Albers WH, Tyler CW & Boxerbaum B. Asymptomatic bacteremia in the newborn infant. *J Pediatr* 1966; **69**: 193–7.

63 Gin AS & Zhanel GG. Vancomycin-resistant enterococci. *Ann Pharmacother* 1996; **30**: 615–24.

64 Gray JE, Richardson DK, McCormick MC & Goldmann DA. Coagulase-negative staphylococcal bacteremia among very low birthweight infants: relation to admission illness severity, resource use and outcome. *Pediatrics* 1995; **95**: 225–30.

65 Isaacs D, Barfield C, Clothier T *et al.* Late onset infections of infants in neonatal units. *J Paediatr Child Health* 1996; **32**: 158–61.

66 Stoll BJ, Gordon T, Korones SB *et al.* Late-onset sepsis in very low birth weight neonates: a report from the National Institute of Child Health and Human Development Neonatal Research Network. *J Pediatr* 1996; **129**: 63–71.

67 Padovani EM, Khoory BJ, Beghini R, Chiaffoni GP & Fanos V. Teicoplanin: clinical efficacy, antibacterial activity and tolerance in the treatment of staphylococcal infections in the newborn. *Ann Exp Clin Med* 1994; **i**: 111–15.

68 Neumeister B, Kastner S, Conrad S, Klotz G & Bartmann P. Characterization of coagulase-negative staphylococci causing nosocomial infections in preterm infants. *Eur J Clin Microbiol Infect Dis* 1995; **14**: 856–63.

69 Freedman RM, Ingram DL, Gross I *et al.* A half century of neonatal sepsis at Yale. *Am J Dis Child* 1981; **135**: 140–4.

70 Isaacs D, Wilkinson AR & Moxon ER. Surveillance of colonisation and late-onset septicaemia in neonates. *J Hosp Infect* 1987; **10**: 114–19.

71 Nelson JD. Control of infection acquired in the nursery. In: Remington JS & Klein JO (eds) *Infectious Diseases of the Fetus and Newborn Infant*, 2nd edn. Philadelphia: WB Saunders, 1983: 1035–52.

72 Stone JW & Das BC. Investigation of an outbreak of infection with *Acinetobacter calcoaceticus* in a special care baby unit. *J Hosp Infect* 1985; **6**: 42–8.

73 Adams BG & Marrie TJ. Hand carriage of aerobic Gram-negative rods may not be transient. *J Hyg* 1982; **89**: 33–46.

74 Morrison AJ & Wenzel RP. Epidemiology of infections due to *Pseudomonas aeruginosa*. *Rev Infect Dis* 1984; **6** (Suppl): 627–42.

75 Challacombe D. Bacterial microflora in infants receiving nasojejunal tube feeding. *J Pediatr* 1974; **85**: 113.

76 Goldmann DA, Leclair J & Macone A. Bacterial colonization of neonates admitted to an intensive care unit. *J Pediatr* 1978; **69**: 193–7.

77 Coudron PE, Mayhall CG, Facklam RR *et al*. *Streptococcus faecium* outbreak in a neonatal intensive care unit. *J Clin Microbiol* 1984; **20**: 1044–8.

78 Luginbuhl LM, Rotbart HA, Facklam RR *et al*. Neonatal enterococcal sepsis: case–control study and description of an outbreak. *Pediatr Infect Dis J* 1987; **6**: 1022–30.

79 Dobson SRM & Baker CJ. Enterococcal sepsis in neonates: features by age at onset and occurrence of focal infection. *Pediatrics* 1990; **85**: 165–71.

80 Galazka A, Gasse F & Henderson RH. Neonatal tetanus in the world and the global expanded programme on immunisation. In: *Proceedings of the VII International Conference on Tetanus, Leningrad*. Geneva: WHO, 1987.

81 Hinman AR, Foster SO & Wassilak SGF. Neonatal tetanus: potential for elimination in the world. *Pediatr Infect Dis J* 1987; **6**: 813–16.

82 Traverso HP, Bennett JV, Kahn AJ *et al*. Ghee applications to the umbilical cord: a risk factor for neonatal tetanus. *Lancet* 1989; **i**: 486–8.

83 Woody RC & Ross EM. Neonatal tetanus. St Kilda, 19th century. *Lancet* 1989; **i**: 1339.

84 Athavale VB & Pai PN. Tetanus neonatorum – clinical manifestations. *J Pediatr* 1965; **67**: 649–57.

85 Salimpour R. Cause of death in tetanus neonatorum. Study of 233 cases with 54 necropsies. *Arch Dis Child* 1977; **52**: 587–94.

86 Smythe PM, Bowie MD & Voss TJV. Treatment of tetanus neonatorum with muscle relaxants and intermittent positive-pressure ventilation. *BMJ* 1974; **i**: 223–6.

87 Cohen P & Scadron SJ. The placental transmission of protective antibodies against whooping cough by inoculation of the pregnant mother. *JAMA* 1943; **121**: 656–62.

88 Bass JW & Zacher LL. Do newborn infants have passive immunity to pertussis? *Pediatr Infect Dis J* 1989; **8**: 352–3.

89 Granstrom G, Sterner G, Nord CE & Granstrom M. Use of erythromycin to prevent pertussis in newborns of mothers with pertussis. *J Infect Dis* 1987; **155**: 1210–14.

90 Gilbert GL. Chlamydial and mycoplasmal infections. *Semin Neonatol* 1996; **1**: 119–26.

91 Cassell GH, Waites KB & Crouse DT. Perinatal mycoplasimal infection. *Clin Perinatol* 1991; **18**: 241–62.

92 Waites KB, Rudd PT, Crouse DT *et al.* Chronic *Ureaplasma urealyticum* and *Mycoplasma hominis* infections of central nervous system in preterm infants. *Lancet* 1988; **i**: 17–21.

93 Likitnukul S, Nelson JD, McCracken GH *et al.* Role of genital mycoplasma infection in young infants with aseptic meningitis. *J Pediatr* 1987; **110**: 998.

94 Mardh PA. *Mycoplasma hominis* infections of the central nervous system in newborn infants. *Sex Transm Dis* 1983; **10**: 331–4.

95 Heggie AD, Jacobs MR, Butter VT, Baley JE & Boxerbaum B. Frequency and significance of isolation of *Ureaplasma urealyticum* and *Mycoplasma hominis* from cerebrospinal fluid and tracheal aspirate specimens from low birth weight infants. *J Pediatr* 1994; **124**: 956–61.

96 Waites KB, Crouse DT & Cassell GH. Therapeutic considerations for *Ureaplasma urealyticum* infections in neonates. *Clin Infect Dis* 1993; **17** (Suppl 1): S208–12.

97 Farrar HC, Walsh-Sukys MC, Kyllonen K & Blumer JL. Cardiac toxicity associated with intravenous erythromycin lactobionate: two case reports and a review of the literature. *Pediatr Infect Dis J* 1993; **12**: 688.

98 Gouyon JB, Benoit A, Bétremieux P *et al.* Cardiac toxicity of intravenous erythromycin lactobionate in preterm infants. *Pediatr Infect Dis J* 1994; **13**: 840–1.

99 Brus F, van Waarde WM, Schoots C & Oetomo SB. Fatal ureaplasmal pneumonia and sepsis in a newborn infant. *Eur J Pediatr* 1991; **150**: 782–3.

100 Wang EE, Cassell GH, Saucher PJ, Regan JA, Payne NR & Liu PP. *Ureaplasma urealyticum* and chronic lung disease of prematurity: critical appraisal of the literature on causation. *Clin Infect Dis* 1993; **17** (Suppl 1): S112–16.

15 | Fungal infections

INTRODUCTION

As the survival of babies of very low birthweight has improved, fungal infections have become an increasing problem. Fungi are ubiquitous organisms found in soil and decaying organic matter and commonly found colonizing animals, birds and humans. They are organisms of low pathogenicity; they may cause local disease in the face of normal or marginally reduced immunity, but systemic disease usually indicates a profound immune defect.

CANDIDIASIS

THE ORGANISM

Named for the colour of its colonies (from the Latin *candidus* = dazzling white), *Candida* exists mainly as oval yeast cells (blastospores), which bud asexually and can form true filamentous hyphae and chains of elongated budding cells called pseudohyphae. These are seen in tissues during infection. *Candida* species possess a cell wall. There is limited evidence that they can elaborate toxins which could contribute to pathogenicity. *C. albicans* is the most pathogenic species and causes over two-thirds of neonatal cases. *C. parapsilosis* is increasing in frequency and causes most other cases [1,2], but other species (*C. krusei, C. tropicalis, C. pseudotropicalis, C. lusitaniae, C. guilliermondii*) are occasional human pathogens. The most important characteristics associated with virulence seem to be the ability to form pseudohyphae, attachment to epithelial cells of the buccal and vaginal mucosa, and secretion of acid proteinases [3].

C. albicans and other *Candida* species are the most important causes of neonatal fungal infections. Oral candidiasis affects about 4% of all babies [4], many of whom will develop dermatitis of the napkin area, and is particularly likely in babies who have received antibiotics [5].

IMMUNITY

Immunity against deep candidiasis and other deep fungal infections is predominantly mediated by neutrophil leucocytes, and persistently leucopenic patients are at increased risk of systemic fungal infection. T cells are important in mucosal immunity: patients with the most profound T cell defects, as, for example, those with AIDS, develop severe mucosal candidiasis, but systemic infection is relatively rare. Opsonization of *Candida* can be mediated with great efficiency by the alternative pathway of complement in the absence of antibody. *Candida* will elicit secretory and humoral antibodies in adults.

The greatly increased susceptibility of infants of very low birthweight to systemic fungal infection is not completely understood. It probably results from defective function of a number of host defence mechanisms, notably relatively impaired opsonization and less efficient neutrophil phagocytosis.

EPIDEMIOLOGY

Candida species have been demonstrated as commensals and pathogens in many animals and birds, although spread from these to humans has not been described. The organisms readily colonize mucous membranes and skin, but are not found in the air [6]. Transmission of *Candida* usually requires direct proximity of a mucous membrane or skin to a colonized site. Adults are frequently colonized without developing overt disease: about one-third carry *Candida* in the mouth, gastrointestinal tract, vagina or on intertriginous areas of skin. Pregnancy is associated with an increased incidence of colonization with *Candida* [7]. Infection ascending from the vaginal tract, which is frequently colonized in the last trimester, can cause disseminated or mucocutaneous infection in the fetus. Placental infection may occur, but transplacental haematogenous transmission is not thought to occur commonly, if at all. *Candida* may be acquired during parturition or from sucking on an infected nipple. *Candida* can contaminate feeding bottles and dummies and can be carried on the hands of staff, although nosocomial infection is probably far less common than infection following colonization from birth. Bottles of intravenous fluids have occasionally been contaminated in hospital pharmacies by the use of air pumps, and this has resulted in outbreaks of nosocomial candidaemia.

Neonatal systemic candidiasis is increasing in frequency. Weese-Mayer and colleagues described 21 patients in their neonatal unit over a 7-year period with systemic candidiasis, representing 0.9% of all admissions [8]. Significant risk factors are shown in Table 15.1. The most important of these, apart from birthweight which was not specifically evaluated, was duration of previous antibiotic therapy. The presence of intravascular catheters for intravenous feeding is a risk factor for systemic candidiasis, but the duration of central venous or umbilical artery catheterization was not a risk factor in the study of Weese-Meyer and colleagues [8]. Other studies have

---

Very low birthweight (<1500 g)
Prolonged antibiotic therapy
Use of broad-spectrum antibiotics
Prolonged total parenteral nutrition
Prolonged use of fat emulsion in parenteral nutrition
Prolonged endotracheal intubation

Table 15.1 Risk factors for the development of neonatal systemic candidiasis

shown that babies <1500 g are at increased risk of systemic candidiasis, with an incidence of about 3–5% [9–12]. Fat emulsions such as Intralipid may encourage growth of *Candida,* although they have been particularly associated with infection with another fungus, *Malassezia furfur. Candida* will grow well in parenteral nutrition fluid containing 20–40% glucose. Prolonged parenteral nutrition, particularly when fat emulsions are used, is an independent risk factor for systemic candidiasis [8]. The same risk factors generally apply to babies who develop infection with *C. albicans* and with *C. parapsilosis* [13]. However, Welbel and colleagues described an outbreak of *C. parapsilosis* infection in which epidemiological studies suggested a common source was liquid glycerin suppository from a multidose bottle [2].

Other risk factors have been the use of broad-spectrum antibiotics [9] and the duration of endotracheal intubation [8,10]. Rabalais and co-workers described 17 babies with birthweight over 2500 g who developed invasive candidiasis [14]; all had a condition causing prolonged NICU hospitalization, 13 had a major congenital malformation, and the urinary tract (70%) was the commonest site involved.

The mechanisms by which antibiotics increase susceptibility to fungal infections is not clear. Although the suppression of normal flora permitting proliferation of fungi is often quoted, even relatively narrow-spectrum antibiotics may lead to fungal infection. Other possibilities are that antibiotics might remove competition for nutrients or might remove antifungal substances elaborated by bacteria. The suggestion that antibiotics might stimulate fungal growth by some unknown direct effect has never been substantiated experimentally.

PATHOLOGY AND PATHOGENESIS

Candida blastospores attach to the mucosa or skin, and pseudohyphae, chains of elongated yeast forms, develop. Invasion of the mucosal surface or epidermis results in formation of a pseudomembrane of epithelial cells, leucocytes and *Candida* yeast cells, both blastospores and pseudohyphae. Ulcers may form on mucosal surfaces, and have a sharp edge and a base of granulation tissue with fibrin, neutrophils and *Candida*.

When disseminated infection occurs there may be haematogenous spread to multiple sites with the formation of microabscesses in brain, lung, liver, spleen and kidney. Endocarditis may occur. Organisms may embolize to bone or joint, causing osteomyelitis or septic arthritis. Deep subcutaneous abscesses, indistinguishable clinically from staphylococcal abscesses, may develop in neonates; these contain abundant hyphae. Granulomata are rare in neonatal *Candida* infections.

The mechanism by which *Candida* causes damage is poorly understood. Some workers have proposed that surface proteins may stimulate histamine release, and others have emphasized the role of putative toxins from the organisms, but no cause of tissue damage has been shown consistently. What is clear is that *Candida* is of low pathogenicity in normal hosts. Neonates seem to be at particular risk because of their impaired host defences and possibly also because they may be exposed to a large number of organisms.

CLINICAL FEATURES

Congenital candidiasis is a rare but distinctive clinical entity, associated with the presence of a retained intrauterine contraceptive device (IUCD) or cervical suture [15,16], while the mother often gives a history of vaginal candidiasis in pregnancy [12].

Whyte and colleagues described 18 babies with congenital candidiasis [15]: in 8 the mother had a retained IUCD and in 5 a cervical suture. The placenta shows characteristic discrete yellow plaques on the membranes and cord.

Babies are asymptomatic at birth in over 40% of cases [17]. They may be born with the characteristic rash or develop it within 72 hours. Lesions may be vesicular or pustular with an erythematous base (Colour plate 15.1). They may form bright red patches like scalds, sometimes with satellite lesions, or discrete small lesions of the face and trunk, or generalized pustulosis [15,16,18,19]. In some babies the disease remains localized to the skin and topical therapy clears the infection. In others, there may be lung involvement with pneumonia which can be severe [12,15]. In the series of Whyte and colleagues, 18 babies were described with a median birth weight of 860 g and gestation of 25 weeks [15]. Five died, three within an hour of birth, but the mortality rate was no greater than in age-matched controls. Four developed skin rash and five developed pneumonia. One baby had an intestinal perforation which may not have been due to *Candida*, but resulted in *Candida* septicaemia. None of the other babies had *Candida* in urine, blood or CSF cultures.

The diagnosis is readily made by microscopy of scrapings from the placenta or baby's skin which show numerous yeasts and pseudohyphae.

Oral candidiasis, which often appears at about 1 week of age, causes distinctive white plaques with underlying erythema on the tongue, buccal, palatal, gingival and pharyngeal mucosa. Candidiasis of the skin is common, causing vesicles or pustules which frequently coalesce to form patches of thickened skin. These are commonest in the napkin area, but may occur also around the umbilicus, in skin folds such as the axillae and over the trunk and face. The angry red napkin rash often has a white edge, involves the skin creases and discrete satellite lesions may be seen.

Systemic involvement usually presents acutely and the signs and symptoms mimic bacterial sepsis and can rarely be distinguished clinically. One or several organs may be involved. *Candida* meningitis may be present in babies without obvious neurological impairment and lumbar puncture should always be considered. Isolated renal candidiasis may lead to huge fungal balls in the pelvis of one or both kidneys, causing obstruction (Figure 15.1); if bilateral, the baby may present with oliguria or anuria and renal enlargement.

Fundoscopy should always be performed in suspected candidiasis, because endophthalmitis may be present, causing fluffy white exudates in the retina or floating in the vitreous humour [9]. Skin abscesses may develop as the first presenting

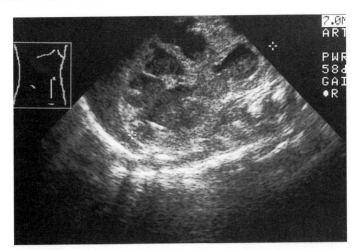

Figure 15.1a

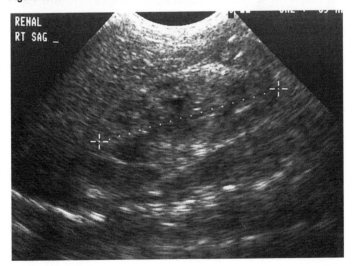

Figure 15.1b

Figure 15.1 Hydronephrosis in a neonate with obstructive uropathy due to *Candida albicans*. (a) Ultrasonographic scan on day 41 shows an enlarged right kidney with particulate matter in the pelvis and calyces. (b) Ultrasonographic scan on day 47 shows resolution of hydronephrosis

sign and resemble staphylococcal abscesses, so that fungal infection can be diagnosed only by microscopic examination and culture of the pus. Arthritis, osteomyelitis and endocarditis are very occasionally described. Brain abscess has been described in the absence of meningitis, usually as an autopsy finding. Pulmonary candidiasis can occur as part of congenital candidiasis. However, babies may also develop later pulmonary infection which presents as pulmonary consolidation with increasing ventilatory requirements. These features are very non-specific and *Candida* is a common commensal isolate in endotracheal cultures, perhaps from oral contamination. Nevertheless, *Candida* pneumonia has been shown at autopsy to be present in some cases [12].

DIAGNOSIS

The diagnosis of systemic candidiasis is notoriously difficult to make, with a mean delay of 11 days (range 2–32 days) between onset of symptoms and starting antifungal therapy [9]. The organism may grow slowly if at all in blood cultures, taking up to 11 days to grow, and cultures may be intermittently positive [20]. Thrombocytopenia is very common in neonatal candidiasis [21,22], but it also occurs in about 50% of babies with bacteraemia, which is much more common than fungaemia.

A common scenario would be a very low birthweight baby who becomes unwell at 10–28 days of age, perhaps older [23], is thought to be septic and is found to be thrombocytopenic. After 3 or 4 days of appropriate antibacterial therapy, the baby remains unwell, the thrombocytopenia persists or is worse, and cultures are negative. We now advocate giving serious thought to doing appropriate investigations (cultures of blood, urine, and CSF, and renal and cerebral ultrasonography) and commencing empirical antifungal treatment [24].

As the clinical features of candidiasis are non-specific, a laboratory diagnosis should be made whenever possible by obtaining clinical specimens. *Candida* species grow readily on Sabouraud dextrose media; they will also grow in blood culture bottles.

Scrapings or swabs from skin or mucosal lesions should be examined for fungal elements using a potassium hydroxide preparation. Some laboratories use calciflor white instead of KOH to stain for yeasts. Cottonwool swabs are not the best to use, as *Candida* sticks to the cottonwool. Pus from skin abscesses and 'septic' arthritis should always be examined by wet-mount microscopy and cultured for fungi. *Candida* meningitis causes a CSF pleocytosis and fungal elements are usually seen on Gram staining or wet-mount microscopy.

There are particular problems with the clinical diagnosis of *Candida* pneumonia and UTI. The isolation of *Candida* from an endotracheal aspirate is probably clinically significant only when there is associated radiological and clinical deterioration. Even when the baby has clinical pneumonia and *Candida* is found in endotracheal secretions, it may not be the cause of the pneumonia. Confirmation should be sought by obtaining cultures of any pleural fluid present and of blood and urine before starting treatment. Similarly, bag urine specimens may frequently become contaminated with *Candida*, and urine cultures positive for *Candida* should be repeated, with a very low threshold for suprapubic aspiration of urine. Indeed, if renal candidiasis is suspected, this is the investigation of choice.

Candida is a rare contaminant of blood cultures in neonates. In neonates, it is extremely unwise to ignore the growth of *Candida* from a blood culture, even if taken through an umbilical or central catheter. Repeat blood cultures may be negative, yet the baby progresses to fulminant systemic *Candida* infection [8]. We, too, have mistakenly dismissed growth of *Candida* from one of two blood culture bottles as a contaminant, and have been reassured by a sterile repeat blood culture, only for the baby to develop *Candida* meningitis 1 week later. In suspected fungaemia, blood cultures should always be performed, and a single positive culture is a strong indication for starting antifungal treatment. Ascuitto and colleagues detected fungal elements in Gram stains of buffy coat smears from three babies with fungaemia [25].

Antibody tests and skin tests are of no value in deciding whether or not a baby is infected with *Candida*. Antigen detection has occasionally been of value [26], but remains to be more completely evaluated.

Case history 15.1

A 27-week gestation, 660-g boy developed respiratory distress from birth, requiring artificial ventilation. He was extubated and in air by 7 days. On day 14, he developed a fluctuant swelling above the left ankle, not involving the joint.

The aspirated pus contained neutrophils and Gram-positive cocci and grew a heavy growth of MRSA and a few colonies of *Candida albicans*. He was treated with i.v. vancomycin. Four days later, he became systemically unwell with increasing apnoea and bradycardia. The CSF contained 90×10^9/L WBCs (72% neutrophils) and 10×10^9/L RBCs. No organisms were seen on Gram staining, but the CSF grew a scanty growth of *C. albicans*. Blood cultures were sterile, but urine contained yeasts and grew a heavy pure growth of *Candida*. Cerebral ultrasonography and computed tomography of the brain showed rounded lesions in the brain parenchyma, ventricular dilatation and early cerebral atrophy. Renal ultrasonography showed similar lesions in both kidneys. He was treated with i.v. amphotericin B and flucytosine for 30 days with no toxicity, and with clinical and radiological resolution of the meningeal, cerebral and renal lesions.

TREATMENT

The treatment of local skin conditions and mucocutaneous candidiasis in the neonatal period is with topical and oral preparations of nystatin, miconazole or clotrimazole. Whenever possible, antibacterial antibiotics should be stopped when candidiasis, either local or systemic, is diagnosed. Systemic candidiasis is usually treated with amphotericin B, with or without flucytosine (5-fluorocytosine).

Amphotericin B is a polyene macrolide which acts by

binding to ergosterol in the fungal cell wall. Levels in CSF are 40–90% of serum levels, but little is recovered in the urine. Amphotericin B has to be given by intravenous infusion, although it can be effective topically for some local infections. Amphotericin B causes significant renal toxicity in a proportion of patients. In the study by Baley and colleagues, seven of ten babies of very low birthweight treated with amphotericin B developed 'severe renal toxicity', defined as oliguria (<1 mL/kg per hour) or anuria for 18 hours, while five had a rise in serum creatinine concentration and five (all of whom died) had hypo- or hyperkalaemia [9]. On the other hand, some of the babies had renal candidiasis, the criteria for severe renal toxicity were somewhat dubious and only two babies had raised urea levels. Faix reported similar renal toxicity [27], but other workers have reported far less toxicity with amphotericin B [11,12], although anaemia and hypokalaemia may occur as well as renal toxicity. In older children and adults, it is recommended that a test dose of 0.1 mL/kg be given. If no reaction occurs, treatment is begun at 0.25 mg/kg per day, then increased by daily increments of 0.25 to 1.0 mg/kg per day, at which dose it is continued. This is because adverse reactions such as fever, chills, headache, nausea and vomiting often develop. These have not been reported in neonates, however, and we begin treatment at the full dose of 1 mg/kg per day without a test dose. Baley and co-workers have examined the pharmacokinetics and toxicity of amphotericin B and have come, via a more scientific approach, to the same conclusion [28]. If renal toxicity does develop, we reduce the dose or stop the drug, but in our experience significant toxicity is extremely rare.

Amphotericin B must be diluted in 5% dextrose, because saline causes precipitation; it should be infused over 4–6 hours and the solution should be protected against the light. It is recommended that a total dose of 25–30 mg/kg amphotericin be given, equating to about 4 weeks' treatment.

Flucytosine, also called 5-fluorocytosine (5-FC), is a fluorinated pyrimidine antimetabolite that competitively inhibits fungal nucleic acid synthesis. It is well absorbed orally and has excellent CSF penetration, with CSF levels up to 88% of serum levels [29]. It cannot be used alone, as resistance rapidly develops. It can accumulate and cause bone marrow toxicity with neutropenia and also hepatotoxicity. For this reason, and to monitor oral absorption, blood levels should be monitored during treatment, usually weekly.

Some use flucytosine as well as amphotericin B for treating *Candida* meningitis because of the superior CSF penetration of flucytosine. If flucytosine is also used, there is no need to use intrathecal amphotericin B, as sometimes advocated, which can cause marked toxicity. For fungaemia without meningitis, amphotericin B alone may suffice. Butler and colleagues used amphotericin B alone for all neonatal fungal infections including meningitis, and report results similar to those reported by others who also use flucytosine [30].

Fluconazole is a broad-spectrum bistriazole which binds to fungal cytochrome P450 and interferes with ergosterol synthesis. It is related to ketoconazole, but has less hepatic toxicity. It can be given intravenously and is well absorbed orally. CSF penetration is good and fluconazole is excreted in the urine. Indeed a case of fungal obstructive uropathy has been described in which medical treatment with fluconazole produced resolution of the obstruction [31].

The duration of therapy and optimal route of administration of fluconazole is yet to be determined, but fluconazole can be used as monotherapy and oral therapy can be a very useful option when there is a problem obtaining venous access. Side-effects include rash, hepatotoxicity and thrombocytopenia, but are uncommon.

Driessen and colleagues compared the use of amphotericin B with fluconazole in 23 South African babies with fungal septicaemia, 16 with *C. albicans* [32]. Amphotericin B 1 mg/kg per day was given and 5-FC was added if CSF cultures were positive. Fluconazole 10 mg/kg loading dose i.v. or oral was followed by 5 mg/kg once daily i.v. or oral. Antifungals were given until the baby was well and cultures had been negative for a week. Bilirubin and alkaline phosphatase levels were higher in the amphotericin group. Amphotericin B was given for a mean of 14 days and fluconazole for a mean of 21 days, only 5 of which were i.v. on average. No babies on fluconazole needed a central venous catheter. Fluconazole caused fewer side-effects and the mortality rate was comparable (33% in the fluconazole group and 45% in the amphotericin B group). Fluconazole is a convenient alternative to amphotericin B, although not yet the antifungal treatment of choice.

In vitro sensitivities of fungi to antifungals are notoriously unreliable. *C. albicans* is universally sensitive to amphotericin B, but *C. parapsilosis* may not respond clinically to amphotericin B. Most, but not all, infections with *C. parapsilosis* are sensitive to fluconazole.

Miconazole used to be used occasionally to treat systemic candidiasis, but experience is extremely limited compared with that of amphotericin B and flucytosine. Clarke and colleagues reported intermittent ventricular tachycardia which resolved when miconazole was stopped and did not recur when the drug was re-started [33].

McDougall and colleagues reported its use in two babies, one of whom relapsed after stopping miconazole, although only 10 days' treatment was given, and the other who deteriorated on miconazole [34]. Both babies responded to amphotericin B and flucytosine. Miconazole is no longer used systemically, but topical preparations are still in use.

It is generally believed that it is not possible to treat systemic fungal infections successfully without removing intravascular catheters, because these are always colonized during fungaemia [35]. It has sometimes been thought sufficient to remove central venous or umbilical artery catheters in babies with isolated fungaemia and not to start antifungal treatment. The number of days that catheters were in place was not a risk factor in the study of Weese-Mayer *et al.*, although their presence or absence could not be assessed as a risk factor [8]. The same authors removed catheters without initiating antifungals in 12 babies out of 21 with confirmed fungaemia: nine of these were cured, and the authors considered the treatment was particularly successful in babies with birthweight >2000 g and those not critically ill. However, two of the three babies unsuccessfully managed this way died from systemic fungal infection and one relapsed 36 days later. Thus, antifungal therapy should always be started, as well as removing central intravascular catheters. Most reports of neonatal fungal infection have emphasized that the high mortality rate was in part attributable to delayed diagnosis and failure to recognize the seriousness of positive fungal cultures.

PREVENTION

In the only controlled study of prophylactic oral nystatin, Sims and co-workers showed that oral nystatin, 1 ml 8-hourly until 1 week after extubation, reduced the proportion of babies <1250 g birthweight colonized with fungi from 44% to 6% [36]. Renal candidiasis was reduced from 32% to 6% of the babies. What is more, colonized babies remained on the ventilator longer, had central venous catheters longer, and their mortality rate was higher than that of controls, although this does not prove cause and effect. It is possible that colonization is a marker for particularly sick babies. Nevertheless, oral nystatin is a cheap, non-toxic intervention, and we use it routinely for all ventilated babies under 1500 g birthweight until 1 week post-intubation.

Other equally important preventive measures are to attempt to reduce the use of antibiotics and parenteral nutrition. Rational antibiotic use is discussed in Chapter 6, and depends on the use of narrow-spectrum antibiotics, which should be stopped after 2–3 days if systemic cultures are negative. In the series reported by Baley and colleagues, the mean duration of prior antibiotics for babies developing systemic candidiasis was 23.9 days [9].

Early enteral feeding, with associated reduction in duration of parenteral nutrition and with early removal of central venous catheters, will reduce the risk of systemic candidiasis further.

PROGNOSIS

The mortality rate from systemic candidiasis is high, in part at least because of the high-risk population with compounding problems. The mortality rate from untreated disease is nearly 80%, whereas that from disease treated with antifungal agents is about 25–30%, although it is >60% for babies of very low birthweight [9,11]. In up to 30% of cases the diagnosis of fungal infection is not made until autopsy. Long-term renal damage from renal candidiasis is not usually a major problem. Survivors of *Candida* meningitis may have hydrocephalus or neurological impairment, but other factors may contribute to the adverse outcome.

OTHER FUNGI

There have been few reports of other fungi causing problems in the neonatal period. *Malassezia furfur* appears to thrive on fat emulsions and has been associated with total parenteral nutrition. Murphy and colleagues reported an outbreak of and infection with *Hansenula anomala*, a yeast usually encountered as a contaminant in the brewing industry [37]. The origin of the outbreak was never established, despite close scrutiny of the doctors' drinking habits. Seven of eight babies with systemic infection weighed <1500 g and all had multiple problems of prematurity. *Coccidioides immitis*, which is endemic in parts of North, Central and South America, is a very rare neonatal cause of patchy pneumonic infiltration and disseminated coccidiomycosis. *Cryptococcus neoformans*, which is found worldwide, is an equally rare cause of disseminated disease: it can cause hepatosplenomegaly, jaundice, hydrocephalus, intracranial calcification and chorioretinitis, a spectrum of disease suggesting congenital infection, although the mother is usually asymptomatic. Fewer than 10 neonatal cases of infections with each of these organisms have been documented.

Infections due to the bread moulds often found in refrigerators – the Zygomycetes (which include *Mucor*, *Absidia* and *Rhizopus*) – are equally rare. Dennis and colleagues reported isolating *Rhizopus* from the plaster dressing on an abdominal wound [38], while Mitchell and co-workers reported four cases of *Rhizopus* infection associated with the use of wooden tongue depressors as arm splints: one baby died from systemic *Rhizopus* infection and one had an arm amputated because of necrotizing cellulitis [39]. The Zygomycetes are ubiquitous and can cause enterocolitis with diarrhoea, often bloody, and abdominal distension. *Aspergillus* infection, resulting in pneumonia and disseminated aspergillosis involving the brain and most other organs, has been described in only seven babies, aged 2–7 weeks.

SUMMARY

- Systemic candidiasis affects primarily very low birthweight babies.

- Prolonged antibiotic therapy with broad-spectrum antibiotics, prolonged use of parenteral feeding, particularly with fat emulsions, and prolonged endotracheal intubation are additional risk factors.

- Positive culture of fungi from blood should not be dismissed as a contaminant.

- Most babies with fungaemia are thrombocytopenic.

- Empirical antifungal therapy should be considered early for clinically septic, very-low-birthweight babies who are thrombocytopenic.

- Infections with *Candida albicans* should be treated with amphotericin B, but *Candida parapilosis* may only respond to fluconazole.

- Measures to prevent systemic candidiasis include rational use of narrow-spectrum antibiotics, prophylactic oral nystatin, and early enteral feeding.

References

1 Saxen H, Virtanen M, Carlson P *et al.* Neonatal *Candida parapsilosis* outbreak with a high case fatality rate. *Pediatr Infect Dis J* 1995; **14**: 776–81.

2 Welbel SF, McNeil MM, Kuykendall RJ *et al. Candida parapsilosis* bloodstream infections in neonatal intensive care unit patients: epidemiologic and laboratory confirmation of a common source outbreak. *Pediatr Infect Dis J* 1996; **15**: 998–1002.

3 Odds FC. The pathogenesis of candidosis. *Hospital Update* 1981; **7**: 935–45.

4 Kozinn PJ, Taschdjian CL, Wiener H *et al.* Neonatal candidiasis. *Pediatr Clin North Am* 1958; **5**: 803–15.

5 Seelig MS. The role of antibiotics in the pathogenesis of *Candida* infections. *Am J Med* 1966; **40**: 887–917.

6 Nilsby I & Norden A. Studies of occurrence of *Candida albicans. Acta Med Scand* 1949; **133**: 340–5.

7 Pedersen GT. Yeasts isolated from the throat, rectum and vagina in 60 women examined during pregnancy and half to one year after labour. *Acta Obstet Gynaecol Scand* 1964; **42** (Suppl 6): 47–51.

8 Weese-Mayer DE, Fondriest DW, Brouillette RT & Shulman ST. Risk factors associated with candidemia in the neonatal intensive care unit: a case–control study. *Pediatr Infect Dis J* 1987; **6**: 190–6.

9 Baley JE, Kliegman RM & Fanaroff AA. Disseminated fungal infections in very low birth-weight infants: clinical manifestations and epidemiology. *Pediatrics* 1984; **73**: 144–52.

10 Faix RG, Kovarik SM, Shaw TR & Johnson RV. Mucocutaneous and invasive candidiasis among very low birth weight (<1500 grams) infants in intensive care nurseries: a prospective study. *Pediatrics* 1989; **83**: 101–7.

11 Johnson D, Thompson T, Green T & Ferrieri P. Systemic candidiasis in very low-birth-weight infants, less than 1500 grams. *Pediatrics* 1984; **73**: 138–43.

12 Loke HL, Verber I, Szymonowicz W & Yu VYH. Systemic candidiasis and pneumonia in preterm infants. *Aust Paediatr J* 1988; **24**: 138–42.

13 Faix RG. Invasive neonatal candidiasis: comparison of *albicans* and *parapsilosis* infection. *Pediatr Infect Dis J* 1992; **11**: 88–93.

14 Rabalais GP, Samiec TD, Bryant KK & Lewis JJ. Invasive candidiasis in infants weighing more than 2500 grams at birth admitted to a neonatal intensive care unit. *Pediatr Infect Dis J* 1996; **15**: 348–52.

15 Whyte RK, Hussain Z & de Sa D. Antenatal infections with *Candida* species. *Arch Dis Child* 1982; **57**: 528–35.

16 Hood IC, de Sa D & Whyte RK. The inflammatory response in candidal chorioamnionitis. *Hum Pathol* 1983; **14**: 984–90.

17 Gilbert GL. *Infectious Disease in Pregnancy and the Newborn Infant*. Harwood: Chur, 1991.

18 Dvorak AM & Gavaller B. Congenital systemic candidiasis: report of a case. *N Engl J Med* 1966; **274**: 540–3.

19 Chapel TA, Gagliardi C & Nicholas W. Congenital cutaneous candidiasis. *J Am Acad Dermatol* 1982; **6**: 926–8.

20 Smyth H & Congdon P. Neonatal systemic candidiasis. *Arch Dis Child* 1985; **60**: 365–9.

21 Dyke MP & Ott K. Severe thrombocytopenia in extremely low birthweight infants with systemic candidiasis. *J Paediatr Child Health* 1993; **29**: 298–301.

22 Gray PH, Dawson C & Tan W. Severe thrombocytopenia in ELBW infants with systemic candidiasis. *J Paediatr Child Health* 1994; **30**: 557.

23 Isaacs D, Barfield C, Clothier T *et al*. Late onset infections of infants in neonatal units. *J Paediatr Child Health* 1996; **32**: 158–61.

24 McDonnell M & Isaacs D. Neonatal systemic candidiasis. *J Paediatr Child Health* 1995; **31**: 490–2.

25 Ascuitto RJ, Gerber MA, Cates KL & Tilton RC. Buffy coat smears of blood drawn through central venous catheters as an aid to rapid diagnosis of systemic fungal infections. *J Pediatr* 1985; **106**: 445–7.

26 Schreiber JR, Maynard E & Lew MA. *Candida* antigen detection in two premature neonates with disseminated candidiasis. *Pediatrics* 1984; **74**: 838–41.

27 Faix RG. Systemic candida infections in infants in intensive care nurseries: high incidence of central nervous system involvement. *J Pediatr* 1984; **105**: 616–22.

28 Baley JE, Meyers C, Kliegman RM *et al*. Pharmacokinetics, outcome of treatment, and toxic effects of amphotericin B and 5-fluorocytosine in neonates. *J Pediatr* 1990; **116**: 791–7.

29 Steer PL, Marks MI, Klite PD & Eickhoff TC. 5-Fluorocytosine: an oral antifungal compound. A report on clinical and laboratory experience. *Ann Intern Med* 1972; **76**: 15–22.

30 Butler KM, Rench MA & Baker CJ. Amphotericin B as a single agent in the treatment of systemic candidiasis in neonates. *Pediatr Infect Dis J* 1990; **9**: 51–6.

31 Morris SA, Bailey CJ & Cartledge JMcP. Neonatal renal candidiasis. *J Paediatr Child Health* 1994; **30**: 186–8.

32 Driessen M, Ellis JB, Cooper PA *et al*. Fluconazole vs. amphotericin B for the treatment of neonatal fungal septicaemia: a

prospective randomized trial. *Pediatr Infect Dis J* 1996; **15**: 1107–12.

33 Clarke M, Davies DP, Odds F & Mitchell C. Neonatal systemic candidiasis treatment with miconazole. *BMJ* 1980; **281**: 354.

34 McDougall PN, Fleming PJ, Speller DCE *et al.* Neonatal systemic neonatal candidiasis: a failure to respond to intravenous miconazole in two infants. *Arch Dis Child* 1982; **57**: 884–6.

35 Sadiq HF, Devaskar S, Keenan WJ & Weber TR. Broviac catheterisation in low birth weight infants: incidence and treatment of associated complications. *Crit Care Med* 1987; **15**: 47–50.

36 Sims ME, Yoo Y, You H, Salminen C & Walther FJ. Prophylactic oral nystatin and fungal infections in very-low-birthweight infants. *Am J Perinatol* 1988; **5**: 33–6.

37 Murphy N, Buchanan CR, Damjanovic V *et al.* Infection and colonisation of neonates by *Hansenula anomala*. *Lancet* 1986; **i**: 291–3.

38 Dennis JE, Rhodes KH, Cooney DR *et al.* Nosocomial *Rhizopus* infection, zygomycosis; in children. *J Pediatr* 1980; **96**: 824–8.

39 Mitchell SJ, Gray J, Morgan MEI, Hocking MD & Durbin GM. Nosocomial infection with *Rhizopus microsporus* in preterm infants: association with wooden tongue depressors. *Lancet* 1996; **348**: 441–3.

16 | Viral infections

INTRODUCTION

Viruses cause relatively few neonatal infections, yet these can be severe and often fatal. Their recognition is important because of the increasing potential to prevent or treat such infections and because the diagnosis often has important implications for the management of other babies in the nursery.

HERPES SIMPLEX VIRUS

Herpes simplex virus (HSV), like the other herpesviruses, has the ability to remain latent for months or years and to reactivate periodically. HSV is a DNA virus. Two major subtypes, HSV-1 and HSV-2, are recognized: HSV-1 primarily causes oral and pharyngeal lesions, whereas HSV-2 usually affects genital areas and is thus a commoner cause of neonatal infections (85%), but both subtypes can affect the genital area and cause neonatal infections. The presence of HSV-1 antibodies provides some limited protection against acquisition of HSV-2, and vice versa.

EPIDEMIOLOGY

Neonatal HSV infection has a reported incidence of 50 per 100 000 live births in the USA [1], whereas it is only 1.7 per 100 000 in the UK [2]. In the USA, about 5% of women of child-bearing age give a history of genital herpes, but 20–30% are seropositive for HSV-2 [3].

Neonatal HSV infection is acquired at the time of delivery, from a woman who is shedding the virus in genital secretions. In most cases, the woman has been infected in the past (secondary infection), but gives no history of genital herpes (75–80% of women), and has no visible lesions at the time of delivery. There is a 1% chance that a woman with past genital herpes will be shedding HSV on the day of delivery [4,5]. Women with active primary genital herpes also may be asymptomatic. Screening of pregnant women for antibodies to HSV or for virus shedding is impractical in view of the very low yield, although peripartum examination for genital lesions is still important.

TRANSMISSION

About 5% of babies with HSV infection have true congenital HSV infection, acquired transplacentally following primary maternal HSV in the first trimester [6].

About 85–90% of babies with neonatal HSV infection acquire infection 'vertically' by passage through an infected birth canal or, more rarely, by ascending infection through ruptured or even intact membranes. An unknown proportion of babies with neonatal HSV infection, perhaps as many as 10%, acquire HSV nosocomially from asymptomatic shedders or people with cold sores (staff, relatives, visitors) or carried on the hands of staff from other babies. Light could find only 24 documented cases of nosocomial neonatal HSV infection in 26 years from 1951 to 1977 [7], but neonatal unit outbreaks have since been described in which DNA fingerprinting was used to show that outbreak isolates were identical [8–10].

Transplacentally acquired maternal immunoglobulin G (IgG) antibody is the most important protection against neonatal infection. The risk of neonatal infection during primary maternal HSV infection, when the baby acquires lots of virus and very little or no IgG, is 30–50% [5,11,12], whereas the risk in secondary maternal infection (less virus, plenty of IgG) is much lower: it is 0.04% of all deliveries to seropositive women, but up to 3% of asymptomatic seropositive women shedding virus at the time of delivery [5,12]. The risks are summarized in Table 16.1.

Caesarean section reduces the risk of neonatal HSV infection if primary maternal lesions are present at delivery, and is indicated even if a woman has been in labour for up to 24 hours. The earlier it is performed the better, and known primary HSV genital lesions are an indication for elective lower segment caesarean section (LSCS). LSCS does not abolish the risk completely, and babies will need to be followed closely (see below).

Maternal infection	Risk of neonatal HSV infection	References
Active primary genital lesion	50%	13,14
Asymptomatic primary infection	33%	4,5
Recurrent lesion	4%	4,12,15
Asymptomatic with history of past genital herpes	0.04%	16

Table 16.1 Risks of neonatal HSV infection in relation to maternal genital herpes infection

CLINICAL FEATURES

Very few babies have been reported with features such as microcephaly and keratoconjunctivitis that are suggestive of true congenital HSV infection attributable to transplacental transmission [6]. There is an increased risk of spontaneous abortion in mothers with genital herpes, and HSV has occasionally been isolated from abortuses.

Neonatal HSV can present as infection: (1) localized to the skin, eye or mouth (SEM); (2) generalized, involving the liver, adrenals, lungs and many other organs including the brain as well as skin, eye and mouth; (3) localized to the lung (pneumonitis); or (4) localized to the central nervous system (meningoencephalitis).

Involvement of the skin, eye or mouth may be an isolated finding or part of disseminated disease. It can present at, or soon after, birth and usually in the first week of life, but skin lesions may present for the first time up to 3 weeks after birth, and should be treated urgently with i.v. aciclovir. If untreated, up to 80% of cases of localized disease will progress to involve the CNS or other organs [17].

With improved awareness, an increasing proportion of babies are being diagnosed with localized infection, and early recognition and treatment of localized disease has been paralleled by a fall in the proportion of infected babies with disseminated disease (see Table 16.2). This provides strong, if

Years	Distribution of neonatal HSV infection		
	Localized to skin, eye and/or mouth (SEM)	Generalized infection	Encephalitis alone
1973–80	18%	50%	32%
1981–87	43%	23%	34%
From ref. [18].			

Table 16.2 Change in relative proportions of distribution of neonatal HSV infection in the USA over time, attributed to early diagnosis and treatment of localized (SEM) infection

historical, evidence of the efficacy of early recognition and treatment of babies with localized infection.

Skin involvement is the commonest manifestation of HSV infection. There may be only one or two vesicles, or crops of vesicles that sometimes are quite large and bullous (Figure 16.1 and Colour plate 16.1). Rarer skin lesions are zosteriform eruptions, which are easily misdiagnosed as due to varicella-zoster virus, a generalized petechial rash, areas of denuded skin or erythema multiforme.

The most common eye lesion is keratoconjunctivitis with characteristic dendritic conjunctival or corneal ulcers (see Colour plates 16.2 and 16.3). Chorioretinitis may be seen at birth or complicating keratoconjunctivitis. Uveitis and cataracts may also develop. Microphthalmia and optic atrophy have been described as sequelae of eye infection.

The mouth, tongue, palate (Colour plate 16.4) and occasionally the larynx may be involved with classic herpetic ulceration, which is also often seen as part of disseminated disease.

Disseminated disease usually presents in the first week of life, although occasionally at birth or even after 2 weeks of age. The presentation is usually non-specific with fever, vomiting, lethargy and poor feeding. Other variable features are jaundice, hepatomegaly, purpura or generalized erythema, apnoeic episodes, acidosis, cyanosis and respiratory distress. Convulsions or irritability may be the presenting feature if there is concomitant CNS involvement, which is present in about one-

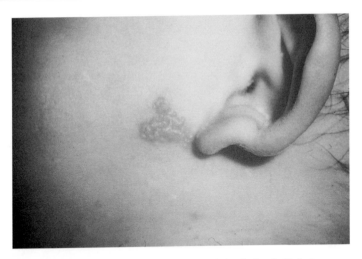

Figure 16.1 Herpes simplex virus infection. Blistering (bullous) skin lesions

half. Pneumonitis may be the sole presenting feature, usually at 3–7 days (Figure 16.2), and HSV infection is rarely considered in the initial differential diagnosis [19]. Prompt treatment prevents HSV pneumonitis progressing to disseminated disease. About one-quarter of patients with disseminated HSV develop a bleeding diathesis with disseminated intravascular coagulopathy (DIC) and shock, which usually is rapidly fatal. Disseminated disease is often fulminant with death within hours, and before specific antiviral therapy the mortality rate was >80% [17]; even with the newer antiviral drugs (aciclovir and vidarabine) the mortality rate is 15–20%.

Localized meningoencephalitis presents later, at a mean age of 11 days, but with a range of 7–30 days [17,20]. The clinical features are those of meningitis, although focal seizures and absent gag reflex are particularly suggestive of HSV encephalitis. The seizures rapidly become generalized and intractable. The CSF usually contains only 50–200 white cells per ml, mostly lymphocytes, although occasionally up to 2500. Red cells in the CSF are only occasionally found, suggesting haemorrhagic

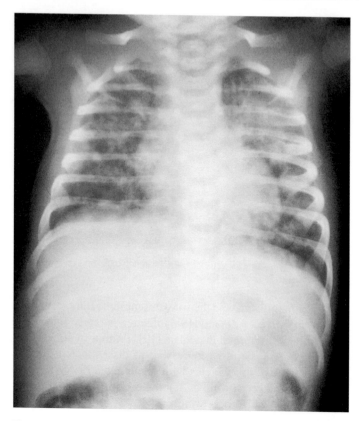

Figure 16.2 Herpes simplex virus pneumonitis. Full-term baby with symptoms from day 3 (see Case history 16.1)

necrosis, but no more commonly than in other forms of neonatal meningoencephalitis. The CSF protein concentration is usually high and glucose levels are normal or slightly low.

HSV can be grown from the CSF in about 50% of cases of meningoencephalitis [21].

DIAGNOSIS

Considering the high rate of dissemination if localized HSV infection is untreated (approximately 80%), and the high mortality rate from disseminated disease, early diagnosis is essential, especially as effective antiviral therapy is now available.

HSV infection often resembles bacterial sepsis clinically. However, the timing of symptoms may suggest a diagnosis of HSV infection. A history of primary or recurrent HSV infection or clinical evidence of maternal genital infection is obtained in <30% of cases of neonatal HSV infection [22].

The timing of symptoms may help to distinguish HSV infection from bacterial sepsis. Pneumonitis presents at 3–7 days with respiratory distress and radiographic appearance of perihilar streaky shadowing (Figure 16.2) progressing to a 'white-out'. Disseminated disease tends to present somewhat later than early-onset bacterial sepsis. Focal fits and absent gag reflex may suggest HSV encephalitis. The baby should be examined carefully with special reference to skin, eyes and mouth.

If vesicular lesions are seen in isolation or as part of generalized disease, every effort should be made to obtain some vesicle fluid for electron microscopy or immunofluorescence and viral culture. Electron microscopy will not distinguish HSV from other herpesviruses, such as varicella-zoster virus, but in the absence of a history of maternal chickenpox, neonatal zosteriform eruptions should be presumed to be due to HSV. The presence of intranuclear inclusions and giant cells on Papanicolau staining of cell scrapings from the base of skin vesicles, oral ulcers or the cervix is only 60–75% sensitive in diagnosing HSV infection [17]. If the roof of a vesicle is removed with a needle, the base can be vigorously swabbed and the swab smeared on a slide for immunofluorescent staining (see Figure 16.3). Immunofluorescence is more sensitive than electron microscopy and has replaced it in many laboratories, but is only 80–90% sensitive compared with culture [23]. The same swab can be used for viral culture, but must be placed in viral transport medium, not Stuart's medium.

Viral cultures take 1–4 days to show the classic cytopathic effect and can be extremely useful. Cultures should be taken from the nasopharynx in all suspected cases (a nasopharyngeal

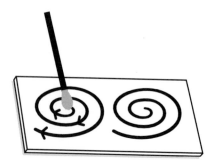

Figure 16.3 Technique for making slide for immunofluorescent stain for HSV and/or VZV. Vigorous swabbing of a de-roofed vesicle, vesicle fluid placed on glass slide, snail-shaped circular smear made out from centre and transported to laboratory

aspirate is best), and from any skin lesions, the conjunctiva and CSF where clinically indicated.

Serology is generally unhelpful. Serum IgM responses are often delayed: Sullender and colleagues found an IgM response in neither of two babies tested <10 days after onset of symptoms, in three of six tested at 10–12 days, and in 13 of 17 tested after 14 days [24]. Serum IgG can be used only to attempt to make a retrospective diagnosis of HSV infection and neonates often produce no IgG antibodies or the titre does not rise fourfold [25]. The use of CSF antibodies to HSV is controversial because IgG may diffuse passively into the CSF rather than being synthesized intrinsically [20]. However, occasionally HSV-specific IgM may appear early in the CSF, allowing rapid early diagnosis [26].

In the past, brain biopsy was advocated, particularly in the Untied States, to make a definitive diagnosis of HSV encephalitis (HSVE). Brain biopsy has been completely superseded by the use of the polymerase chain reaction (PCR) on CSF to detect HSV nucleic acid sequences. PCR is extremely sensitive in most hands and, although contamination can result in false-positive PCR results, a positive PCR is obviously an indication for urgent treatment. Does a negative PCR exclude

HSVE? The problem is that there have been reports of negative PCRs early in HSVE [27], and in practice almost all babies with an encephalopathic illness compatible with HSVE are treated with aciclovir, at least until the clinical and laboratory picture is clearer. The clinical picture and CSF findings of HSVE may be supported by an EEG showing a temporal or parieto-temporal focus, albeit a non-specific finding, and neonatologists would treat on suspicion of HSVE regardless of PCR results. The CT scan is often normal early in the disease, but within days may show unilateral or bilateral temporal lobe changes, cerebral atrophy and loss of grey–white matter differentiation. The CT scan may rarely progress to calcification of the gyrae. Levels of CSF antibodies may take 6–8 weeks to rise, so repeat lumbar puncture for a retrospective diagnosis should be postponed until then.

TREATMENT

Aciclovir and adenosine arabinoside (vidarabine, ara-A) are equally effective in neonatal HSV infection [28]. The daily dose of both drugs is 30 mg/kg, aciclovir being given intravenously 8-hourly and vidarabine 12-hourly, for 14–21 days. Whitley and colleagues found no difference in mortality, morbidity or drug toxicity for aciclovir and ara-A in treating babies with localized, disseminated disease or encephalitis [28]. However, because of the large volume of fluid needed to administer ara-A, aciclovir is the drug of choice to treat neonatal HSV infection. The current recommendation for treating established HSV infection [29] is aciclovir i.v. 30 mg/kg per day in three divided doses for 14–21 days. Eye lesions should also be treated with topical antivirals such as 1% idoxuridine (IDU) under the supervision of an ophthalmologist.

Even with early treatment, which has been shown to reduce significantly the mortality rate from HSV infection, one-half of the survivors of meningoencephalitis and 86% of the survivors of disseminated disease have major sequelae. Relapses can occur after stopping treatment.

Cases of aciclovir-resistant HSV have been reported, either

naturally occurring and apparently of low virulence, or after prolonged aciclovir therapy. So far, there have not been any failures of therapy of neonatal HSV infection attributed to aciclovir-resistant strains.

A small proportion, about 5–10%, of babies with HSV infection apparently localized to skin, eye and mouth (SEM) nevertheless develop long-term neurological sequelae. It is unclear whether these babies had unrecognized CNS involvement in the neonatal period or deteriorated from progressive HSV replication in the CNS over a period of months. Whitley and colleagues found that all babies with fewer than three skin recurrences in the first 6 months were normal, but only 79% of those with three or more recurrences [30]. Kimberlin and colleagues showed that 13 of 16 babies (81%) given suppressive oral aciclovir (300 mg/m^2 per dose three times daily) developed no skin lesions, compared with 54% in a previous study [31]. Nearly half the babies treated with aciclovir developed neutropenia and the study had insufficient power to look at neurodevelopmental outcome.

Gutman and colleagues reported six babies with neonatal HSVE, two of whom had recurrence or worsening of disease immediately after initial parenteral therapy, two of whom had late developmental deterioration, and two seemed to do better on long-term oral aciclovir [32].

As yet, there is insufficient evidence to recommend long-term suppressive oral aciclovir therapy for any babies with HSV infection, although it might be considered for those with frequent skin recurrences.

The prognosis of babies with disseminated disease and those with intractable convulsions from meningoencephalitis is so poor that failure to respond rapidly to treatment should be seen as grounds for considering withdrawing intensive care.

PREVENTION

Babies of women with active genital herpes lesions are at greatest risk (Table 16.3). If the mother has active, primary genital herpes, a caesarean section should be performed as soon as

Maternal infection	Risk to fetus/baby	Management of mother	Management of baby
Primary genital herpes in first trimester	?20% of abortion or intrauterine infection	No action	As for recurrent herpes
Genital lesions present at delivery			
(a) Proven primary maternal	About 50% risk of neonatal HSV	Caesarean section (LSCS)	Cultures[a], if LSCS done Prophylactic aciclovir if vaginal delivery
(b) Proven secondary maternal	About 4% risk of neonatal HSV	Caesarean section (LSCS) or vaginal delivery	Cultures[a], if LSCS done Prophylactic aciclovir if vaginal delivery
(c) Unknown if primary or secondary maternal	About 30% chance that first lesion in woman is primary	Caesarean section (LSCS)	Cultures[a], if LSCS done Prophylactic aciclovir if vaginal delivery
Asymptomatic woman with no visible lesions, but history of genital herpes	About 0.04% risk of neonatal HSV (2% if mother shedding HSV asymptomatically)	Vaginal delivery	Cultures[a], and treat if positive

Adapted from ref. [140].

[a]Cultures = nasopharyngeal and conjunctival samples taken from baby at age 24–48 hours for HSV immunofluorescence and culture. Treat with i.v. aciclovir, 15 mg/kg per day ÷ 3 if either positive.

Table 16.3 Management of HSV infection in pregnancy

possible after membrane rupture and certainly within 6 hours, if possible. Nasopharyngeal viral cultures should be taken after 24 hours to identify infected babies. Should a mother with active primary genital herpes deliver vaginally, especially after prolonged rupture of the membranes, strong consideration should be given to starting the baby on anticipatory (prophylactic) aciclovir. Treatment of the symptomatic mother around the time of delivery with aciclovir has not been evaluated, but Greffe and colleagues have documented modest transplacental passage of aciclovir [33].

Neonates with confirmed or suspected HSV infection should be isolated whenever possible and vigorous attention paid to handwashing. Staff or mothers with cold sores present particular problems. We recommend that the lesions be treated with topical 35% IDU in DMSO cream or topical aciclovir cream 5–6 times a day for up to 3 days. Staff are not allowed to handle babies for 24 hours. Mothers are not separated from their babies, but wear a mask for 24 hours. These recommendations are empirical and based on the potential severity of infection.

COMMON CLINICAL SCENARIOS

Asymptomatic mother with history of recurrent genital herpes

If the mother has no visible lesions at the time of delivery, the risk to the fetus is about 0.04% [3], far too low to justify LSCS. Vaginal delivery is advised. Cultures from the baby taken within 24 hours may merely reflect surface contamination. Nasopharyngeal aspirate and conjunctival swab are, therefore, taken from the baby 24–48 hours after birth and examined for HSV by immunofluorescence and culture. If HSV grows in tissue culture, cytopathic changes are evident within 2–3 days, before any clinical manifestations are at all likely. If either immunofluorescence or culture is positive, the baby should probably be treated with i.v. aciclovir, 30 mg/kg per day in three divided doses for 5–7 days [34]. If both are negative, then no treatment is indicated unless the baby develops lesions.

Baby with blistering lesions

A baby with blistering lesions whose mother has a history of genital herpes should obviously be treated with i.v. aciclovir. If, however, there is no positive maternal history, the presence of blistering lesions in a neonate should be treated as an emergency. It is imperative that a vigorous swab of the lesion be put onto a glass slide, making one or two snail-shaped smears (see Figure 16.3), which can be used for immunofluorescence for HSV (and VZV). A swab should also be sent in viral transport medium for culture.

Babies with positive HSV immunofluorescence and those in whom there is doubt about the quality of the specimen, e.g. no cells, should be treated as above with i.v. aciclovir.

Case history 16.1

A boy was born at 37 weeks' gestation weighing 2360 g after a normal pregnancy. Neither mother nor father gave a history of genital herpes. The baby was breastfed. From 3 days of age, he developed low-grade fever and tachypnoea, but continued to feed well and a chest radiograph on day 3 was normal. He was commenced on antibiotics. His tachypnoea increased and he developed increasing oxygen requirement and, on day 6, pneumonic changes (Figure 16.2). On day 8, he was referred and had developed thrombocytopenia and required artificial ventilation. HSV was detected in nasopharyngeal secretions by immunofluorescence, but, despite intravenous aciclovir, the baby died from disseminated HSV infection.

It is important to remember that postnatal respiratory distress with pneumonitis may be due to HSV. Without treatment, HSV pneumonitis is almost always fatal. If HSV had been suspected early, a positive HSV immunofluorescence on a nasopharyngeal aspirate would have led to aciclovir treatment, which is curative [19].

Case history 16.2

A full-term baby boy was delivered vaginally to an 18-year-old mother after normal pregnancy and labour. On day 5, the baby developed blistering lesions on the scalp and axilla. These were diagnosed as impetigo and treated by the local doctor with topical antibiotics. They gradually dried up. On day 19, the baby became febrile, lethargic and developed intractable seizures. The CSF had 100×10^6/L white blood cells, 1000×10^6/L red cells, protein 1.4 g/L and glucose 3.8 mmol/L. Serum HSV IgM was detected in mother's and baby's blood. HSV could not be grown.

Blistering or vesicular skin lesions developing postnatally may be due to HSV. Early treatment with i.v. aciclovir can prevent the very high risk of progression to encephalitis and/or disseminated HSV infection.

SUMMARY OF HSV INFECTION

- Neonatal HSV infection is usually acquired at the time of delivery from the maternal genital tract.
- Neonatal HSV infection can result either from primary maternal or secondary genital infection.
- Most babies with neonatal HSV infection are born to women with no history of ever having genital herpes.
- There is a high risk that neonatal HSV infection localized to skin, eye or mouth (SEM) will disseminate; this risk can be greatly reduced by prompt diagnosis and treatment.
- Respiratory distress developing at 3–7 days may be due to HSV pneumonitis, which requires immediate diagnosis and treatment.

VARICELLA-ZOSTER VIRUS

Only about 5% of women of child-bearing age in industrialized countries have not had chickenpox. Varicella-zoster virus (VZV) infection affects about 3 per 1000 pregnancies in the UK [35] and 0.7 per 1000 pregnancies in the USA [36]. Its effects on mother, fetus and baby can sometimes be disastrous.

VZV AND THE IMMUNE SYSTEM

Protection against VZV infection is dependent largely on IgG antibody: at-risk patients exposed to someone with chickenpox or shingles can be protected against infection, or at least against severe infection, by the administration of passive IgG antibodies in the form of zoster immune globulin (ZIG). In contrast, boys with agammaglobulinaemia recover normally from chickenpox, showing that antibody is not important for recovery.

Recovery from VZV infection is dependent on cellular immunity, i.e. T cells. Those most at risk from VZV are children and adults with congenital or acquired T cell defects: notably children with congenital immunodeficiency, HIV infection and oncology patients on immunosuppressive drugs. Pregnant women are relatively immunocompromised by pregnancy and can develop severe, even fatal, pneumonitis. Neonates are at risk, not so much because of impaired T cell function, but when they are infected peripartum with high titres of virus in the absence of antibody.

EFFECT ON MOTHER OF GESTATIONAL CHICKENPOX

A high incidence of life-threatening pneumonitis in women with gestational chickenpox (but not zoster) has been reported [37,38]. In one North American study, 24 of 118 pregnant women with chickenpox developed pneumonia and 11 died [38], a mortality rate far in excess of that expected. Pregnant women, particularly those in the first trimester, who are in contact with chickenpox and have no past history of having had chickenpox, should be given varicella-zoster immune globulin (ZIG). The rationale is to modify the severity of disease in the mother and to decrease the risk of congenital varicella syndrome. Women who develop varicella in pregnancy should be treated with aciclovir, because of their own risk of severe disease.

LONG-TERM EFFECTS OF EXPOSURE *IN UTERO* TO VARICELLA-ZOSTER VIRUS

There is very limited evidence that intrauterine chickenpox could lead to an increased risk of leukaemia (two fatal cases in 270 exposures [39]) and of other cancers. Fine and colleagues reported the incidence of cancer to be 2.3-fold greater than expected in a follow-up study of babies exposed *in utero* to VZV or CMV [40].

The basis for this slight increase in risk of malignancy could be the chromosome abnormalities, usually transient, that VZV can induce *in vitro* in tissue culture and *in vivo* in peripheral blood leukocytes from children with chickenpox [41].

CONGENITAL VARICELLA SYNDROME

First-trimester maternal chickenpox may result in characteristic congenital malformations sufficient to be termed a syndrome [42]. There are cicatricial skin lesions of a limb, usually the leg (Figure 16.4), often with hypoplasia and paresis of that limb. This is thought to result from intrauterine zoster, and occasionally a zoster-like lesion is found on the body (Colour plate 16.5). Brain (microcephaly, cortical atrophy, cerebellar hypoplasia) and eye lesions (microphthalmia, optic atrophy, lenticular cataracts, chorioretinitis, nystagmus) are usual. Multiple other lesions have been described as less common features, including hypoplasia of digits, renal, genital, bowel and auditory lesions [35]. The risk of congenital varicella syndrome in the baby of a mother with first-trimester chickenpox was estimated from prospective studies at 2.2% with a range of 0–9% and 95% confidence intervals of 0–4.6% [37,43–46]. Women with varicella infection have more preterm births than controls (14.3% versus 5.6%) [46]. In a large prospective 13-year study in Germany and the UK, the risk of congenital varicella syndrome (CVS) was highest at 2.0% (7 of 351 pregnancies) between 13 and 20 weeks' gestation. Before 13 weeks, the incidence of CVS was 0.4% (2 of 472) while there were no cases in 477 pregnancies in which maternal varicella occurred after 20 weeks' gestation [47]. However, the risk is

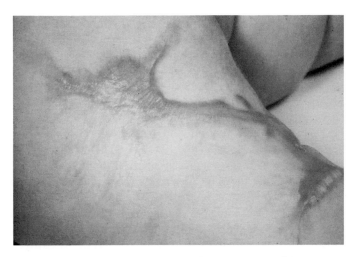

Figure 16.4 Congenital varicella syndrome. Cicatricial scarring of the leg

not zero, as occasional cases of CVS have followed maternal varicella in the second [48] or third trimester [49].

Enders and colleagues reported no cases of CVS in 366 women who had herpes zoster in pregnancy [47], but occasional affected babies have been described [50].

Diagnosis of CVS is primarily clinical. Enders *et al.* found VZV-specific IgM in only 25% (4 of 16) of babies with CVS, although 5 of 7 had persistent VZV-specific IgG on subsequent testing [47]. VZV DNA has been detected by DNA probe [51] and VZV DNA sequences by PCR [52] in autopsy tissues from babies with CVS.

PERINATAL MATERNAL CHICKENPOX

The spectrum of illness in the neonatal period varies from a well baby with a few spots to a fulminant illness with rash, visceral lesions and pneumonitis with extensive exudation of fluid from the lungs followed by pulmonary necrosis (Colour plate 16.6).

When maternal chickenpox occurs around the time of delivery, the baby may develop life-threatening illness. Only about one-quarter of the babies whose mothers develop chickenpox at any time during pregnancy will be infected [53]; however, the timing of illness in mother and baby is critical to the severity. Erlich and colleagues noted that, if the baby's rash was present at birth or appeared within 4 days, the baby survived; if, however, the baby's rash developed 5 or more days after birth, fatalities occurred (Table 16.4) [54].

The incubation period for congenital varicella (time between mother's and baby's rash) is about 9–15 days, although if maternal viraemia is massive, this may be shortened to 3 days or the baby's rash may very occasionally occur simultaneously with the mother's. The corollary of the timing of the baby's rash is that, if the mother's rash appeared 5 or more days before delivery, the baby survives, whereas if the mother's rash appeared 4 days before to 2 days after delivery, then without intervention the mortality rate is approximately 30% (Table 16.4 [55]).

The reason for the importance of the timing appears to be that severely affected babies acquire a large transplacental inoculum of virus before maternal antibody has crossed the placenta. Babies whose mother's rash develops more than 5 days before delivery all have detectable antibody, whereas if the mother's rash develops within 5 or fewer days of delivery, antibody is often undetectable [56].

Zoster immune globulin (ZIG), an immunoglobulin preparation from donors with a high antibody titre to VZV, is gener-

Onset of mother's rash in relation to delivery	Onset of baby's rash in relation to delivery (days after)	Died (n)	Survived (n)	Neonatal mortality (%)
5–21 days before	0–4	0	27	0
4 days before to 2 days after	5–10	7	16	30
From ref. [55].				

Table 16.4 Timing of chickenpox in mother and baby in relation to severity

ally effective in ameliorating the severity of infection, although often it does not actually prevent infection.

Hanngren and colleagues gave ZIG to 95 babies with perinatal exposure and 45 (50%) developed chickenpox [57]. Of the 41 babies in the maximum risk group (mother's chickenpox 4 days before to 2 days after delivery), 21 became infected, of which two cases were severe. ZIG has not been standardized and the effective dose is not known. When 100–125 mg was being given in the UK, three babies died from neonatal chickenpox in 5 years, despite early prophylactic ZIG [58], and the recommended dose was increased to 250 mg. The UK was then free of fatalities for some years [56]. Nevertheless, babies do sometimes develop severe varicella despite ZIG [58,59] and the incidence of 'severe disease' is suggested by the data of Hanngren et al. to be about 5% of ZIG-treated babies who develop varicella [57]. This means that babies treated with ZIG should be carefully observed, although not necessarily in hospital, since only half will develop varicella. If they develop a varicella rash, they should be reviewed. Some authors have advocated treating all babies who develop varicella with i.v. aciclovir, and, even more controversial, giving prophylactic aciclovir at the same time as ZIG, a regimen for which there are no data. We prefer to review a baby given ZIG who develops varicella, and observe closely at home or in hospital for poor feeding, tachypnoea or other signs of more severe illness.

Which babies should be given ZIG? The serological data of Miller et al. suggest that babies whose mothers developed their rash 6 or more days before delivery do not need ZIG, whereas those whose mother's rash appeared 0–5 days before delivery should be given ZIG [56]. There are fewer data for babies whose mother's rash develops after delivery: these babies have no antibody, but the viral inoculum may not be as great, although the mother may well have been viraemic before delivery. Rubin and co-workers reported a case of severe neonatal varicella in a baby aged 15 days whose mother developed varicella 8 days after delivery [60]. It is, perhaps, reasonable to give ZIG to babies whose mother's rash develops up to

30 days after delivery, as suggested by Rubin, although there are no data to support such a recommendation.

The antiviral treatment of babies with severe varicella infection is with aciclovir (30–60 mg/kg per day, 8-hourly, i.v.), but this is not always successful [58].

Given the importance of the timing of the maternal rash, it may be worth attempting to delay labour for a few days when a mother has had recent chickenpox. This is obviously easier in spontaneous or elective preterm labour, but consideration could be given to trying to prevent spontaneous term labour from progressing.

There have been no controlled studies of aciclovir treatment for mothers with peripartum chickenpox. In view of the report of Greffe *et al.* that aciclovir may sometimes cross the placenta, this approach, aimed at decreasing maternal and fetal viraemia, may be worth further study [33].

Babies exposed *in utero* or perinatally to chickenpox, even if they do not have clinical infection, have an increased risk of developing zoster infection early in childhood. Nb: if ZIG is unavailable, normal human immunoglobulin i.m. is one alternative and intravenous immunoglobulin is another.

POSTNATAL EXPOSURE TO CHICKENPOX

Neonates exposed to chickenpox postnatally as opposed to perinatally, usually when a sibling develops the infection, may be at slightly increased risk of severe infection if the mother has not had chickenpox [60–62], although the risk is difficult to quantify because of selective reporting. Rubin and colleagues reviewed the literature and found four babies with severe postnatally acquired neonatal chickenpox, one of whose mother had a history of past chickenpox [60]. This does not necessarily indicate that neonates who acquire infection postnatally are at increased risk of severe disease, since severe VZV may occur at any age. Thus, there may be reporting bias.

A common situation is that a sibling at home has chickenpox at the time that a well mother and term baby are due to be discharged from hospital. If the mother has had chickenpox, there is virtually no risk, and mother and baby should be sent home.

If the mother gives no history of having had chickenpox, she may have had subclinical infection and blood should be sent for urgent testing for VZV-IgG. If the mother has no anti-bodies to VZV or testing is unavailable, it seems reasonable to give the baby ZIG and to send mother and baby home. The alternatives, which are unacceptable, would be to split up the family, give impossible advice to keep the infected sibling away from the baby, or not to intervene at all, in which case the baby would almost certainly develop chickenpox with a risk of severe infection [60].

BREASTFEEDING

When mothers develop varicella, the question of breastfeeding always arises. If the baby has been given ZIG there is no rea-son to prevent breastfeeding. The virus has already been acquired transplacentally, the baby has been protected with ZIG, and there is no known added risk from breastfeeding.

If mother acquires varicella postnatally, her baby is bound to be heavily exposed from mother or siblings. In normal fam-ilies, VZV is highly contagious with a transmission rate of over 90%. Preventing breastfeeding is unlikely to reduce the risk of transmission to the baby to any significant effect and breast milk might even reduce the severity of neonatal varicella.

Occasionally, varicella lesions of the breast render breast-feeding too painful for the mother to continue, and she has to postpone breastfeeding. In general, maternal varicella is not a contraindication to breastfeeding.

ISOLATION

Mothers and/or their babies with varicella lesions are highly contagious and should be isolated from other babies in a side-room whenever possible. Occasionally, a baby is too sick to be isolated, and requires mechanical ventilation in the neonatal unit. In this case, the situation should be managed as described under Nursery outbreaks below (p. 326).

There is never any indication to separate a mother from her own baby because of varicella. The baby has always been exposed to VZV transplacentally or is bound to be heavily exposed postnatally. Similarly, there is little point, and a lot of unnecessary trauma, in trying to prevent exposure of a baby to his or her siblings with chickenpox. Either the baby already has maternal antibodies or should be given ZIG, both of which are highly protective against severe varicella.

NURSERY OUTBREAKS

Most nursery outbreaks are characterized by very little spread of chickenpox, probably because of the high proportion of babies with maternal antibody and very mild disease. However, one baby with Turner's syndrome exposed at 7 days developed fatal chickenpox pneumonitis at 21 days despite maternal antibody [63]. Because of reduced transplacental transfer of IgG, very preterm babies (less than 30 weeks' gestation) are likely to have low or undetectable levels of antibody even if the mother has had chickenpox. If such babies are exposed to chickenpox, they should be given ZIG, as should other preterm babies with no maternal history of VZV infection. Infected babies and mothers should be isolated and nursed by immune staff.

SUMMARY OF VZV INFECTION

- The risk of congenital varicella syndrome is about 2.0% if maternal varicella occurs between 13 and 20 weeks' gestation, but only 0.4% before 13 weeks.
- Maternal varicella after 20 weeks' gestation and maternal zoster at any stage are associated with a very low risk of congenital varicella.
- Babies whose mothers develop varicella 5 or fewer days before, or up to 2 days after, delivery are at high risk of severe varicella and should be given zoster immune globulin (ZIG) at birth.
- Non-immune babies exposed to varicella up to 30 days after delivery should be given ZIG.

- If a newborn baby's siblings have chickenpox, the baby should be given ZIG if the mother is non-immune, but does not need to be separated from mother or siblings.
- Maternal varicella is not a contraindication to breastfeeding.

ENTEROVIRUSES

The enteroviruses (echoviruses, coxsackieviruses and polioviruses) are small RNA viruses for which humans are the only natural host. Spread in older children and adults is primarily by the faecal–oral route, although respiratory spread may also occur. However, in the neonatal period, aspiration or ingestion of infected maternal blood or cervical secretions at the time of delivery (vertical infection) can result in severe, often fatal, infection and usually causes more fulminant disease than infection acquired 'horizontally' from baby-to-baby spread.

EPIDEMIOLOGY

In temperate climates, enterovirus infections peak in the summer and autumn months although they may occur at any time of the year. Neonatal poliomyelitis is rare in both developed and developing countries. Echovirus and coxsackievirus infections have been reported worldwide, although coxsackievirus outbreaks have been described in South Africa in particular [64]. The incidence of neonatal enterovirus infection is unknown because many cases are asymptomatic and because often the appropriate viral cultures are not performed. Prospective studies carried out in neonatal units over 1–2 years may detect no cases of enterovirus infection, whereas in other years there may be an outbreak with several cases. We detected 18 enterovirus infections in 5 years on the neonatal unit in Oxford, either babies with symptoms or well contacts of symptomatic babies, which is an incidence of 0.7 per 1000 live births, and almost certainly an underestimate.

TRANSMISSION

There is a biphasic presentation of neonatal enteroviral infections [65–67]. Babies developing symptoms within 7 days of birth usually have more severe disease, and are thought usually to have been infected 'vertically' at the time of delivery from maternal faeces or genital secretions, or possibly even transplacentally. In contrast, babies infected 'horizontally' after 7 days, for example in nursery outbreaks, may be asymptomatic or have relatively mild disease.

There is some evidence that polioviruses can cross the placenta, particularly late in pregnancy, and cause abortion, stillbirth or neonatal infection. First-trimester intrauterine infection probably does not occur. Live oral polio vaccines given in the first trimester have not caused congenital abnormalities. It has been suggested that coxsackieviruses can cause placental and transplacental infection in the third trimester as babies are sometimes born with rash, although probably not in the first or second trimesters. Echoviruses probably do not cause transplacental infection to the same extent as the other enteroviruses, although occasional cases have been described.

The most common mode of neonatal echovirus and coxsackievirus infection, based on the time of presentation, is almost certainly contact with infected maternal blood or cervical secretions during delivery. Following oral or respiratory acquisition there is local spread to regional lymph nodes within 24 hours. After about 3 days there is minor viraemia with spread to multiple sites. Symptoms start when viral multiplication occurs in these sites at 4–5 days and leads to major viraemia. Some infections have followed caesarean delivery, even with intact membranes, suggesting that infection has occurred from maternal blood or that the viruses can cross intact membranes.

Outbreaks of echovirus and coxsackievirus infections frequently occur on neonatal units. Usually, a baby presents with the features of perinatally acquired ('vertical') infection and spread occurs to other babies ('horizontal' infection) via secretions carried on the hands of staff or when staff members become infected. Sometimes there is no clear index case and infection presumably started with an ill member of the family or the staff. Horizontal infections are nearly always far milder, presumably because the babies receive less virus and perhaps also because many have passively acquired maternal antibody.

MATERNAL SYMPTOMS

When babies develop early enteroviral infections, a history of peripartum maternal illness can be obtained in about half of all cases. This illness may be a mild respiratory or gastrointestinal infection.

One well-recognized maternal enteroviral syndrome is the sudden onset of severe cramping abdominal pains [68]. These pains are often diagnosed as due to placental abruption, leading to an urgent caesarean section. The baby is thus born at a time of high viral load before maternal IgG antibodies have been produced and crossed the placenta, i.e. a time of high risk to the baby.

CLINICAL MANIFESTATIONS

It is now clear that babies infected at delivery (vertical infection) generally have a different and more fulminant clinical course than those infected horizontally. However, at any age, neonatal enteroviral infections can mimic bacterial infections and be difficult to diagnose [67].

Echoviruses

Babies with vertically acquired echovirus infection tend to present at 3–5 days, although very occasionally at birth or as late as 7 days. In about one-half of the cases, there is a history of peripartum maternal illness (see above). The most common neonatal clinical manifestation is a sepsis-like picture, sometimes with rash, progressing rapidly to fulminant hepatic necrosis with a severe bleeding disorder due to disseminated intravascular coagulopathy (DIC) and decreased levels of clotting factors [66]. The liver may be enlarged and ascites, often heavily bloodstained, develops. Bleeding becomes generalized and may cause haemopericardium. The haemoglobin concentration often falls by several grams in a few hours. The mortality rate from this condition is 80% [66]. Liver histology at autopsy shows centrilobular necrosis suggestive of ischaemia as well as hepatitis, a picture also seen in yellow fever. As most babies who die have had catastrophic bleeding and hypotension, ischaemia is not surprising, and virus can be readily grown from the liver. It is not clear whether the primary insult to the liver is infection (hepatitis) or ischaemia, or perhaps both.

In fulminant echovirus infection there may also be meningitis, myocarditis, pneumonitis and gastroenteritis, and virus can easily be cultured from stool, throat swab or nasopharyngeal aspirate as well as urine, CSF, ascitic fluid, pleural fluid and multiple organs including the adrenal glands.

In contrast, horizontal infection is usually relatively mild, even in very preterm infants [66,69]. More than one-half of the babies are symptom-free. Most babies present after 7 days of age and often after 14 days. Babies may develop meningitis (with a presentation similar to that of bacterial meningitis), myocarditis, pneumonia, gastroenteritis, or a non-specific illness with fever, irritability and apnoeic episodes.

Any echovirus serotype can probably cause severe infection, although the most commonly reported serotypes are echoviruses 11, 6 and 7, presumably reflecting their frequency of circulation in the population.

Coxsackieviruses

A less clear distinction can be drawn between vertical and horizontal infections for cocksackie than for echoviruses, although for both, horizontal are usually milder than vertical infections [65]. In South Africa, there have been neonatal unit outbreaks in which babies who were thought to be horizontally infected developed fatal myocarditis [64]. Neonatal coxsackie A virus infections have rarely been reported. Coxsackie B virus infections most commonly result in either meningitis or myocarditis, or sometimes both [70]. A macular rash, occasionally petechial, is a common accompaniment. Rarer manifestations include hepatitis, pancreatitis, enterocolitis, fever, paralysis and bronchitis.

Babies with myocarditis may present suddenly with listlessness, poor feeding, tachycardia and fever. Murmur is often absent or unremarkable and the diagnosis is made by finding cardiomegaly and ECG changes and by echocardiography. Babies may recover gradually, may die rapidly from circulatory failure, may make an apparent recovery, but then collapse in terminal heart failure, or may deteriorate relentlessly despite inotropic support [65]. Occasionally, pericardial calcification develops. The presentation of coxsackievirus B meningitis is clinically similar to that of bacterial meningitis.

Polioviruses

Symptomatic neonatal poliovirus infection is uncommon, and probably over 90% of neonatal poliovirus infections are asymptomatic. Bates described 58 cases of symptomatic infections: about one-half were secondary to maternal infection, 15% were due to nosocomial infection and the rest were of unknown origin [71]. The initial presentation was non-specific with fever, anorexia and irritability, although rarely diarrhoea.

All but one of the 44 with adequate clinical data developed paralytic poliomyelitis, of whom one-half died, one-quarter recovered and one-quarter had residual paralysis. Poliovirus immunization is effective in the neonatal period and is recommended at birth in developing countries.

DIAGNOSIS

The diagnosis of neonatal enteroviral infections is largely based on appropriate viral cultures. If there is a suspicious peripartum maternal illness, stool and throat swabs from the mother should be cultured, and at least stool and nasopharyngeal aspirate or throat swab from the baby. A viral cytopathic effect is usually seen in tissue culture within 2–4 days. Rapid viral diagnosis will soon be freely available. RNA probes have been developed which can detect enterovirus genome by hybridization, very much a research tool at present. Similarly, enterovirus PCR can detect either echovirus or coxsackievirus infections and may be very useful, for example in suspected enteroviral meningitis. Serology is not generally helpful because of the large numbers of serotypes that can cause similar disease. However, specific IgM against coxsackie B viruses may be detected in myocarditis, as only B2–B5 have been associated frequently with myocarditis [67,70].

TREATMENT

The treatment of severe enterovirus infections is supportive. Immunoglobulins are highly unlikely to modify the illness once established. We have unsuccessfully given intravenous human immunoglobulin in a vain attempt to treat babies with massive bleeding from hepatic necrosis. Blood transfusions and replacement of clotting factors with fresh frozen plasma and vitamin K are the mainstay of attempted management for hepatic necrosis. Myocarditis may require digitalization and possibly additional inotropic support if heart failure develops or progresses, and antiarrhythmics for arrhythmias. Digitalis should be used with caution and initially at low doses because of possible increased sensitivity during enterovirus infection.

PREVENTION

It has been advocated that, when there is evidence or even suspicion of an outbreak of enterovirus infection on a neonatal unit, the unit should be closed to outside admissions and all babies in contact with infected babies, including all new admissions, should be given prophylactic immunoglobulin [72]. We have questioned the wisdom of such a policy, because (a) most horizontal infections are relatively mild, (b) closing units may lead to babies receiving suboptimal care, and (c) human immunoglobulins, being blood products, are not completely without risk. In an outbreak in Oxford, there were two simultaneous 'index' cases, both with meningitis and both thought to have been horizontally infected [69]. At this time spread had already occurred to eight other babies, all but one being at 27–30 weeks' gestation. Five were symptom-free and one each had pneumonia, gastroenteritis and apnoeic episodes. With no intervention other than to reinforce the importance of hand-washing there was further spread to only two babies, both symptom-free.

Because of the evidence that horizontal infections with coxsackieviruses are more severe than horizontal echovirus infections, coxsackievirus outbreaks should be managed more aggressively. In a coxsackievirus outbreak, especially if there is more than one case of myocarditis, i.m. or i.v. immunoglobulins should be given to all unaffected babies to attempt to lessen the severity of subsequent infection.

When perinatal enterovirus infection is strongly suspected on clinical grounds (we were recently consulted on twins delivered to a mother with hand, foot and mouth disease), or if virus has been isolated from the mother, the baby should be given 400 mg/kg of immunoglobulin by i.v. infusion immediately after birth. Poliovirus infections are preventable by immunization. Whenever possible, we isolate babies with known or suspected enterovirus infection and cohort the staff.

PROGNOSIS

Vertically transmitted echovirus infection has a high mortality rate (over 60%), and if hepatic necrosis develops the rate is over 80% [66]. Horizontal echovirus infections have occasionally been fatal in neonates, as they have in infants, older children and adults. In general, however, death from horizontal infection is extremely rare. There have been contrasting reports on the long-term outcome of enteroviral meningitis with estimates of the incidence of residual neurological sequelae ranging from none [73] to up to 15% [74–76]. Myocarditis usually responds to conservative management or digitalization. Coxsackievirus myocarditis has a high mortality rate, particularly if the disease is vertically acquired [65].

SUMMARY OF ENTEROVIRUS INFECTION

- Babies infected with coxsackievirus or echovirus around delivery (vertically infected) usually have worse disease than those infected horizontally.

- Babies with perinatal echovirus infection usually present at 3–5 days with 'sepsis' progressing to fulminant hepatitis, liver failure and DIC.

- The mothers of babies with perinatal enterovirus infection may present with severe abdominal pain mimicking abruption.

- Babies with either vertical or horizontal coxsackievirus infection can develop myocarditis.

- Enteroviruses are the commonest cause of neonatal viral meningitis.

HEPATITIS B VIRUS

Hepatitis B is a highly infectious DNA virus which can cause severe to fulminant hepatitis, but also has the important ability to cause a chronic carrier state lasting many years. There are over 200 million carriers in the world. Carriers are at greatly increased risk (approximately tenfold) of cirrhosis and hepatocellular carcinoma.

STRUCTURE

The hepatitis B virus comprises an inner core, which contains the DNA, a DNA polymerase and an antigen called the core antigen (HBcAg), and an outer coat of lipid, glycoprotein and the surface antigen (HBsAg). An additional antigen, the e antigen (HBeAg), is seen during acute infections, but also in some asymptomatic carriers, and is an important marker of infectivity (Figure 16.5).

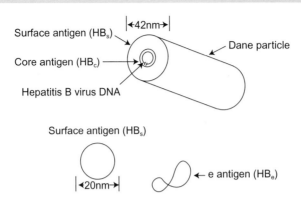

Figure 16.5 Diagrammatic representation of the electron microscopic appearance of the hepatitis B virus (Reproduced with permission from ref. [140].)

EPIDEMIOLOGY

In Taiwan, China, South-East Asia, Japan and parts of Africa, hepatitis B infection is endemic, with up to 15% of the population being chronic carriers (surface antigen positive). In the UK, Europe and America, it is people whose families originate from those areas who are most likely to be chronically infected with hepatitis B. Other high-risk groups are intravenous drug abusers, male homosexuals, people regularly receiving blood or blood products such as those on haemodialysis (particularly if the donors are not screened), and medical and nursing staff. There is increasing evidence of spread occurring within families, mainly to siblings [77].

TRANSMISSION

The most important method of transmission of hepatitis B virus in the neonatal period is vertical transmission from an infected mother. This is also the most common method of transmission worldwide, being the major factor in maintaining endemicity in Asian populations. Transmission could be transplacental or at the time of delivery. The success of immunoglobulin and vaccine in preventing transmission suggests that most neonatal infections occur around delivery, presumably by contact with infected maternal secretions. In Africa, in contrast, most hepatitis B infection is transmitted horizontally during childhood, and not vertically.

The e antigen is an important determinant in transmission to neonates and particularly in the development of the chronic carrier state. Babies of asymptomatic carrier mothers who are e antigen positive and have no detectable antibody to the e antigen (HBeAg⁺) nearly all become infected and 85% will become chronic carriers [78,79]. In contrast, babies of mothers with antibody to e antigen (HBeAb⁺) virtually never become carriers. Polakoff found that none of 71 babies of HBeAb⁺ mothers became carriers [80], while Stevens and colleagues found 3 of 14 such babies were infected, but none became carriers [78].

In South-East Asia, a high proportion (up to 50%) of surface antigen-positive carrier women of child-bearing age are e antigen positive with no antibody, whereas in the UK, Europe and America, most carriers are either e antibody positive or have no detectable e antigen or e antibody (i.e. they are just surface antigen positive). This explains the fact that the vertical transmission rate in Japan, Taiwan and South-East Asia from all surface antigen-positive mothers is 40–80%, whereas in Britain, Europe and the USA, the transmission rate is usually <5%.

Some babies become infected and may develop acute hepatitis (although they do not become carriers), despite their mothers being e antigen negative or e antibody positive. It may be that the demonstration of hepatitis B virus DNA in the mother's blood will prove a good indicator of whether such neonatal infection is likely to occur [81].

If women develop acute hepatitis B infection in pregnancy or up to 2 months after delivery, about one-half of their babies become infected [82]. Neonatal infection is most likely (>70%) if the mother's hepatitis is in the third trimester or early puerperium, but only 10% in the first or second trimesters [83].

Hepatitis B surface antigen can be detected in breast milk by radioimmunoassay, but not by less sensitive techniques.

Studies have not shown any difference in transmission rates between breastfed and bottlefed babies, so breast milk is probably an uncommon mode of transmission. It is not known, however, whether breast milk infects a small number of babies who would not otherwise have been infected. Transmission of hepatitis B from breast milk could be important where wet nursing is practised.

DIAGNOSIS

Traditional diagnostic tests for hepatitis B antigens were superseded initially by radioimmunoassay and subsequently by enzyme-linked immunosorbent assays (ELISAs), which can also be used to detect antibody. Hepatitis B virus DNA can be detected by hybridization [84] and, although this is primarily a research tool, the presence of hepatitis B virus DNA may correlate with those babies who develop infection [81].

CLINICAL FEATURES

Most babies who become chronic carriers are asymptomatic, although they may have persistently raised serum levels of transaminases and liver biopsy may show chronic persistent or chronic active hepatitis [83].

Acute icteric hepatitis develops in a small number of infected babies, but does not usually present until 2–5 months of age [85]. This may be fulminant with massive hepatic necrosis, or may progress to cirrhosis.

PREVENTION

Ideally, all pregnant women should be screened for HBsAg, but if this is impossible, women with risk factors for hepatitis B, as outlined above, should be tested.

Passive immunization with hepatitis B immunoglobulin is 70–80% effective in preventing perinatal transmission of hepatitis B from both e- antigen-positive and surface antigen-positive mothers [86,87]. The first dose needs to be given within hours of birth.

Active immunization with plasma-derived vaccines is 80

to 95% effective in preventing perinatal transmission [88,89]. The new hepatitis B vaccines derived by recombinant DNA technology, such as the recombinant yeast vaccines where yeasts produce surface antigen, are equally effective.

Combined passive–active prophylaxis using both hepatitis B immunoglobulin and hepatitis B vaccine gave a protective efficacy of 85–95% in Taiwan [89] and Hong Kong [90], whereas >70% of untreated babies became chronic carriers. Presumably, some babies still become chronic carriers despite prophylaxis, because of intrauterine transmission.

There have been occasional reports of babies of e antibody-positive mothers developing severe acute hepatitis B [91,92], as well as babies whose mothers were e antigen and antibody negative, but surface antigen positive [93]. In the USA, it is recommended that all babies of women who are surface antigen positive be given 0.5 mL of hepatitis B immunoglobulin (HBIg) as soon as possible after birth and 10 µg hepatitis B vaccine at birth, 1 and 6 months [94].

Universal neonatal hepatitis B immunization is a recommendation of the World Health Organization for all non-industrialized countries. It is also being adopted by an ever-increasing number of industrialized countries (see Chapter 21).

Breastfeeding is considered to be indicated in developing countries where the risks of bottlefeeding outweigh the very small risk of transmitting hepatitis B, but is not advised in developed countries where the relative risks may be reversed.

All medical and nursing staff should be immunized against hepatitis B.

HEPATITIS C VIRUS

Hepatitis C virus (HCV) is the virus responsible for the post-transfusion hepatitis, previously called non-A, non-B hepatitis. The virus was identified in the late 1980s and is a flavivirus, a small RNA virus, related to yellow fever virus.

HCV is primarily transmitted in blood and blood products.

Around the world, from 2 in 1000 to 2 in 100 blood donors are found to be HCV antibody positive. Since screening of blood and blood products for HCV antibody was introduced, the major mode of transmission in industrialized countries has been found to be by intravenous drug use. The approximate seroprevalence of HCV in different situations is shown in Table 16.5. These figures suggest that transmission by blood products is common, but that sexual transmission is rare.

At least 200 million people in the world have been infected with HCV. HCV persists in about 80% of infections [95]. There is a substantial risk of progression to chronic liver disease with cirrhosis, although this risk varies according to different epidemiological and virological factors [96]. About half of all patients with chronic HCV infection show an initial response to interferon α therapy, but the response is sustained in a minority [96]. Similar results have been found in a small study of children and young adults [97]

In a number of relatively small follow-up studies of babies of HCV-positive women, the risk of transmission from mother to baby has been about 5–10% [98–100]. The risk is highest if the mother has active viral replication, as shown by the detection of HCV RNA in blood by PCR, and is particularly high for women who have both HIV and HCV infection.

Hepatitis C virus RNA cannot be detected by PCR in breast milk of seropositive mothers, although it can be detected in saliva in about 50% [101]. Breastfeeding is believed to be

Population	HCV seropositive
Healthy blood donors	0.2–2%
Post-transfusion non-A, non-B hepatitis	75–85%
Intravenous drug users (IVDUs)	50–80%
Haemophiliac (factor VIII dependent)	60–85%
Haemodialysis patients	5–20%
Homosexual men (excluding IVDUs)	4–8%
Prostitutes (excluding IVDUs)	4–6%

Table 16.5 Approximate seroprevalence of anti-HCV antibodies in different populations

safe, and almost all authorities counsel HCV-positive women that breastfeeding does not appear to increase the risk of their babies being infected.

It is impossible to tell whether newborn babies of HCV-seropositive women are infected. They will have passively acquired HCV IgG antibodies, and PCR is insufficiently reliable to be used to diagnose or exclude infection. Babies should be followed with serial blood tests. The mean age of loss of maternal antibody in babies who became seronegative was 5 months in one study [97], but can be up to 15 months of age, so a firm diagnosis of infant infection cannot be made until antibodies have persisted for 15 months.

PARVOVIRUS B19

Human parvovirus B19 (HPV B19) derives its name from *parvo* (= small) and B19, the serum sample in which the virus was first serendipitously identified by electron microscopy by Yvonne Cossart in 1975. HPV B19 is the cause of the childhood exanthem called variously fifth disease, 'slapped cheek' syndrome or erythema infectiosum. This is a contagious febrile illness with rash, lymphadenopathy and, in women and older girls, arthropathy, which mimics rubella. It causes epidemics in school-aged children.

The virus classically infects erythroid precursors in the bone marrow, causing transient reticulocytopenia lasting about 1–2 weeks. In normal children and adults, this results in an asymptomatic fall in haemoglobin level of about 1 g/dL, whereas in those with shortened red cell survival, it can cause significant anaemia due to red cell aplasia. In children with sickle cell disease or haemoglobinopathies such as thalassaemia, HPV B19 infection can cause transient aplastic crises. The virus can cause persistent infection with anaemia in patients with congenital or acquired immune deficiency.

The fetus has a shortened red cell survival, and fetal infection can result in hydrops fetalis, due to severe anaemia, resulting in cardiac failure (Figure 16.6) [102]. Congenital

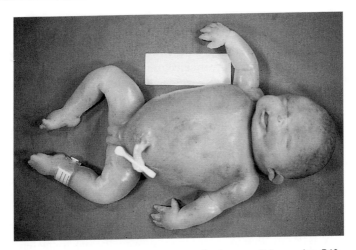

Figure 16.6 Stillborn baby with fetal hydrops due to congenital parvovirus B19 infection

parvovirus B19 infection is one of the commonest causes of non-immmune (i.e. non-Rhesus) hydrops.

In industrialized countries, about 50% of adults are seronegative, and the estimated incidence of HPV B19 infection during pregnancy is 0.3–3% [102]. When maternal infection does occur, most fetuses are unaffected. The PHLS Working Party studied 186 pregnant women with confirmed HPV B19 infection: only two babies developed hydrops [103].

There are no recognized congenital malformations consistently associated with fetal HPV B19 infection, although encephalopathy with cerebral calcification has been described in three liveborn infants [104,105].

There is an excess fetal loss of about 5–10% associated with maternal HPV, mainly in the second trimester [103].

For neonatologists and paediatricians, congenital HPV B19 infection is most important in four settings: the neonate with hydrops fetalis, the neonate with encephalopathy and cerebral calcification, the pregnant woman exposed to proven or suspected HPV B19 infection, and the pregnant woman with a clinical illness consistent with or shown to be due to HPV B19.

HPV B19 cannot be grown in normal tissue culture, so diagnosis is by serology, by electron microscopy or by detection of nucleic acid by *in situ* hybridization or polymerase chain reaction (PCR). The sensitivity of serum IgM for detecting fetal HPV B19 infection is about 90%, but there is cross-reaction with other viruses such as rubella. PCR on fetal blood or amniotic fluid is now the diagnostic modality of choice for antenatal diagnosis [102].

A pregnant woman in contact with a child with fifth disease or who herself develops a consistent clinical illness should have acute and convalescent sera taken looking for IgM or seroconversion to HPV B19 and also rubella serology. Even if HPV B19 infection in pregnancy is proven, the risk to the fetus is very low, at under 2% [102], while diagnosis of fetal infection by PCR on amniotic fluid or fetal blood is in its infancy and is anyway risky.

After counselling the parents, we strongly discourage termination of pregnancy, since malformations/deformations probably do not occur and hydrops is potentially curable. We recommend performing immediate fetal ultrasonography, followed by weekly ultrasonography until delivery, looking for hydrops. The maximum risk period for hydrops is 4–6 weeks after maternal infection. If hydrops develops, then assessment for possible intrauterine blood transfusion should be made at a specialized obstetric centre.

RESPIRATORY SYNCYTIAL VIRUS

Respiratory syncytial virus (RSV) occasionally causes neonatal unit outbreaks of infection, nearly always during the winter epidemic season, and predominantly affecting babies >3–4 weeks old. The clinical features of neonatal RSV infection are non-specific and may include rhinitis, apnoeic episodes, irritability, lethargy, poor feeding, fever, tachypnoea, pulmonary infiltrates and increased requirements for respiratory support.

Lower respiratory involvement is more often seen in older babies, but chest signs (crackles, wheezes, intercostal recession) are not often present [106–108]. Younger babies may have merely cough or coryza. Asymptomatic infection is not uncommon.

Hall and co-workers reported that 23 of 82 babies (28%) on a neonatal unit studied during a community outbreak developed RSV infection [106]. Four babies died in association with RSV infection: one was already terminally ill; one had bronchopulmonary dysplasia decompensated, and two died suddenly and unexpectedly. This was an early report of babies studied in 1977. Nowadays, with better intensive care and greater awareness of RSV infection, the mortality rate from neonatal RSV infection is considerably lower.

Certain groups of patients are at increased risk from RSV infection, particularly babies with cyanotic congenital heart disease and bronchopulmonary dysplasia.

The American Academy of Pediatrics [29,109] recommended that the antiviral agent ribavirin should be *considered* for high-risk patients, including babies with congenital heart disease or bronchopulmonary dysplasia, 'certain premature infants' and severely ill infants. However, there is no evidence that ribavirin prevents the need for mechanical ventilation in high-risk babies, and there are considerable concerns, albeit theoretical, about potential teratogenicity to pregnant staff exposed to ribavirin. There are considerable problems in delivering ribavirin to ventilated babies because it precipitates in ventilator tubing and there is no evidence that it reduces mortality. The drug is also extremely expensive [110]. We do not routinely use ribavirin for preterm or high-risk babies infected with RSV, but 'consider' it for critically ill babies and those with cyanotic congenital heart disease or bronchopulmonary dysplasia, though virtually never use it.

High-dose RSV immunoglobulin administered i.v. to 'high-risk' infants (mean age of 8 months, with chronic lung disease, congenital heart disease or prematurity) significantly reduced the incidence of RSV-related infections the following winter [111]. However, this is a high-cost preventive measure that has not been shown to be cost effective.

Handwashing is the most important way of preventing spread of RSV in the neonatal unit, which occurs predominantly via infected nasal secretions, either carried from baby-to-baby on the hands of staff or via the staff themselves becoming infected [112].

OTHER RESPIRATORY VIRUSES

Parainfluenza, influenza and rhinoviruses can cause sporadic infections or neonatal unit outbreaks in which babies characteristically develop rhinitis, cough, fever, apnoeic episodes, pulmonary infiltrates and feeding difficulties. These signs and symptoms are similar to those of RSV infection. In simultaneous outbreaks of RSV and rhinovirus [113] and of RSV and parainfluenza type 3 [114], babies infected with RSV were clinically indistinguishable from those infected with the other respiratory viruses. The clustering of cases in the second outbreak strongly suggested patient-to-patient spread.

Most mothers have antibodies to measles. Measles is rare in pregnancy and does not cause a recognized syndrome of congenital infection, although there have been reports of sporadic fetal abnormalities in association with gestational measles. Gestational measles is associated with a high risk of spontaneous abortion. Neonatal unit outbreaks are extremely rare. Postnatal measles with rash occurring at 14–30 days, and usually resulting from postnatal maternal infection or from a sibling, is generally mild. However, congenital measles, in which the rash is present at birth or appears in the first 10 days, may be severe, and dominated by pneumonia or pneumonitis. There is an obvious parallel with perinatal chickenpox, although less is known about transfer of maternal antibody. The mortality rate appears to be the same, whether rash is present at birth or appears in the next 10 days [115,116], and in one report 7 of 16 preterm babies exposed to measles died from pneumonitis without developing a rash [117]. In Greenland, however, none of 13 babies whose mothers had measles at delivery developed congenital measles [118]. The age of these reports should be emphasized and the mortality rate of 30–44% almost certainly no longer applies; there is no information on the current mortality rate from congenital measles. Given the potential severity, it would seem wise to give hyperimmune measles gammaglobulin to babies of mothers with peripartum measles and to neonates whose siblings have measles and whose mothers are non-immune.

First-trimester maternal mumps carries a modestly increased risk of abortion [119]. There is also a possible slightly increased long-term risk of the baby later developing diabetes [120]. No consistent congenital syndrome has been described, although attempts have been made to link gestational mumps with endocardial fibroelastosis, Down's syndrome and other malformations. Even if the mother has mumps at the time of delivery, neonatal illness is rare, and parotitis exceedingly so. Jones *et al.* [121] and Reman *et al.* [122] reported babies aged 7 and 3 days respectively with mumps pneumonitis.

EPSTEIN–BARR VIRUS

Primary maternal Epstein–Barr virus (EBV) infection is rare in pregnancy, and there is no firm evidence of the existence of a congenital EBV syndrome.

Early descriptions of associations with congenital heart disease have not been confirmed by any consistent disease associations. Evidence of intrauterine exposure may be shown by detecting maternal serum IgM to EBV and evidence of infection by detecting IgM in the newborn baby's serum. Some babies with detectable EBV IgM have had multiple congenital anomalies with no consistent syndrome. Two babies had serological evidence of simultaneous congenital CMV and congenital EBV infection, but with clinical findings more suggestive of CMV [123]. As the use of PCR for EBV becomes more widely available it may become easier to prove or disprove possible links between EBV infection and abortion, congenital anomalies and other possible disease associations.

HUMAN IMMUNODEFICIENCY VIRUS (HIV)

STRUCTURE

The virus that causes the acquired immunedeficiency syndrome (AIDS), the human immunodeficiency virus (HIV), is a lentivirus, which is a subfamily of the retroviruses. The great majority of cases are caused by subtype 1 (HIV-1), although HIV-2 causes some cases in Africa. Although these are RNA viruses, they can code for DNA synthesis directly by transcribing the RNA using an enzyme, reverse transcriptase. The virus consists of a central core of RNA and reverse transcriptase surrounded by two protein membranes (Figure 16.7). The detection of circulating p24 antigen and of antibodies to p24 is often used in serological tests. The outer lipid bilayer contains the envelope (env) protein and from the bilayer protrude glycoproteins.

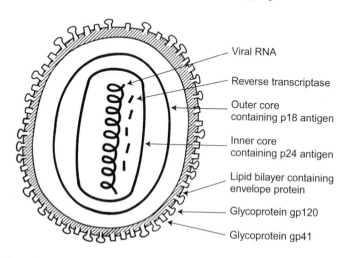

Viral RNA

Reverse transcriptase

Outer core containing p18 antigen

Inner core containing p24 antigen

Lipid bilayer containing envelope protein

Glycoprotein gp120

Glycoprotein gp41

Figure 16.7 Diagrammatic representation of the human immunodeficiency virus (HIV)

EPIDEMIOLOGY

The HIV pandemic probably began in the late 1970s. The World Health Organization has estimated that, within 20 years, over 20 million adults and 1.5 million children in the world have been infected, most of them in sub-Saharan Africa and southern Asia [124]. By the year 2000, 15 million women in the world will have been infected and up to 10 million children will be AIDS orphans, having lost one or both parents [125].

Perinatal transmission now represents the major mode of HIV infection in childhood. In Europe, the prevalence of HIV in women of child-bearing age is from 0.0002% to 0.26%, whereas it is often 30% or higher in major cities in sub-Saharan Africa [125]. In Africa and Asia, most HIV transmission is via heterosexual spread and the prevalence is equal for men and women.

MOTHER-TO-INFANT TRANSMISSION

Newborns may be infected at the time of delivery or transplacentally. HIV can be detected in cervical and vaginal secretions, and neonatal rhesus monkeys can be infected orally with simian immunodeficiency virus (SIV). Peripartum transmission is thought to cause about two-thirds of neonatal HIV infection [125]. The rest of the cases are caused by intrauterine transmission: HIV can be detected in first- and second-trimester fetuses, as well as in amniotic fluid and placenta.

First-born twins are more likely to be infected with HIV than second-born. This discordance is thought to be due to greater exposure of the first-born twin to infected maternal secretions at the time of delivery, and the risk can be reduced by caesarean delivery [126].

In the past, neonates have been infected postpartum through blood transfusions, but screening of the blood supply for HIV antibodies has effectively eliminated this risk.

BREASTFEEDING

It was initially appreciated that babies could be infected via breast milk when HIV was diagnosed in the breastfed baby of a woman infected postnatally by contaminated blood transfusion [127]. Mothers thus infected have high-level viraemia, increasing the risk to the baby. The risk of infection to the breastfed baby of a seroconverting woman has been estimated at 29% [128].

The risk to the breastfed baby of a woman with established HIV infection is harder to estimate, because intrauterine and peripartum routes are the major routes of transmission. The risk is generally lower than for seroconverting women, because maternal viraemia is at a lower level. Dunn and colleagues estimated the additional transmission risk from breastfeeding to be 14% (range 7–22%) [128]. In the Côte d'Ivoire, the risk of late postnatal transmission, i.e. due to breastfeeding, was 12% for HIV-1-positive mothers and 6% for mothers with both HIV-1 and HIV-2 infection [129].

In developing countries, the risk of HIV-positive mothers *not* breastfeeding is considered to exceed the additional risk of HIV transmission, so breastfeeding by HIV-positive mothers is encouraged. In industrialized countries, bottlefeeding is safer and is preferred to breastfeeding.

RATE OF TRANSMISSION

The rate of transmission from an HIV-positive pregnant woman to her baby has varied from a low of 13% in some countries in western Europe [130] to over 40% in parts of Africa, with intermediate transmission rates of 20–30% in the USA, Australia, France and Italy [125].

As might be expected, the rate of transmission is highest when the mother has more advanced disease, as determined by high viral load, measured by plasma HIV RNA concentration, and low CD4 counts [131]. The rate of transmission is also higher for preterm babies and for first-born twins.

CLINICAL FINDINGS

A distinctive HIV embryopathy described by Marion *et al.* [132,133] and Iosub *et al.* [134], characterized by a prominent forehead and large, widely spaced eyes, was not confirmed by subsequent investigators [135].

Children with HIV infection occasionally are born with lymphadenopathy, hepatomegaly or splenomegaly, and with haematological abnormalities such as thrombocytopenia [125]. Babies with HIV infection in Zaire are born smaller than the babies of non-infected control mothers, but are not smaller than the non-infected babies of HIV-positive mothers [136]. This suggests that the low birthweight is due to maternal malnutrition, not intrauterine growth retardation secondary to HIV.

In general, it is rare for HIV-infected babies to present with opportunistic infections such as *Pneumocystis carinii* infection or oral candidiasis in the neonatal period, although such presentations have occasionally been described.

INVESTIGATION

Babies born to HIV-positive women may or may not be infected. The presence of HIV IgG antibody cannot distinguish infected from non-infected babies, since it is acquired transplacentally. IgG disappears from the bloodstream of uninfected babies by a median of 9 months of age, although occasionally may be detected up to 15 months of age. Thus, only if HIV IgG antibody is detected 15 months after birth can it be said to indicate certain infection.

Other tests now available include viral isolation from blood, polymerase chain reaction (PCR) for HIV RNA and the presence of p24 antigen in the baby's blood. Using these three tests, together with HIV IgA antibody, it is almost always possible to tell by 6 months whether or not a baby is infected.

The tests should be sent within 48 hours of birth, since *in utero* transmission is defined as detection of HIV by PCR or virus isolation within 48 hours of birth, while intrapartum transmission is defined as negative tests under 7 days of age, followed by tests becoming positive (PCR, isolation or p24 antigen) from 7 to 90 days of age [125].

TREATMENT OF MOTHER AND BABY

The current trend in HIV treatment is to use multiple anti-retroviral drugs, to attempt to reduce viral load to undetectable levels and limit the emergence of resistance. Monotherapy with zidovudine (AZT) is considered outmoded.

Nevertheless, the most exciting development in preventing paediatric HIV infection, at least for industrialized countries which can afford it, is the dramatic reduction in perinatal transmission achieved by treating mother and baby with zidovudine. The AIDS Clinical Trials Group (ACTG) Trial 076, was a randomized, double-blind, placebo-controlled trial of the use of AZT 100 mg × 5 orally for the last 6 weeks of pregnancy, i.v. treatment with AZT in labour, and treatment of the baby with AZT orally for the first 6 weeks [137]. The reduction in infection rate from 25.5% to 8.3% (shown in Table 16.6) was highly significant ($P = 0.0006$), but it should be remembered that the mothers were a highly selected group of HIV-positive women who had not previously been on antivirals during the pregnancy, were well and whose CD4 count was over 200 per µL.

PNEUMOCYSTIS PROPHYLAXIS

It is controversial which babies should be given cotrimoxazole prophylaxis against *Pneumocystis carinii* pneumonia (PCP). Most PCP in children occurs in infants, and CD4 counts are not entirely reliable at predicting which babies will develop CD4 [125]. Some authorities recommend that PCP prophylaxis be

Treatment	No. of babies treated	No. of babies infected	Infection rate	95% confidence intervals
Placebo	184	47	25.5%	18.3–33.7%
Zidovudine	180	15	8.3%	3.8–33.8%
From ref. [137].				

Table 16.6 Summary of ACTG Trial 076 results

given to all babies of HIV-positive mothers, until they are proven to be uninfected or unless they reach 1 year of age with normal CD4 counts. Ziegler suggests that PCP prophylaxis might be withheld unless the mother herself requires PCP prophylaxis, or the baby is shown to be HIV infected, or has a low or falling CD4 count [125].

PREVENTION

Clearly, treatment of mother and baby according to the protocol used in ACTG Trial 076 is, at the time of writing, the most effective means of preventing maternal–infant transmission of HIV. Bottlefeeding, as discussed above, is indicated in industrialized countries. These interventions will have no impact whatsoever in developing countries where AZT is unaffordable and breastfeeding is clearly preferred to bottlefeeding.

In developing countries, are there any options apart from preventing women becoming infected by interventions such as the use of condoms and the treatment of other genital tract infections? One study from Malawi showed an inverse relationship between maternal serum vitamin A levels and transmission rate [138]. The effect of vitamin A supplementation of pregnant women in reducing transmission has not yet been reported, and low maternal vitamin A levels may merely reflect maternal malnutrition due to more advanced disease.

References
1 Prober CG & Arvin AM. Genital herpes and the pregnant woman. *Curr Clin Top Infect Dis* 1989; **10**: 1–26.
2 Tookey P & Peckham CS. Neonatal herpes simplex virus infection in the British Isles. *Paediatr Perinatal Epidemiol* 1996; **10**: 432–42.
3 Scott LL. Perinatal herpes: current status and obstetric management strategies. *Pediatr Infect Dis J* 1995; **14**: 827–32.
4 Prober CG, Hensleigh PA, Boucher FD, Yasukawa LL, Au DS & Arvin AM. Use of routine viral cultures at delivery to identify neonates exposed to herpes simplex virus. *N Engl J Med* 1988; **318**: 887–91.
5 Brown ZA, Benedetti J, Ashley R *et al.* Neonatal herpes simplex

virus infection in relation to asymptomatic maternal infection at the time of labour. *N Engl J Med* 1991; **324**: 1247–52.

6 Hutto C, Arvin A, Jacobs R *et al.* Intrauterine herpes simplex infections. *J Pediatr* 1987; **110**: 97–101.

7 Light IJ. Postnatal acquisition of herpes simplex virus by the newborn infant: a review of the literature. *Pediatrics* 1979; **63**: 480–2.

8 Linnemann CC, Buchman TG, Light IJ & Ballard JL. Transmission of herpes-simplex virus type 1 in a nursery for the newborn. Identification of viral isolates by DNA 'fingerprinting'. *Lancet* 1978; **i**: 964–6.

9 Halperin SA, Hendley JO, Nosal C & Roizman B. DNA fingerprinting in investigation of apparent nosocomial acquisition of neonatal herpes simplex. *J Pediatr* 1980; **97**: 91–3.

10 Hammerberg O, Watts J, Chernesky M *et al.* An outbreak of herpes simplex virus type 1 in an intensive care nursery. *Pediatr Infect Dis* 1983; **2**: 290–4.

11 Brown ZA, Vontver LA, Benedetti J *et al.* Effects on infants of a first episode of genital herpes during pregnancy. *N Engl J Med* 1987; **317**: 1246–51.

12 Prober CG, Sullender WM, Yasukawa LL *et al.* Low risk of herpes simplex virus infections in neonates exposed to the virus at the time of vaginal delivery to mothers with recurrent genital herpes simplex virus infection. *N Engl J Med* 1987; **316**: 240–4.

13 Nahmias AJ & Roizman B. Infection with herpes-simplex viruses 1 and 2. *N Engl J Med* 1973; **289**: 781–9.

14 Nahmias AJ, Josey WE, Naib ZM, Freeman MG, Fernandez RJ & Wheeler JH. Perinatal risk associated with maternal genital herpes simplex virus infection. *Am J Obstet Gynecol* 1971; **110**: 825–37.

15 Arvin AM, Hensleigh PA, Prober CG *et al.* Failure of antepartum maternal cultures to predict the infant's risk of exposure to herpes simplex virus at delivery. *N Engl J Med* 1986; **315**: 796–800.

16 Whitley RJ & Kimberlin DW. Treatment of viral infections during pregnancy and the newborn period. *Clin Perinatol* 1997; **24**: 267–83.

17 Nahmias AJ, Keyserling HL & Kerrick GM. Herpes simplex. In: Remington JS & Klein JO (eds) *Infectious Diseases of the Fetus and Newborn Infant*, 2nd edn. Philadelphia: WB Saunders, 1983: 636–78.

18 Whitley RJ, Corey L, Arvin A *et al.* Changing presentation of herpes simplex virus infection in neonates. *J Infect Dis* 1988; **158**: 109–16.

19 Barker JA, McLean SD, Jordan GD, Krober S & Rawlings JS. Primary neonatal herpes simplex virus pneumonia. *Pediatr Infect Dis J* 1990; **9**: 285–9.

20 Nahmias AJ, Whitley RJ, Visitine AN *et al.* Herpes simplex virus encephalitis: laboratory evaluations and their diagnostic significance. *J Infect Dis* 1982; **145**: 829–36.

21 Whitley RJ, Nahmias AJ, Visintine AM *et al.* The natural history of herpes simplex virus infection of mother and newborn. *Pediatrics* 1980; **66**: 489–94.

22 Yeager A & Arvin A. Reasons for the absence of a history of recurrent genital infections in mothers of neonates infected with herpes simplex virus. *Pediatrics* 1984; **73**: 188–93.

23 Gilbert GL. *Infectious Disease in Pregnancy and the Newborn Infant.* Harwood: Chur, 1991.

24 Sullender WM, Miller JL, Yasukawa LL *et al.* Humoral and cell-mediated immunity in neonates with herpes simplex virus infection. *J Infect Dis* 1987; **155**: 28–37.

25 Kahlon J & Whitley RJ. Antibody response of the newborn after herpes simplex virus infection. *J Infect Dis* 1988; **158**: 925–33.

26 Dwyer DE, O'Flaherty S, Packham D & Cunningham AL. Herpes simplex encephalitis in infants. *Med J Aust* 1986; **144**: 714–15.

27 Uren EC, Johnson PDR, Montanaro J & Gilbert GL. Herpes simplex virus encephalitis in pediatrics: diagnosis by detection of antibodies and DNA in cerebrospinal fluid. *Pediatr Infect Dis J* 1993; **12**: 1001–6.

28 Whitley RJ, Arvin A, Prober C *et al.* Predictors of morbidity and mortality in neonates with herpes simplex virus infections. *N Engl J Med* 1991; **32**: 450–4.

29 American Academy of Pediatrics. Committee on Infectious Diseases. Ribavirin therapy of respiratory syncytial virus disease. *Pediatrics* 1987; **79**: 475–8.

30 Whitley RJ, Arvin A, Prober C *et al.* A controlled trial comparing vidarabine with aciclovir in neonatal herpes simplex virus infection. *N Engl J Med* 1991; **324**: 444–9.

31 Kimberlin D, Powell D, Gruber W *et al.* Administration of oral aciclovir suppressive therapy after neonatal herpes simplex virus disease limited to the skin, eyes and mouth: results of a phase I/II trial. *Pediatr Infect Dis J* 1996; **15**: 247–54.

32 Gutman LT, Wilfert CM & Eppes S. Herpes simplex virus encephalitis in children. Analysis of cerebrospinal fluid and progressive neurodevelopmental deterioration. *J Infect Dis* 1986; **154**: 415–21.

33 Greffe BS, Dooley SL, Deddish RB & Krasny HC. Transplacental passage of aciclovir. *J Pediatr* 1986; **108**: 1020–1.

34 Overall JC Jr, Whitley RJ, Yeager AS, McCracken GH Jr & Nelson JD. Prophylactic or anticipatory antiviral therapy for newborns exposed to herpes simplex infection. *Pediatr Infect Dis* 1984; **3**: 193–5.

35 Miller E, Marshall R & Vurdien JE. Epidemiology, outcome and control of varicella infection. *Rev Med Microbiol* 1993; **4**: 222–30.

36 Sever JA & White LR. Intrauterine viral infections. *Annu Rev Med* 1968; **19**: 471–86.

37 Paryani SG & Arvin AM. Intrauterine infection with varicella-zoster virus after maternal varicella. *N Engl J Med* 1986; **314**: 1542–6.

38 Gershon AA. Chickenpox, measles and mumps. In: Remington JS & Klein JO (eds) *Infectious Diseases of the Fetus and Newborn Infant*, 3rd edn. Philadelphia: WB Saunders, 1990: 395–44.

39 Adelstein AM & Donovan JW. Malignant disease in children whose mothers had chickenpox, mumps, or rubella in pregnancy. *BMJ* 1972; **4**: 629–31.

40 Fine PEM, Adelstein AM, Snowman J *et al.* Long term effects of exposure to viral infection *in utero*. *BMJ* 1985; **290**: 509–11.

41 Aula P. Chromosomes and viral infections. *Lancet* 1964; **i**: 720–1.

42 Alkalay AL, Pomerance JJ & Rimoin D. Fetal varicella syndrome. *J Pediatr* 1987; 111: 320–3.

43 Siegel M. Congenital malformations following chickenpox, measles, mumps and hepatitis. *JAMA* 1973; **226**: 1521–4.

44 Enders G. Varicella-zoster virus infection in pregnancy. *Prog Med Virol* 1984; **29**: 166–96.

45 Preblud SR, Cochi SL & Orenstein WA. Varicella-zoster infection in pregnancy. *N Engl J Med* 1986; **315**: 1416–17.

46 Pastuszak A, Levy M, Schick B *et al.* Outcome after maternal vari-cella infection in the first 20 weeks of pregnancy. *N Engl J Med* 1994; **330**: 901–5.

47 Enders G, Miller E, Cradock-Watson J, Bolley I & Ridehalgh M. Consequences of varicella and herpes zoster in pregnancy: prospective study of 1739 cases. *Lancet* 1994; **343**: 1547–50.

48 Brice JEH. Congenital varicella resulting from infection during second trimester of pregnancy. *Arch Dis Child* 1976; **51**: 474–6.

49 Bai PVA & John TJ. Congenital skin ulcers following varicella in late pregnancy. *J Pediatr* 1979; **94**: 65–7.

50 Webster MH & Smith CS. Congenital abnormalities and maternal herpes zoster. *BMJ* 1977; **2**: 1193.

51 Scharf A, Scherr O, Enders G & Helftenbein E. Virus detection in the fetal tissue of a premature delivery with a congenital varicella syndrome – a case report. *J Perinat Med* 1990; **18**: 317–20.

52 Puchhammer-Stockl E, Kunz C, Wagner G & Enders G. Detection of varicella zoster virus DNA in fetal tissue by polymerase chain reaction. *J Perinat Med* 1994; **22**: 65–9.

53 Myers JD. Congenital varicella in term infants: risks reconsidered. *J Infect Dis* 1974; **129**: 215–17.

54 Erlich RM, Turner JAP & Clarke M. Neonatal varicella. *J Pediatr* 1958; **53**: 139–47.

55 de Nicola LK & Hanshaw JB. Congenital and neonatal varicella. *J Pediatr* 1979; **94**: 175–6.

56 Miller E, Cradock-Watson JE & Ridehalgh MKS. Outcome of newborn babies given anti-varicella-zoster immunoglobulin after perinatal maternal infection with varicella-zoster virus. *Lancet* 1989; **ii**: 371–3.

57 Hanngren K, Grandien M & Granstrom G. Effect of zoster immunoglobulin for varicella prophylaxis in the newborn. *Scand J Infect Dis* 1985; **17**: 343–7.

58 Holland P, Isaacs D & Moxon ER. Fatal neonatal varicella infection. *Lancet* 1986; **ii**: 1156.

59 Bakshi SS, Miller TC, Kaplan M, Hammerschlag MR, Prince A & Gershon AA. failure of varicella-zoster immunoglobulin in modification of severe congenital varicella. *Pediatr Infect Dis J* 1986; **5**: 699–702.

60 Rubin L, Leggiadro R, Elie MT & Lipsitz P. Disseminated varicella in a neonate: implications for immunoprophylaxis of neonates exposed to varicella. *Pediatr Infect Dis J* 1986; **5**: 100–2.

61 Preblud SR, Bregman DJ & Vernon LL. Deaths from varicella in infants. *Pediatr Infect Dis J* 1985; **4**: 503–7.

62 Preblud SR, Orenstein WA & Bart KJ. Varicella: clinical manifestations, epidemiology and health impact in children. *Pediatr Infect Dis J* 1984; **3**: 505–9.

63 Gustafson TL, Shehab Z & Brunell PA. Outbreak of varicella in a newborn intensive care nursery. *Am J Dis Child* 1984; **138**: 548–50.

64 Editorial. Avoiding the danger of enteroviruses in newborn babies. *Lancet* 1986; **i**: 194–6.

65 Kaplan MH, Klein SW, McPhee J & Harper RG. Group B coxsackievirus infections in infants younger than three months of age: a serious childhood illness. *Rev Infect Dis* 1983; **5**: 1019–32.

66 Modlin JF. Perinatal echovirus infection: insights from a literature review of 61 cases of serious infection and 16 outbreaks in nurseries. *Rev Infect Dis* 1986; **8**: 918–26.

67 Haddad J, Gut JP, Weinling M *et al.* Enterovirus infections in neonates. A retrospective study of 21 cases. *Eur J Med* 1993; **2**: 209–14.

68 Feldman RG, Bryant J, Ives KN & Hill NCW. A novel presentation of coxsackie B2 virus infection during pregnancy. *J Infect* 1987; **15**: 73–6.

69 Isaacs D, Dobson SRM, Wilkinson AR *et al.* Conservative management of an echovirus 11 outbreak in a neonatal unit. *Lancet* 1989; **i**: 543–5.

70 Daley AJ, Isaacs D, Dwyer DE & Gilbert GL. A cluster of cases of neonatal coxsackievirus B meningitis and myocarditis. *J Paediatr Child Health* 1998; **34**: 196–8.

71 Bates T. Poliomyelitis in pregnancy, fetus and newborn. *Am J Dis Child* 1955; **90**: 189–95.

72 Nagington J, Gandy G, Walker J & Gray JJ. Use of normal immunoglobulin in an echovirus 11 outbreak in a special-care baby unit. *Lancet* 1983; **ii**: 443–6.

73 Bergman I, Painter MJ, Wald ER *et al.* Outcome in children with enteroviral meningitis during the first year of life. *J Pediatr* 1987; **110**: 705–9.

74 Farmer K, MacArthur BA & Clay MM. A follow-up study of 15 cases of neonatal meningoencephalitis due to coxsackie B5. *J Pediatr* 1975; **87**: 568–71.

75 Sells CJ, Carpenter RL & Ray CG. Sequelae of central nervous system enterovirus infections. *N Engl J Med* 1975; **293**: 1–4.

76 Wilfert CM, Thompson RJ Jr, Sunder TRO *et al.* Longitudinal assessment of children with enterovirus meningitis during the first three months of life. *Pediatrics* 1981; **67**: 811–15.

77 Szmuness W, Prince AM, Hirsch RL & Brotman B. Familial clustering of hepatitis B infection within families. *N Engl J Med* 1973; **289**: 1162–6.

78 Stevens CE, Neurath RA, Beasley P & Szmuness W. HBeAg and anti HBe detection by radioimmunoassay – correlation with vertical transmission of HBV in Taiwan. *J Med Virol* 1979; **3**: 237–41.

79 Stevens CE, Beasley RP, Tsui J *et al.* Vertical transmission of hepatitis B antigen in Taiwan. *N Engl J Med* 1975; **292**: 771–4.

80 Polakoff S. Hepatitis B virus DNA and e antigen in serum from blood donors positive for HBsAg. *BMJ* 1985; **290**: 1211–12.

81 de Virgilis S, Frau F, Sanna G *et al.* Perinatal hepatitis B virus detection by hepatitis B virus-DNA analysis. *Arch Dis Child* 1985; **60**: 56–8.

82 Schweitzer IL, Wing A, McPeak C & Spears RL. Hepatitis and hepatitis-associated antigen in 56 mother–infant pairs. *JAMA* 1972; **220**: 1092–5.

83 Schweitzer IL, Dunn AE, Peters RL & Spears RL. Viral hepatitis B in neonates and infants. *Am J Med* 1973; **55**: 762–71.

84 Scotto J, Hadchouel M & Hery C. Detection of hepatitis B virus DNA in serum by a simple spot hybridization technique. Comparison with results for other viral markers. *Hepatology* 1983; **3**: 279–84.

85 Dupuy JM, Frommel D & Alagille D. Severe viral hepatitis in infancy. *Lancet* 1975; **i**: 191–4.

86 Beasley RP, Hwang LY, Stevens CE *et al.* Efficacy of hepatitis B immune globulin for prevention of perinatal transmission of the hepatitis B virus-carrier state: final report of a randomized, double-blind, placebo-controlled trial. *Hepatology* 1983; **3**: 135–41.

87 Beasley RP, Hwang L-Y, Lin C-C *et al.* Hepatitis B immune globulin. HBIG; efficacy in the interruption of perinatal transmission of hepatitis B carrier state. *Lancet* 1981; **ii**: 388–93.

88 Maupas P, Chiron J-P, Barim F *et al.* Efficacy of hepatitis B vaccine in prevention of HBsAG carrier state in children. Controlled trial in an endemic area. *Lancet* 1981; **i**: 289–92.

89 Beasley RP, Hwang LY, Lee GCY *et al.* Prevention of perinatally transmitted hepatitis B virus infections with hepatitis B immune globulin and hepatitis B vaccine. *Lancet* 1983; **ii**: 1099–102.

90 Wong VCW, Ip HMH, Reesink HW *et al.* Prevention of the HBsAG carrier state in newborn infants of mothers who are chronic carriers of HBsAG and HBeAG by administration of hepatitis B vaccine and heptatitis B immunoglobulin. *Lancet* 1984; **i**: 921–6.

91 Shiraki K, Yoshi N, Sakurai M *et al.* Acute hepatitis B in infants born to carrier mothers with the antibody to hepatitis B e antigen. *J Pediatr* 1980; **97**: 768–70.

92 Sinatra FR, Shah P, Weissman JY *et al.* Perinatal transmitted acute icteric hepatitis B in infants born to hepatitis B surface antigen-positive and anti-hepatitis Be-positive carrier mothers. *Pediatrics* 1982; **70**: 557–9.

93 Tong MJ, Sinatra FR, Thomas DW *et al.* Need for immunoprophylaxis in infants born to HBsAg-positive carrier mothers who are HBeAg negative. *J Pediatr* 1984; **105**: 945–7.

94 Brunell PA, Bass JW, Daum RS *et al.* Prevention of neonatal hepatitis B virus infections. *Pediatrics* 1985; **75**: 362–4.

95 van der Poel CL, Cuypers HT & Reesink HW. Hepatitis C virus six years on. *Lancet* 1994; **344**: 1475–9.

96 Preston H & Wright TL. Interferon therapy for hepatitis C. *Lancet* 1996; **348**: 973–4.

97 Marcellini M, Kondili LA, Comparcola D *et al.* High dosage alpha-interferon for treatment of children and young adults with chronic hepatitis C disease. *Pediatr Infect Dis J* 1997; **16**: 1049–53.

98 Weintrub PS, Veereman-Wauters G, Cowan MJ & Thaler MM. Hepatitis C virus infection in infants whose mothers took street drugs intravenously. *J Pediatr* 1991; **119**: 869–74.

99 Reinus JF, Leikin EL, Alter HJ *et al.* Failure to detect vertical transmission of hepatitis C virus. *Ann Intern Med* 1992; **117**: 881–6.

100 Wejstal R, Widell A, Persson A-S, Hermodsson S & Norkrans G. Mother-to-infant transmission of hepatitis C. *Ann Intern Med* 1992; **117**: 887–90.

101 Ogasawara S, Kage M, Kosai K-I, Shimamatsu K & Kejiro M. Hepatitis C virus RNA in saliva and breast milk of hepatitis C carrier mothers. *Lancet* 1993; **341**: 561.

102 Gilbert GL. Congenital fetal infections. *Semin Neonatal* 1996; **1**: 91–105.

103 Public Health Laboratory Service (PHLS). Working Party on Fifth Disease. Prospective study of human parvovirus (B19) infection in pregnancy. *BMJ* 1990; **300**: 1166–70.

104 Tiessen RG, van Elsacker Niele AM, Vermeÿ Keers C, Oepkes D, van Roosmalen J & Gorsira MC. A fetus with a parvovirus B19 infection and congenital anomalies. *Prenat Diagn* 1994; **14**: 173–6.

105 Conry JA, Toroy TJ & Andrews PI. Perinatal encephalopathy secondary to *in utero* human parvovirus B19 (HPV) infection. *Neurology* 1993; **43** (Suppl A): 346.

106 Hall CB, Kopelman AE, Douglas RG *et al.* Neonatal respiratory syncytial virus infection. *N Engl J Med* 1979; **300**: 393–6.

107 Mintz L, Ballard RA, Sniderman SH *et al.* Nosocomial respiratory syncytial virus infections in an intensive care nursery: rapid diagnosis by direct immunofluorescence. *Pediatrics* 1979; **64**: 149–53.

108 Rudd PT & Carrington D. A prospective study of chlamydial, mycoplasmal and viral infections in a neonatal intensive care unit. *Arch Dis Child* 1984; **59**: 120–5.

109 American Academy of Pediatrics. Committee on Infectious Diseases. Use of ribavirin in the treatment of respiratory syncytial virus infection. *Pediatrics* 1993; **92**: 501–4.

110 Isaacs D, Moxon, ER, Harvey D *et al.* Ribavirin in respiratory syncytial virus infection. *Arch Dis Child* 1988; **63**: 986–90.

111 Groothuis JR, Simoes EAF, Levin MJ *et al.* Prophylactic administration of respiratory syncytial virus immune globulin to high-risk infants and young children. *N Engl J Med* 1993; **329**: 1524–30.

112 Hall CB & Douglas RG. Modes of transmission of respiratory syncytial virus. *J Pediatr* 1981; **99**: 100–2.

113 Valenti WM, Clarke TA, Hall CB *et al.* Concurrent outbreaks of rhinovirus and respiratory syncytial virus in an intensive care nursery. *J Pediatr* 1982; **100**: 722–6.

114 Meissner HC, Murray SA, Kiernan MA *et al.* A simultaneous outbreak of respiratory syncytial virus and parainfluenza virus type 3 in a newborn nursery. *J Pediatr* 1984; **104**: 680–4.

115 Dyer I. Measles complicating pregnancy. Report of 24 cases with three instances of congenital measles. *South Med J* 1940; **33**: 601–6.

116 Kohn JL. Measles in newborn infants (maternal infection). *J Pediatr* 1933; **3**: 176–9.

117 Richardson DL. Measles contracted *in utero. Rhode Island Med J* 1920; **3**: 13–16.

118 Christensen PE, Schmidt H, Bang HO *et al.* An epidemic of measles in southern Greenland, 1951. *Acta Med Scand* 1953; **144**: 430–6.

119 Siegel M, Fuerst HT & Peress NS. Comparative fetal mortality in maternal virus diseases. A prospective study on rubella, measles, mumps, chickenpox and hepatitis. *N Engl J Med* 1966; **274**: 768–71.

120 Fine PEM, Adelstein AM, Snowman J *et al.* Long term effects of exposure to viral infection *in utero. BMJ* 1985; **290**: 509–11.

121 Jones JF, Ray GG & Fulginiti of VA. Perinatal mumps infection. *J Pediatr* 1980; **96**: 912–14.

122 Reman O, Freymuth F, Laloum D & Boute JP. Neonatal respiratory distress due to mumps. *Arch Dis Child* 1986; **61**: 80–1.

123 Arvin AM & Maldonado YA. Other viral infections of the fetus and newborn. In: Remington JS & Klein JO (eds) *Infectious Diseases of the Fetus and Newborn Infant*, 4th edn. Philadelphia: WB Saunders, 1995: 746–7.

124 Quinn TC. Global burden of the HIV pandemic. *Lancet* 1996; **348**: 99–106.

125 Ziegler JB. HIV infection. *Semin Neonatal* 1996; **1**: 127–39.

126 Duliege AM, Amos CI, Felton S *et al.* Birth order, delivery route and. concordance in the transmission of human immunodeficiency virus type 1 from mothers to twins. *J Pediatr* 1995; **126**: 625–32.

127 Ziegler JB, Cooper DA, Johnson RO & Gold J. Postnatal transmission of AIDS-associated retrovirus from mother to infant. *Lancet* 1985; **i**: 896–8.

128 Dunn DT, Newell ML, Ades AE & Peckham CS. Risk of human immunodeficiency virus type 1 transmission through breast feeding. *Lancet* 1992; **340**: 585–8.

129 Ekpini ER, Wiktor SZ, Satten GA *et al.* Late postnatal mother-to-child transmission of HIV-1 in Abidjan, Cote d'Ivoire. *Lancet* 1997; **349**: 1054–9.

130 European Collaborative Study. Children born to women with HIV-1 infection: natural history and risk of transmission. *Lancet* 1991; **337**: 253–60.

131 Sperling RS, Shapiro DE, Coombs RW *et al.* Maternal viral load,

zidovudine treatment, and the risk of transmission of human immunodeficiency virus type 1 from mother to infant. *N Engl J Med* 1996; **335**: 1621–9.

132 Marion RW, Wiznia AA, Hutcheon RG & Rubinstein A. Human T-cell lymphotropic virus type III. HTLV-III; embryopathy: a new dysmorphic syndrome associated with intrauterine HTLV-III infection. *Am J Dis Child* 1986; **140**: 638–40.

133 Marion RW, Wiznia AA, Hutcheon RG & Rubinstein A. Fetal AIDS syndrome score: correlation between severity of dysmorphism and age at diagnosis of immunodeficiency. *Am J Dis Child* 1987; **141**: 429–31.

134 Iosub S, Bamji M, Stone RK *et al.* More on human immunodeficiency virus embryopathy. *Pediatrics* 1987; **80**: 512–16.

135 Qazi QH, Sheikh TM, Fikrig S & Menikoff H. Lack of evidence for craniofacial dysmorphism in perinatal human immunodeficiency virus infection. *J Pediatr* 1988; **112**: 7–11.

136 Ryder RW, Nsa W, Hassig SE *et al.* Perinatal transmission of the human immunodeficiency virus type 1 to infants of seropositive women in Zaire. *N Engl J Med* 1989; **320**: 1637–42.

137 Connor EM, Sperling RS, Gelber R *et al.* Reduction of maternal–infant transmission of human immunodeficiency virus type 1 with zidovudine treatment. *N Engl J Med* 1994; **331**: 1173–80.

138 Semba RD, Miotti PG, Chiphangwi JD *et al.* Maternal vitamin A deficiency and mother-to-child transmission of HIV-1. *Lancet* 1994; **343**: 1593–7.

139 Campbell AGM & McIntosh N. *Forfar & Arneil's Textbook of Pediatrics*, 5th edn. New York: Churchill Livingstone, 1998.

140 Isaacs D. Infections due to viruses and allied organisms. In: Campbell AGM, McIntosh N (eds) *Forfar & Arneil's Textbook of Pediatrics*, 5th edn. New York: Churchill Livingstone, 1998.

17 | Congenital infections

INTRODUCTION

It was only in 1941 that the connection between maternal infection in pregnancy and damage to the fetus caused by that infection was first recognized by Sir Norman Gregg, when he described congenital rubella syndrome. The terminology used to describe congenital infections can be confusing. Babies are 'born with' congenital infections, which are infections transmitted 'vertically' from the mother to her newborn. The infection may be transmitted transplacentally in the first trimester at the time of maximum organogenesis, and result in *malformations*, as in congenital rubella syndrome. The infection may be transmitted transplacentally, at almost any time in pregnancy, and attack organs or tissues already formed, causing *deformations*, as with some of the features of congenital cytomegalovirus (CMV) infection and congenital varicella syndrome. In both these last two conditions, brain malformations may also occur, so malformation and deformation can coexist.

Infection may be acquired at the time of labour and delivery, i.e. peripartum, and result in damage after an incubation period of a few days (e.g. enteroviruses) or weeks (e.g. hepatitis B virus). Some congenital infections (e.g. CMV, HIV) are usually asymptomatic at birth, but progressive infection leads to effects months or years later. Some infections can be acquired in different ways. Most babies acquire HSV infection peripartum, but there is a rare congenital HSV infection acquired transplacentally (see Chapter 16). Similarly, hepatitis B virus and HIV are predominantly acquired at parturition, but some cases of each infection are thought to be transmitted transplacentally.

Some congenital infections will be considered under separate chapter headings, e.g. HSV (Chapter 16), HIV (Chapter 16), enteroviruses (Chapter 16), group B streptococcal infections (Chapter 14) and *Listeria* (Chapter 14), while others will be considered here.

It is perhaps surprising that infection with a range of organisms so disparate as protozoan parasites (*Toxoplasma gondii*), viruses (rubella, CMV, HSV), mycobacteria (*Mycobacterium tuberculosis*) and treponemes (*Treponema pallidum*) can result in clinical syndromes that overlap and may be difficult to distinguish.

TESTS

Simply ordering a 'TORCH' test is no longer acceptable practice [1]. In the past, if any baby was thought to have possible congenital infection, a TORCH test was sent. This test looked for antibodies to Toxoplasma, Rubella, CMV and HSV. What is so wrong with this?

First, true intrauterine or transplacental congenital HSV infection (as opposed to HSV acquired peripartum) is very rare, and many laboratories omit HSV serology from the 'TORCH' screen, which has become 'TORC'. Secondly, because IgM antibody assays are expensive, many laboratories perform an initial immunoglobulin G (IgG) screen, and proceed to look for specific IgM only if specific IgG is present, showing evidence of past maternal infection. Thirdly, additional tests may be indicated, such as viral culture of urine and/or respiratory secretions if CMV is suspected, which might be neglected if a TORCH request is sent as a knee-jerk response.

Finally, there are a number of organisms, old and new, as well as the TORCH group, that should be considered in many babies with suspected congenital infection. Examples are *Treponema pallidum*, parvovirus B19, enteroviruses and HIV.

TOXOPLASMOSIS

Congenital infection with the protozoan parasite *Toxoplasma gondii*, can result in severe manifestations at birth, but babies are often asymptomatic. However, progressive chorioretinitis, even years later, may develop.

TRANSMISSION

Toxoplasmosis is a zoonosis. The parasite was first identified in 1908 in rabbits and rodents. It is commonly found in cats, dogs, pigs, sheep and cattle. The cat is the definitive host. Other hosts, including humans, catch the organism by accidental ingestion of faeces containing oocysts, or tissue pseudocysts in meat. Desmonts and colleagues showed that 9% of children in a TB hospital in Paris seroconverted to *Toxoplasma* every month when fed undercooked mutton [2]. They also showed that about 1% of young married women in Paris seroconverted each year at the time that they started keeping house and preparing food. Toxoplasmosis has been caused by eating undercooked meat from sheep, cows and pigs, including hamburgers. It also occurs in strict vegetarians, in whom ingestion of cysts from cat, dog or other animal faeces is a likely mode of transmission. Other postulated modes such as milk, eggs, chicken and blood transfusion have not been confirmed.

INCIDENCE

In the UK, congenital toxoplasmosis is diagnosed in approximately 0.2 per 1000 pregnancies, although this is probably an underestimate. Prospective studies in the USA and Europe have shown the incidence of maternal infection in pregnancy to vary from 2 to 12 per 1000 and the incidence of congenital infection, diagnosed by cord blood IgM, from 1 to 7 per 1000 live births. Most women who have an affected baby are asymptomatic in pregnancy, but 10–20% report an episode of lymphadenopathy or a flu-like illness. It is controversial whether maternal toxoplasmosis can cause recurrent abortion.

Congenital infection can be demonstrated serologically, with increasing frequency the later in pregnancy that infection occurs (Figure 17.1). In contrast, the severity of fetal infection is greater the earlier in pregnancy that maternal infection occurs (Figure 17.1). Severe fetal infection will occur in about 6% of first-trimester infections, 2% of second-trimester infections and in no third-trimester infections.

CLINICAL FEATURES

Sabin described a tetrad of clinical features of congenital toxoplasmosis: internal hydrocephalus or microcephaly, chorioretinitis, convulsions or other signs of CNS involvement and intracerebral calcification [3]. Since then, a wide range of other clinical manifestations has been described. Neonates may present early with features of generalized infection or with predominantly neurological manifestations. In generalized infection there may be hydrops fetalis from anaemia; rash due to thrombocytopenic purpura or to the 'blueberry muffin' appearance of dermal erythropoiesis (Figure 17.2) which occurs in 25% of such cases, although in less than 10% of all cases of congenital toxoplasmosis; jaundice, which may appear late; hepatosplenomegaly; lymphadenopathy; and pneumonitis. There may be systemic symptoms such as vomiting, diarrhoea,

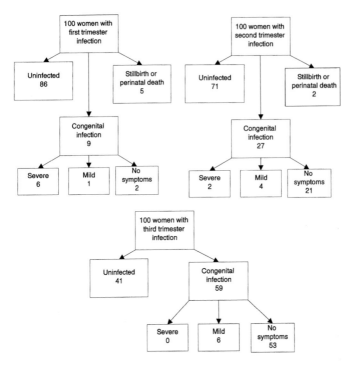

Figure 17.1 Natural history of maternal and fetal infection with *Toxoplasma gondii*. No symptoms = serological infection only. Mild = retinal scars or intracerebral calcification; child neurologically normal. Severe = chorioretinitis and intracerebral calcification or child abnormal

fever or hypothermia and neurological signs and symptoms, as described below.

Sometimes, neurological signs and symptoms are the only clue to neonatal infection. These include convulsions, bulging fontanelle, nystagmus, chorioretinitis (Colour plate 17.1), microphthalmia, cataracts, and microcephaly or hydrocephalus. Alford and co-workers described 'CSF abnormalities' in all eight subclinical cases examined, with 10–110 lymphocytes per mL (which might be considered normal) and protein levels of 1.5–10 g/L (150–1000 mg/100 mL) [4]. Thus,

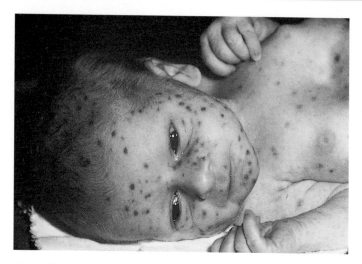

Figure 17.2a

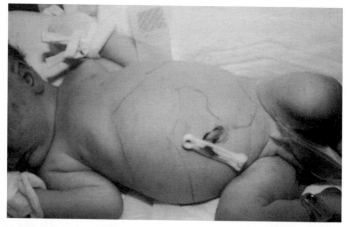

Figure 17.2b

Figure 17.2 Congenital toxoplasmosis: (a) 'blueberry muffin' appearance of dermal erythropoiesis; (b) hepatosplenomegaly

CSF abnormalities, of which raised CSF protein concentration is the commonest, may or may not be present and, if so, are presumably attributable to meningoencephalitis.

Infected babies may be normal at birth, but develop problems, often severe, weeks or months later. These are usually caused by eye involvement (chorioretinitis) presenting as nystagmus, strabismus or blindness (Figure 17.3), but may also be due to CNS involvement (hydrocephalus) causing convulsions, bulging fontanelle or enlarging head circumference, or to generalized infection causing late jaundice, hepatosplenomegaly or lymphadenopathy.

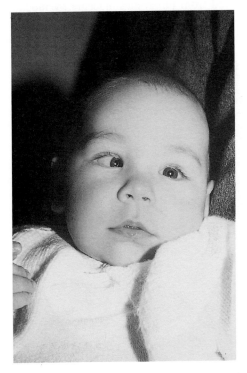

Figure 17.3 Congenital toxoplasmosis: presenting at 4 months of age with strabismus and blindness due to chorioretinitis

Choroidoretinitis may be delayed in onset until school age and ocular lesions may recur in childhood or adolescence. Occasionally, hydrocephalus may occur *de novo* in later childhood due to aqueduct stenosis.

DIAGNOSIS

Diagnosis of baby

The diagnosis of congenital toxoplasmosis is confirmed by detecting specific IgM by immunofluorescence or ELISA in the cord or baby's blood. Detection of specific IgA is also highly suggestive, but IgG is of maternal origin. The organism can also be cultured from blood and placenta by inoculation into mice. Cerebral ultrasonography scan may show hydrocephalus, and this and intracranial calcification may be seen on skull radi-

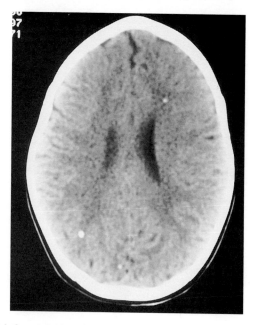

Figure 17.4 Congenital toxoplasmosis: punctate areas of cerebral calcification and mild ventricular dilatation

ographs, but is far better seen by CT scan. Calcification occurs classically as discrete foci (Figure 17.4) but very occasionally may be periventricular, as in congenital CMV infection.

Maternal diagnosis

IgM to *Toxoplasma* can persist for months or even years. Therefore, IgM alone is not a good screening test for recent maternal infection, and its detection suggests maternal toxoplasmosis only if there is a convincing clinical illness or there is a significant rise in IgG (fourfold or greater) or sero-conversion from IgG negative to positive in paired sera. Other helpful tests are serum IgA, serum IgG avidity testing and differential agglutination test [5].

It is not uncommon that positive serology is discovered in the mother or baby almost by mistake, when serum is sent on dubious grounds. The doctor then has to make a difficult decision of whether or not to treat, and has to seek confirmatory evidence, if possible, on which to base this decision (Case history 17.2).

Antenatal diagnosis

If first-trimester maternal toxoplasmosis is confirmed or highly likely, fetal infection can be diagnosed by isolation of *T. gondii* from amniotic fluid or fetal blood or by detection by PCR of *T. gondii* DNA in amniotic fluid taken at about 20 weeks' gestation [6,7].

The French recommend treating women with proven first-trimester infection with spiramycin until antenatal diagnosis can be performed at 20 weeks. Because of the high risk of severe disease, they recommend termination of fetuses proven to have first-trimester infection. For fetal infection after the first trimester they recommend treating the mother with pyri-methamine and sulphadiazine which are thought to be too toxic for first trimester use [5].

Case history 17.1

A baby girl was noted at 2 months of age to have a squint (Figure 17.3). She had been born at term, weighing 3200 g, after a normal pregnancy and labour, and her neonatal examination was normal. The family kept cats. Ophthalmological examination revealed chorioretinitis (Colour plate 17.1). An immediate CT scan of the brain (Figure 17.4) showed punctate calcification and mild ventricular dilatation. Her *Toxoplasma* IgM test was strongly positive. She was treated with alternating courses of spiramycin and with pyrimethamine, sulphadiazine and folinic acid for 1 year. She is partially sighted, but of normal intellect and attends normal school.

Case history 17.2

A baby girl aged 7 days was investigated for jaundice, in retrospect almost certainly due to delayed establishment of breastfeeding. As part of the investigations, a TORCH screen was sent and the baby was found to have serum IgM to *Toxoplasma gondii*. Physical examination was normal, including formal ophthalmological examination. Blood count, liver function test results, skull radiograph and head ultrasonographic scan were normal.

It was the mother's first baby. Mother had a flu-like illness at 12 weeks' gestation, but early sera were not available. Serum taken from the mother at term was *Toxoplasma* IgM negative, but IgG was strongly positive. Repeat serology on the baby showed specific IgA to *Toxoplasma* as well as IgM and IgG. This was believed to be confirmatory evidence of true infection.

After much discussion it was considered that the risk of the child developing later chorioretinitis or brain lesions outweighed the risk of treatment. Spiramycin was unavailable, and she was treated with 12 months of pyrimethamine, sulphadiazine and folinic acid. Development was normal, but at 10 months of age she had an afebrile convulsion and CT scan showed areas of punctate calcification, similar to Figure

17.4. She is now on anticonvulsants and developing normally.

TREATMENT

For babies with congenital toxoplasmosis, the recommended treatment is three or four 21-day courses of pyrimethamine (1 mg/kg orally, once daily) and sulphadiazine (50–100 mg/kg per day, orally 12-hourly), which act synergistically, together with folinic acid 1 mg/kg orally twice a week (to counteract the antifolate effects of pyrimethamine), alternating with 30–45-day courses of the erythromycin-like macrolide antibiotic spiramycin (100 mg/kg per day, orally 12-hourly) over the first year of life (Jacques Couvreur, reported in ref. 2). The rationale is to decrease toxicity, predominantly bone marrow suppression and hepatotoxicity, which should be monitored with regular 1–2-weekly blood tests. Where spiramycin is not available, continuous treatment with pyrimethamine, sulphadiazine and folinic acid can be given, if the above monitoring is maintained. Indeed, McAuley and co-workers reported surprisingly good results using 1 year of pyrimethamine and sulphadiazine plus folinic acid to treat 44 children with congenital toxoplasmosis [8]. Most children did well, despite severe early manifestations of infection. However, three children developed new retinal lesions and three developed new afebrile seizures later in childhood. More controversial are the recommendations that steroids be added for severe infections with evidence of active inflammation, that a single 21-day course of pyrimethamine and sulphadiazine be given for subclinical congenital infection or possible infection, or that spiramycin alone be given to a healthy baby whose mother had a high *Toxoplasma* dye test in pregnancy, but no confirmed infection [2]. There is no controlled evidence for any of these suggestions for treatment of newborn babies and infants.

PREVENTION

As only 10–20% of infected women will have symptoms, any screening programme depends on maternal serology. If infected women are identified, can the babies who are infected be identified antenatally, and is prenatal treatment effective or is termination the only option? It has been suggested that treating infected pregnant women with spiramycin may reduce the incidence and severity of congenital toxoplasmosis [6,7,9,10]. Unfortunately, the studies performed to date have not been adequately controlled, so these claims have not been verified.

About two-thirds of severely affected fetuses have antenatal enlargement of the ventricles detectable by ultrasonography [9]. Antenatal diagnosis is now possible by obtaining fetal blood samples for culture, PCR and IgM. Is screening of pregnant women a realistic proposal?

In France, serological screening to detect and treat women who acquire *Toxoplasma* infection during pregnancy is compulsory and the incidence of congenital toxoplasmosis is apparently falling [6,10]. Desmonts and colleagues studied 278 infected pregnant women: five requested immediate termination despite counselling; of the rest, information was available on 215 pregnancies [9]. All women were treated with spiramycin 3 g daily until the end of pregnancy, and a fetal blood sample was taken at 20–24 weeks' gestation. Nine cases of continuing infection were diagnosed (six with hydrocephalus) and all were terminated. Four mothers requested termination although there was no evidence of continuing infection. Evidence of congenital toxoplasmosis; could be found in only one of 199 babies thought antenatally to be free of infection. In an extension of this study, Daffos *et al.* reported 746 cases of maternal toxoplasmosis; there were 24 therapeutic terminations [6]. Fifteen women with second-trimester infection elected to continue with pregnancy and were given spiramycin 3 g daily until delivery: six babies had mild infection, but all were neurologically normal at follow-up.

It is arguable whether such intensive efforts to prevent congenital toxoplasmosis are justifiable in countries in which the incidence is considerably lower than in France. When the incidence is low, say, 2 per 1000, a screening test with 99% specificity and 100% sensitivity might be expected to identify ten false-positive and two true-positive maternal infections in every 1000 pregnancies. In view of the level of anxiety that this will engender, as shown by requests for immediate termination in Desmont's study, and the risks of fetal blood sampling, the risks of screening may outweigh the benefits, particularly if the incidence is low.

McCabe and Remington called for prospective trials to evaluate maternal serological screening in the USA [11]. They also state that providing information to women on how to avoid infection is the 'simplest, least expensive and ultimately the most efficient and effective means of preventing congenital infection'. Such instructions should be to eat only well-cooked meat, to wash fruit and vegetables before eating, and to wear gloves for gardening and handling cat (or dog) litters, if this is unavoidable. Similarly, Jeannel and co-workers have questioned the validity of the French evidence that treatment of infected pregnant women with spiramycin prevents fetal infection, as no randomized placebo-controlled trial has ever been performed [12]. They argue that the modes of transmission are linked to known living habits, and that health education to prevent maternal toxoplasmosis should be evaluated.

Guerina and co-workers argue that even in a low-risk population, early treatment can avert permanent ophthalmological and central nervous system sequelae [13]. They have used neonatal serological screening to identify subclinically infected babies, rather than maternal screening with its attendant problems.

RUBELLA

In 1941, Sir Norman Gregg, an Australian ophthalmologist, described the association between congenital cataracts and a maternal history of rubella in early pregnancy. He had seen a number of newborns with cataracts, and overheard two mothers discussing how they had both caught German measles in early pregnancy: a classic example of the value of listening to mothers. Children with congenital rubella syndrome are among the most distressing to care for: the combination of deafness and blindness means that it is virtually impossible to communicate with them – the so-called 'locked-in syndrome'. Rubella virus was first isolated in tissue culture in 1962 and this rapidly led to the development of vaccines which can, and should, effectively eliminate congenital rubella syndrome.

EPIDEMIOLOGY

In unimmunized populations, rubella virus circulates readily in young children, particularly those aged 5–9 years. Infection is commonest in the late winter and spring. In unimmunized populations, epidemics occur every 6–9 years, but infections continue to occur at a lower rate in the interval between epidemics.

The attack rate for susceptible adults and children in closed situations, such as military camps or boarding schools, is 90–100%. However, in unimmunized populations, 5–20% of women of child-bearing age are susceptible.

Intrauterine transmission of rubella virus via placental infection occurs in primary maternal rubella. Reinfections with rubella can occur and are usually clinically silent; they occur in 1–3% of the population in natural rubella and at higher rates in immunized populations. Serum IgG concentration rises and IgM sometimes appears. There is brief viral replication and there have been occasional reports of congenital rubella in association with reinfection [14–18]. In most of these cases the original rubella infection was not serologically confirmed, but very occasionally there have been convincing reports of documented reinfections causing congenital infection.

CLINICAL FEATURES

Maternal rubella

Maternal rubella is asymptomatic in about one-third of cases. In adults there is an incubation period of 14–21 days, and a prodromal period of 1–5 days. Prodromal signs and symptoms include fever, headache, sore eyes with conjunctivitis, sore throat, headache and anorexia. Lymphadenopathy, mainly posterior auricular, occipital and cervical, may precede the rash or appear at the same time. The rash, when it occurs, lasts about 3 days, and is fine, pink and maculopapular. It appears first on the face, spreading to the trunk and extremities, and the lesions may coalesce to form a blush. There are many similar rashes caused by other viruses such as parvovirus B19 and enteroviruses, so serological proof of rubella infection should always be sought, by taking acute and convalescent sera. Arthralgia and arthritis may occur before or after the rash. Reinfections are usually asymptomatic [19].

Congenital rubella

Congenital rubella is a chronic infection present from the time of prenatal infection to many months or years after birth. Most congenital infections result from primary maternal infections, but occasional well-documented cases have followed maternal reinfection [19]. The timing of maternal rubella infection is critical, in that infections before 11 weeks almost always cause multiple congenital abnormalities, infections from 11 to 16 weeks may cause deafness, while infections after 17 weeks rarely cause problems [20] (Table 17.1). Almost any organ can be affected in the full congenital rubella syndrome, but some of the commoner manifestations are shown in Table 17.2. The eyes are often cloudy due to corneal opacification (Colour

Timing of maternal rubella in pregnancy (weeks)	Estimated risk of congenital defect (%)	Type of defect
<11	90	Congenital rubella syndrome
11–12	33	Sensorineural deafness
10–14	20	Sensorineural deafness
15–16	10	Sensorineural deafness
17–18	0	–
>18	0	–

Table 17.1 Estimated risk of congenital defect due to maternal rubella occurring at different times in gestation (from [20])

Organ	Defect
Eye	Congenital cataracts
	Cloudy cornea
	Glaucoma
	Choroidoretinitis (salt and pepper)
	Microphthalmia
Ear	Sensorineural deafness
Heart	Pulmonary artery stenosis/hypoplasia
	Persistent ductus arteriosus
CNS	Microcephaly
	Active encephalitis
Growth	Intrauterine growth retardation
Reticuloendothelial	Hepatosplenomegaly
	Lymphadenopathy
Lung	Interstitial pneumonitis
Skin	Thrombocytopenic purpura
Bone	Radiolucencies

Table 17.2 Some of the commoner manifestations of congenital rubella syndrome

plate 17.2) with or without cataracts (Colour plate 17.3). If the retina can be seen there may be 'salt-and-pepper' chorioretinitis (Figure 17.5). The baby may have a purpuric rash due to thrombocytopenia or a 'blueberry muffin' appearance due to dermal erythropoiesis (also sometimes seen in congenital toxoplasmosis, as in Figure 17.2).

The CSF protein level may be high, with or without lymphocyte pleocytosis, suggesting active encephalitis. Cerebral ultrasonography may reveal discrete areas of calcification, previously more classically associated with congenital toxoplasmosis. Pulmonary artery stenosis is the commonest heart lesion, but patent ductus arteriosus is also common, while coarctation of the aorta may occur. The ECG may show an infarct pattern due to necrotic heart lesions. A skeletal survey may reveal bony translucencies. Pneumonitis usually presents postnatally with tachypnoea. Renal abnormalities (polycystic kidney, double ureter, hydronephrosis, renal artery stenosis) may very occasionally occur and babies with proven congeni-

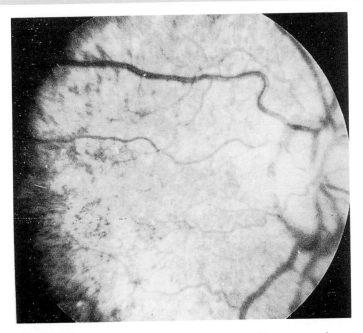

Figure 17.5 Congenital rubella syndrome: 'pepper and salt' appearance of chorioretinitis

tal rubella should have an abdominal ultrasonographic scan. Severely affected babies may die from hepatitis, pneumonitis, cardiac lesions or prematurity.

PROGNOSIS

Babies apparently normal at birth, but with confirmed congenital infection following first- or second-trimester rubella, should be followed closely. Sensorineural deafness may occur in the absence of other clinical features and hearing should be tested regularly, because deafness may be progressive. Hearing loss is easily the commonest manifestation of congenital rubella infection. Other rarer long-term problems from congenital rubella syndrome include a subacute encephalitis resembling subacute sclerosing panencephalitis and usually occurring at 8–14 years, in which CSF and serum levels of antibodies to rubella are raised. Endocrine problems may emerge, including diabetes mellitus, precocious puberty, hyper- and hypothyroidism and growth hormone deficiency. There may be visual deterioration from progressive neovascularization of the retina in babies with choroidoretinitis. Late problems in long-term survivors with congenital rubella syndrome include diabetes mellitus and immune deficiency [21,22].

DIAGNOSIS

Primary maternal infection is ideally diagnosed by showing seroconversion or a rising titre of IgG antibodies to rubella as measured by haemagglutination inhibition, single radial haemolysis, ELISA or radioimmunoassay. If IgG antibodies are detected within 10 days of contact, the woman is immune, but if no antibodies are detected, a second sample should be obtained 2 weeks later. If a woman presents some time after a contact and her previous rubella status is unknown, rubella infection can be diagnosed by looking for IgM antibodies, which appear 5–10 days after the rash and persist for 50–70 days. Antenatal diagnosis by measurement of specific IgM in fetal blood samples is possible in some centres [23], but is insensitive. PCR has been used on amniotic fluid, but its role needs defining. Reinfections are difficult to prove, but can be diagnosed by showing a fourfold rise in IgG titre and/or the appearance of specific IgM in a woman previously shown to have high-titre IgG antibody [19,24]. The risk of congenital rubella syndrome in confirmed maternal reinfection, even first trimester, has been estimated to be below 5% [25], although at least 11 cases have been described [24].

In congenital rubella, the diagnosis can be made by detecting specific IgM in serum or cord blood, or alternatively by culturing rubella virus. The best specimens for virus isolation are nasopharyngeal aspirates, eye swabs, urine, faeces and CSF. Virus may persist in the eye and CSF for a year or more. Babies are infectious and should be isolated from pregnant women.

PREVENTION

In countries such as the USA and Canada, where rubella vaccine (alone or in the form of measles, mumps and rubella (MMR) vaccine) has been given for many years to all children at about 12–15 months, congenital rubella syndrome has virtually disappeared. In the United States, only two cases were reported in 1984 and again in 1985 [26]. This approach to prevention depends on uptake of the vaccine being adequate to prevent exposure of unimmunized non-immune women to the virus. In the USA, where rubella vaccines have been used in this way since 1969, most cases of rubella now occur in adults. It is recommended that non-pregnant susceptible women of child-bearing age also be immunized. The need for this recommendation was illustrated by an increase in the number of cases of congenital rubella syndrome in the USA in the early 1990s. These babies were born to migrant mothers who had never been immunized against rubella.

In the UK and Australia, a different strategy was initially adopted: selective immunization of schoolgirls aged 13–14 years and of non-immune primigravid women after delivery. As rubella virus could then circulate in schoolchildren, this approach depended on an extremely high uptake in schoolgirls. In practice, approximately 2 per 1000 pregnancies in the UK were affected, even in non-epidemic years, resulting in up to 800 terminations of pregnancy and about 80 cases of congenital rubella infection each year. Despite universal antenatal screening of rubella serology, an unacceptably high proportion of cases occurred in second or subsequent pregnancies because, for various reasons, non-immune primigravidas had not been immunized [27]. Since 1988, MMR vaccine has been given to British children at 12 months old, but selective immunization against rubella will also continue indefinitely. The same approach has been adopted in Australia, but, as in the USA, a booster dose of MMR is given later in childhood (either at school entry or at 10–12 years).

There is a small, but definite, risk of congenital rubella syndrome following maternal reinfection, and any woman, even if immune, in contact with rubella in the first 16 weeks of pregnancy should be screened for IgM and rising levels of IgG antibodies to rubella, with acute and convalescent sera.

A large number of terminations of pregnancy are performed each year for inadvertent immunization with rubella vaccine during pregnancy. The vaccine viruses used are live, but attenuated. The situation is not entirely clear because of changes in vaccine strains: in the USA the Cendehill and HPV-77 strains have been completely replaced by RA 27/3 vaccine. There is evidence that the vaccine virus can cross the placenta and infect the fetus in up to 20% of cases, when products of conception have been cultured [28,29]. The vaccine virus has been isolated from the kidney of an abortus [30] and, most worryingly, from the eye of an aborted fetus which had lens abnormalities suggestive of congenital rubella [31]. It is not advisable for women to become pregnant for 3 months after rubella immunization, because virus has been cultured from an abortus when vaccine was given 7 weeks before pregnancy. On the other hand, 364 pregnant women accidentally immunized with rubella vaccine, of whom 112 were known to be non-immune, elected to proceed to term and there were no detectable malformations [29]. There has never been a baby described who was born with vaccine-induced congenital rubella syndrome. The risk that vaccine-associated congenital infection might ever occur appears to be extremely small, almost certainly less than 3%, and pregnant women who are accidentally given the vaccine should be counselled accordingly.

CYTOMEGALOVIRUS

Cytomegalovirus (CMV) is the commonest cause of congenital infection in developed countries, affecting up to 1–2% of all babies, and an important cause of mental retardation and deafness worldwide. Most babies have no symptoms, but congenital CMV infection can at times be devastating. Unlike rubella virus, CMV causes deformation of preformed tissues rather than malformation of developing organs, so CMV can affect fetuses beyond the first trimester, although earlier infection is usually more severe [32]. Primary maternal infection is most likely to cause severe congenital infection, but reactivation may also do so [33]. Postnatal CMV infection may also cause significant problems in preterm neonates and is dealt with here.

THE ORGANISM

CMV is a herpesvirus and has the potential, like the other herpesviruses, to cause persistent infection and to reactivate. It is the largest of the herpesviruses and is an enveloped DNA virus. CMV infection of cells results in large intranuclear inclusions and occasional intracytoplasmic inclusions in enlarged cells (hence the old name, cytomegalic inclusion disease).

TRANSMISSION

CMV can be found in cervical secretions, semen and saliva, and may be transmitted between adults by sexual activity or kissing. In developing countries, most women of child-bearing age have already been infected in childhood, when transmission is probably by respiratory spread of droplets or secretions. The virus can cross the placenta, either during a primary maternal infection or during reactivation, and infect the fetus prenatally. It may also be acquired at delivery from cervical secretions, or postnatally from breast milk [34] or infected blood transfusion [35]. Postnatal infection can be devastating in preterm babies [35], but in term babies, although symptoms (rash, pneumonitis, hepatosplenomegaly, lymphadenopathy) develop in up to one-third [36], it is rarely life-threatening or damaging. In contrast, prenatal infection can have major long-term sequelae.

EPIDEMIOLOGY

Congenital CMV infection, as determined by screening all babies by urine culture and/or cord blood IgM, occurs in around 3 per 1000 live births in Britain [37] and Sweden [38], but in 5 to 25 per 1000 live births in the USA [39,40].

However, only 5–10% of infected infants are symptomatic at birth [41].

The proportion of women of child-bearing age who are seropositive to CMV varies in different populations. In Britain and the USA, about 50% of pregnant women are seropositive, but 80% of girls of low socio-economic status in Alabama were seropositive by puberty [40]. In Japan 65% are seropositive by age 13 [42], while in Africa more than 90% have been infected by puberty [43].

About 1% of non-immune women develop primary CMV infection during pregnancy and around one-half of their babies are infected [37,44–46].

Women who are seropositive at the start of pregnancy may reactivate. About 5% of pregnant women excrete CMV in the urine and CMV may be isolated from the cervix in up to 28% of pregnancies. Serological studies are unhelpful in diagnosing the rate of reactivation, because this may occur at any time during pregnancy, and cultures of urine or cervical secretions suffer from the problem of intermittent excretion of CMV. In Figure 17.6, in which an estimate is made of the relative importance of primary and secondary infections, the rate of reactivation has been given as 10%, which is an approximation. About one-half of the babies will be infected perinatally, from cervical secretions or breast milk, while around 5% will develop intrauterine infections.

Congenital CMV infection can result from primary maternal CMV during pregnancy or from recurrence. The relative importance of these two modes of transmission varies according to the rate of seropositivity of women of child-bearing age. Of 2698 pregnant women of middle or high income, 16 babies (0.6%) had congenital CMV infection, eight due to primary infections and eight due to recurrences, whereas of 1014 women of low income, 16 babies (1.6%) had congenital CMV, but only three were due to primary infections and 13 to recurrences [46]. Primary maternal infection is more likely to lead to severe congenital CMV than reactivation: 25% of babies born to mothers with primary CMV in pregnancy had sequelae,

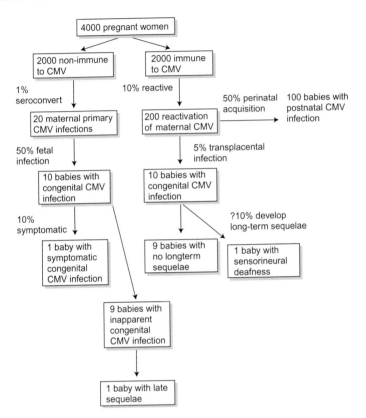

Figure 17.6 Theoretical scheme of outcome of CMV infection in pregnancy. This assumes a country where 50% of women of child-bearing age are immune to CMV and the rate of congenital infection is 5 per 1000 live births

compared to 8% of babies whose mothers had reactivated CMV [33].

It was originally thought that congenital CMV infection with severe sequelae, like congenital infections with toxoplasma and rubella, was likely to follow primary maternal CMV only in the first trimester. Although it is clear that this is the major risk period [32], there is growing evidence that severe sequelae may result from primary infections in the second and third trimesters and from recurrent infections. Stagno and colleagues reported severe handicaps in five of 23 babies with congenital CMV resulting from primary maternal CMV occurring at up to 27 weeks' gestation, whereas the one abnormal baby out of 12 with congenital CMV from late primary infection (28–40 weeks) had only hypoplastic dental enamel [47]. Other studies, however, have shown that at least some babies will have severe sequelae from primary maternal infection occurring in late pregnancy [41,45,48,49].

Although serious handicap is more likely in congenital CMV resulting from primary maternal infection [46,48], such handicap sometimes follows recurrent infection, and these babies [33] may rarely be born symptomatic [41,48,50]. Symptomatic congenital CMV infection may even occur in consecutive pregnancies [51].

The interpretation of follow-up studies of babies with congenital CMV infection is complicated by the finding that most babies are born to young, disadvantaged mothers [46,52].

CLINICAL FEATURES

Only 5–10% of babies with congenital CMV infection are symptomatic at birth. Those with 'cytomegalic inclusion disease' (Colour plate 17.4) typically have a purpuric rash due to thrombocytopenia (usually with pinpoint petechiae), hepatosplenomegaly, jaundice, microcephaly, chorioretinitis and intracerebral calcification. Jaundice may appear within 24 hours of birth and require exchange transfusion, or appear at 2–5 days. The chorioretinitis of CMV resembles that of toxoplasmosis (Colour plate 17.1). Cataracts and microphthalmia are very rare in congenital CMV. Cerebral calcification is classically periventricular, and is found in the subependymal region (Figure 17.7). This appearance may rarely be seen in congenital toxoplasmosis. If the calcification is widespread, it may cause obstructive hydrocephalus.

Pneumonitis may develop as a late manifestation of congenital CMV infection, usually occurring at 1–4 months of age. Preece and colleagues described 6 of 50 children with congenital CMV infection who developed an afebrile pneumonitis at this age, characterized by tachypnoea and hyperinflation [52]. Two children also developed transient hepatosplenomegaly.

Deafness may be present from birth, usually in children who have other manifestations of disease, or may develop as a late sequel which can appear in the first 5 years of life. About 6% of babies with congenital CMV become deaf, making it one of the most important causes of hearing loss in children [41,53–56]. Hearing loss apparently results from viral replication in the inner ear [57].

Yeager and colleagues took viral cultures from 51 preterm babies who were in a neonatal intensive care unit for over 28 days: 16 of the 51 infants began excreting the virus at 1–4 months of age (mean 55 days) and 14 of the 16 babies

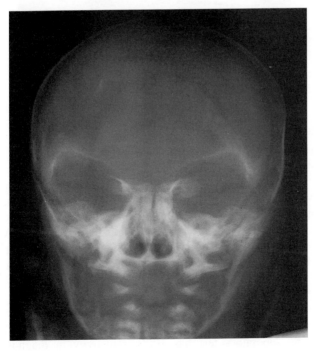

Figure 17.7a

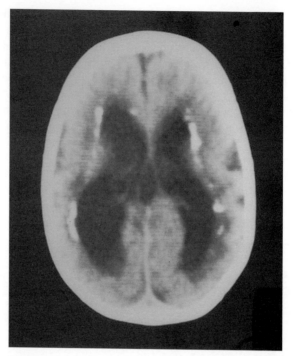

Figure 17.7b

Figure 17.7 Congenital CMV infection: periventricular calcification and ventricular dilatation shown (a) on skull radiograph; (b) on CT scan of brain

developed respiratory deterioration with added pulmonary shadowing, grey pallor, hepatosplenomegaly and atypical lymphocytosis [58]. These 16 babies had apparently acquired CMV infections from blood transfusions. Such infections can be fatal, and are particularly severe in babies of seronegative mothers.

DIAGNOSIS

The best test for congenital CMV infection remains viral culture of urine in the first week after birth.

No laboratory test has 100% sensitivity in diagnosing congenital CMV infection. The newer methods of detecting specific IgM, such as radioimmunoassays and ELISAs, have, however, greatly increased the sensitivity of testing cord or baby's blood. If urine, throat swab or nasopharyngeal aspirate are positive for CMV by culture in the first week of life, this indicates congenital infection. After 1 week of age, the significance of positive cultures and of CMV IgM detection is less clear, as infection may have been acquired postnatally and virus shedding may continue for months.

OUTCOME

It has already been implied that appropriate controls must be included in follow-up studies of babies with congenital CMV infection, because the babies often have a disadvantageous social background. Well-controlled studies now suggest that about 10% of babies with congenital CMV identified by screening at birth will have major neurodevelopmental sequelae. The risk is highest in babies who are symptomatic at birth, but sequelae may occur in babies with inapparent infection. Mental retardation, spastic quadriplegia and deafness are the main problems, but visual impairment may result from chorioretinitis or optic atrophy.

Chorioretinitis, which occurs in 10–15% of symptomatic babies, almost always indicates significant mental impairment. Microcephaly occurs in about 50%, but does not always persist, and does not always result in later handicap. The presence of intracranial calcification or raised CSF protein concentration increases the chance of later mental handicap. The mortality rate associated with symptomatic congenital CMV is about 30% [59].

All babies with congenital CMV infection should be followed until at least school entry, and hearing tests performed regularly to detect late deafness.

TREATMENT

There are now two drugs available with confirmed efficacy against CMV, namely ganciclovir and foscarnet. Neither of these drugs has been evaluated by controlled trial in babies.

Nigro and colleagues reported no effect when six babies were treated with ganciclovir 5 mg/kg per dose twice daily for 2 weeks, but a possible response in six babies given 7.5 mg/kg twice daily for 10 weeks, then 10 mg/kg per dose three times per week for 3 months [60]. On these data, it would be hard to justify the use of ganciclovir, except perhaps in babies with life-threatening CMV pneumonitis or hepatitis, since most damage has been done by birth, and CMV infection cannot be eradicated, only suppressed.

PREVENTION

Screening of pregnant women could not prevent all or even most congenital CMV infections, as cases occur in all trimesters and with recurrences as well as primary infections. Furthermore, the risk to an infected fetus is fairly low, so even if prenatal fetal infection could be reliably diagnosed, many terminations would be of healthy fetuses. It is hard to justify screening pregnant women, even those such as daycare workers at increased risk, with serological tests for CMV (see also 'Staff and CMV' below).

At present there is little prospect of a successful vaccine. Although live, attenuated CMV vaccines have been used in renal transplant patients, the vaccine strain may be able to remain latent and could be oncogenic. Genetically engineered vaccines using viral proteins, but no viral DNA, are a possibility, but it is not known which proteins will induce protective antibody and cell-mediated immune responses.

Yeager and colleagues showed that blood transfusion-acquired CMV infection could be prevented by using only blood from a panel of regularly tested donors who were known to be seronegative to CMV [58]. An alternative approach is to use blood which has been filtered to remove leucocytes, because virus is mainly cell associated, and this approach reduced acquired CMV infection from 21% to zero in one study of neonates [61].

STAFF AND CMV

There are conflicting data on whether female nursing staff working with babies are at increased risk of CMV infection, although the weight of evidence suggests that they are probably at moderately increased risk of primary infection. This is of obvious concern, as many such staff are of child-bearing age. Ahlfors and colleagues found that Swedish nurses were not at increased risk for primary CMV or for having a baby with congenital infection [62]. Dworsky and co-workers similarly found no added risk for health care professionals in Alabama [63]. In contrast, in a small study, Yeager found an annual serconversion rate of 4.1% for Denver neonatal intensive care nurses and 7.7% for general paediatric nurses, but none of 27 staff without patient contact seroconverted [64]. Haneberg and colleagues found that 9.4% of student nurses in Norway serconverted after a 2-month paediatric rotation [65]. Friedman and colleagues in Philadelphia found that 10.9% of intensive care nurses, 18.2% of the venesection/intravenous team, 3.7% of the medical and surgical ward nurses and 2.9% of staff without patient contact seroconverted to CMV in a year [66].

Haldane and colleagues collected data by questionnaire and found a higher rate of congenital anomalies in babies of nurses working with infants than in those working with older patients or off work [67]. However, Ahlfors and co-workers could find no such increased risk [62].

Should female nursing, medical and paramedical staff be screened for CMV antibody status? The objection to this is the same as that to screening all pregnant women: it is difficult to know what advice could usefully be given to seronegative pregnant women, or what course of action to take, should such a woman seroconvert during pregnancy. A Manchester special care baby unit, which adopted a policy of screening staff and advising that seronegative pregnant women should not care for babies with known or suspected CMV infection, abandoned the policy after 18 months. They considered that it was a disaster, having served little useful purpose and generated all sorts of public relation, psychological and management problems [68].

One of the prerequisites of a screening programme is that there should be a clearly accepted course of action for managing those at risk, and screening staff for CMV antibody status does not fulfil these criteria.

TUBERCULOSIS

Virtually all cases of neonatal tuberculosis (TB) result from TB of the mother, although occasionally the baby may be infected by a household contact or even by a member of staff with open TB. The mother most commonly has active pulmonary TB, often asymptomatic, and infects the baby postnatally by the respiratory route. Alternatively, she may have uterine TB which can be due to adjacent spread, such as from tuberculous peritonitis, or due to blood-borne spread to the fallopian tubes; the baby may then aspirate tubercle bacilli *in utero* or at the time of delivery. If the mother is infected during pregnancy, the placenta may be infected, with resultant infection of the amniotic fluid, and the fetus may be infected by transplacental blood-borne spread or by aspiration of contaminated amniotic fluid.

Congenital TB due to early intrauterine infection is very rare and usually results in abortion or stillbirth. Transplacental fetal infection through the portal vein can cause a primary complex in the liver and infection of the portal nodes, leading to hepatomegaly usually accompanied by jaundice, lymphadenopathy, splenomegaly and meningitis. Chorioretinitis may be found on ophthalmological examination [69] and the baby with congenital TB may be thought to have a different congenital infection. Most affected babies, however, are normal at birth, though may be of low birthweight. The mother may have fever before, at or soon after delivery. The baby may fail to thrive and by 3 weeks of age be listless, irritable and anorexic. Very occasionally, however, the baby is well, but has changes visible radiographically (see Figure 17.8). There may be patchy pneumonic changes on the chest radiograph, which progress to mediastinal and hilar lymph node enlargement, with segmental or lobar collapse due to the extrinsic pressure

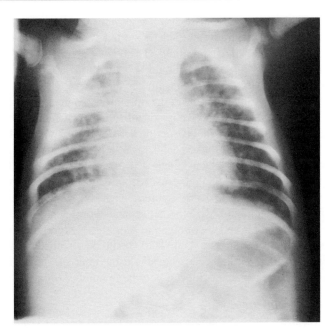

Figure 17.8 Neonatal tuberculosis (see Case history 17.3). Right upper lobe consolidation plus nodular lesions

of the nodes. The baby develops respiratory symptoms with tachypnoea and cyanosis, often intermittent. Acid-fast bacilli are best seen in the gastric aspirate, but may also be found in tracheal aspirates or urine; however, the sensitivity of these tests is less than 10%. Liver ultrasonography and biopsy are helpful if the primary lesion is in the liver. The tuberculin response is unreliable. The mother should be examined and a chest radiograph, tuberculin skin test and other relevant investigations performed if neonatal TB is suspected. The diagnosis of congenital TB will be made only if it is appreciated that the mother comes from a population at high risk of TB.

As it is difficult to prove that the baby has TB, treatment often has to be started empirically, especially when maternal TB has been diagnosed. All the antituberculous drugs are potentially toxic, but neonatal tuberculosis can be devastating and meningeal involvement has a high morbidity. In symptomatic infants, treatment should be started with isoniazid (10 mg/kg per day) and rifampicin (15 mg/kg per day). Pyrazinamide (20 mg/kg per day) should be added for miliary TB or tuberculous meningitis. If the mother has active TB, but the baby is asymptomatic at birth, the options are to give the baby BCG vaccine [70], or to give isoniazid-resistant BCG and treat the baby with isoniazid (10 mg/kg per day) prophylactically [71]; both approaches have been shown to be successful. If the mother has only just been diagnosed, the 'Red Book' of the American Academy of Pediatrics recommends separating her from the baby until she is sputum negative, which occurs rapidly on treatment [72]. Whether separated or not, she should be treated for TB and encouraged to breastfeed, expressing her milk if necessary. Neonatal unit staff should be screened for TB when starting work, because a single member of staff with open TB can expose or infect a very large number of babies.

Case history 17.3

A 3-week-old baby boy was referred by the chest physicians because they had just diagnosed his mother as having sputum-positive pulmonary tuberculosis. The baby had been feeding slightly less well for 2 days, but had good weight gain. He had a staccato cough, but was not tachypnoeic or dyspnoeic, and was afebrile. The remainder of the physical examination was normal. A chest radiograph (Figure 17.8) showed large nodular lesions and right upper lobe consolidation. A Mantoux test was negative, and CSF was normal. A gastric aspirate smear contained acid-fast bacilli, positive for *M. tuberculosis* by PCR, and later grew *M. tuberculosis*. He was treated with rifampicin and isoniazid for 9 months. Mother and baby made complete recoveries.

MOTHER BEING TREATED FOR TUBERCULOSIS

Once a mother has received antituberculous therapy for more than 5 days, she is no longer infectious. If the mother had TB diagnosed and treatment was started before getting pregnant or in the first or second trimester, and the immediate household has been screened, there is no immediate risk to her newborn baby. The American Red Book recommendations are for chest radiography and tuberculin skin testing of the baby at 3–4 months and 6 months [72]. The baby is given isoniazid regardless of the results, since tuberculin reactivity may be delayed. Isoniazid is stopped at 3–4 months if the tests are negative and compliance is good.

There is an antipathy to BCG vaccine in the USA which is hard to fathom. An alternative approach to the above 'wait-and-see' policy is to give neonatal BCG vaccine and to follow the baby clinically and with chest radiographs at, say, 6 and 12 months [70,73]. BCG vaccine gives about 50% protection against any disease and 70% protection against fatal tuberculosis and TB meningitis [74], and the argument that skin testing becomes useless after BCG is not correct: the threshold for positivity just becomes higher.

A minimal amount of antituberculous drugs crosses into breast milk, and breastfeeding by mothers on antituberculous therapy should be encouraged.

SYPHILIS

Untreated latent maternal infection with *Treponema pallidum* in the first 2 years after infection causes fetal or perinatal death in 20% of pregnancies, preterm delivery in 20% and, if pregnancy goes to term, congenital syphilis with resulting handicap in approximately 40% [75]. In most industrialized countries, syphilis serology is included in routine antenatal care; congenital syphilis is seen only, therefore, in the babies of women who do not attend for antenatal care, women who are inadequately treated or those who become reinfected during pregnancy. In many developing countries, congenital syphilis is still one of the commonest and most serious congenital infections. There is evidence of a rising incidence of syphilis amongst disadvantaged groups in the USA and Australia [5].

The mother may often be in the asymptomatic latent stage of syphilis. Infection of the placenta and transplacental spread to the fetus can cause miscarriage, abortion, fetal death, hydrops fetalis, preterm labour and intrauterine growth retardation. The placenta is often enlarged. Babies may be asymptomatic at birth and develop symptoms only later, or may have a wide range of manifestations including fulminant sepsis. The characteristic skin lesion is a maculopapular eruption over the buttocks, back, thighs, soles, palms and perioral area. It is pink, becoming brown, and there may be indurative erythema or desquamation of the soles and palms. Bright red palms and soles can be a useful clinical indicator of congenital syphilis. Sometimes the lesions are bullous (pemphigus syphiliticus) and mimic impetigo, and the desquamation is thought wrongly to be staphylococcal scalded-skin syndrome. There should not be confusion with the vesicular lesions of herpes simplex virus infection. The skin on the trunk is often dry and flakes off when rubbed. Rhinitis ('snuffles') develops at between 1 week and 3 months of age and is initially clear, becoming more purulent or even blood-stained. Ulceration of the nasal mucosa can lead to a 'saddle nose' deformity. Laryngitis may cause a hoarse or aphonic cry. Mucous patches may be seen on the lips, tongue and soft palate. Hepatosplenomegaly is present in up to 90%, and about one-half also have generalized lymphadenopathy. Haemolytic anaemia and thrombocytopenia are common and there may be jaundice with unconjugated and/or conjugated hyperbilirubinaemia. Osteitis of the long bones is usually asymptomatic at birth, although later pain or a pathological fracture may cause pseudoparalysis of a limb (pseudoparalysis of Parrot). Neurological and renal manifestations are rare at birth, although severely affected babies may have signs of meningitis and eye involvement (chorioretinitis, glaucoma, uveitis, chancres of the eyelid). Babies may present at a few weeks of age with pancytopenia, hepatosplenomegaly and oedema, and may be misdiagnosed as having malignancy. Untreated babies are at risk of late manifestations of syphilis: keratitis, deafness, teeth abnormalities and scarring as a result of earlier lesions.

DIAGNOSIS

The most common problem in developed countries is the interpretation of tests in pregnancy before and after treatment, and the management of an asymptomatic seropositive baby. The various tests employed to diagnose syphilis are shown in Table 17.3. Non-treponemal tests (VDRL or RPR) are used to screen women for syphilis and specific treponemal tests are used to confirm (FTA-ABS, TPHA or FIA). If the VDRL/RPR titre is high, it suggests active infection, whereas a low titre suggests successful past treatment or a false positive. Some laboratories use TPHA to screen women for syphilis. A positive TPHA indicates either current or past syphilis, and a VDRL or RPR titre needs to be done to determine which of these is the case.

Type of test	Name of test/Description	Abbreviation
Non-specific screening tests (detect antibodies to cardiolipin)	Venereal Disease Research Laboratory	VDRL
	Wassermann reaction	WR
	Rapid plasma reagin	RPR
	Reagin screen test	RST
Specific antibody tests (detect antibody to *T. pallidum*)	Fluorescent treponemal antibody absorption (absorbed with non-pallidum treponemes)	FTA-ABS
	Fluorescent treponemal antibody absorption double staining	FTA-ABS DS
	Microhaemagglutination assay for *T. pallidum* antibody	MHA-TP
	Haemagglutinating antibody	TPHA (or HATTS)
	Radioimmunoassay	RIA
	Enzyme-linked immunosorbent assay	ELISA
Direct examination of lesion or tissue	Dark-field microscopy	
	Direct fluorescent antibody test for *T. pallidum*	DFA-TP
	Silver stains	
	Haematoxylin and eosin	H & E stains

Table 17.3 Tests for syphilis

Serological testing of the newborn is also problematic. The serum IgM, measured by ELISA, was positive in 88% of babies with congenital syphilis [76] and is the single most useful test, although false negatives occur. The FTA-ABS 19S IgM test is less sensitive at 73% [76]. The other antibody tests described detect IgG antibody which is transplacentally acquired maternal antibody, and reflects maternal infection.

Pregnant women who are seropositive for syphilis, i.e. have positive specific antibody tests, should be treated with penicillin. Even if they give a history of supposed penicillin allergy, skin tests should be performed to confirm or refute this and desensitization performed if positive; penicillin is the only acceptable therapy for syphilis during pregnancy [77]. Maternal erythromycin treatment results in many failures and many cases of congenital syphilis due to poor transplacental passage.

Diagnostic evaluation of the newborn baby of an affected woman (Figure 17.9) should always include a full physical examination and serology on a serum specimen (not cord blood, which may give false-positive reactions). Radiological examination of the long bones for osteitis and CSF examination should be performed for all babies of women not treated before 20 weeks' gestation, for all asymptomatic babies and probably for all babies with a positive Venereal Disease Research Laboratory (VDRL) or RPR test. The CSF of babies with neurosyphilis may have a raised white cell count and protein concentration. A positive CSF VDRL test is diagnostic of neurosyphilis, even if the white cell count and protein level are normal. PCR for *T. pallidum* DNA has been developed, and appears to be a useful test on CSF, with a similar sensitivity to CSF VDRL of about 70% [78]. Babies with negative CSF VDRL or PCR tests, but CSF abnormalities of cells or protein, should be treated for neurosyphilis. Fluorescent treponemal antibody (FTA) tests on CSF have given conflicting results in adults and have not been adequately studied in congenital syphilis. Other tests in the evaluation would include full blood count, liver function tests and urinalysis.

Congenital syphilis is confirmed if *T. pallidum* is identified by direct examination of specimens from lesions, placenta or umbilical cord. Congenital infection is likely if the baby has a positive specific antibody test and is symptomatic or was stillborn, if the baby has a positive CSF VDRL test, if the mother was inadequately treated or if the baby has a fourfold increase in antibody levels over 3 months' follow-up; congenital infection is unlikely if the baby has negative specific serology, if positive tests become negative by 6 months or if the mother was effectively treated (titre fell fourfold or more) and the baby's titre is at least four times lower than the mother's [77]. A working definition is given in Table 17.4.

Treatment of definite or probable congenital syphilis should be with i.v. or i.m. aqueous crystalline penicillin G (50 000 units/kg per day 12-hourly) or with i.m. aqueous procaine penicillin G (50 000 units/kg once daily), given for at least 10 days. Babies in the 'unlikely' category, as defined in the previous paragraph, need not be treated if close follow-up

Confirmed case	*T. pallidum* identified by dark ground microscopy, direct fluorescent antibody or other specific stain in lesions, placenta, umbilical cord or other tissues
Presumptive case	(A) Mother has untreated or inadequately treated (i.e. no penicillin or penicillin given less than 30 days before delivery) syphilis at delivery (B) Infant has positive specific treponemal antibody test and one or more of: (i) clinical evidence of congenital syphilis; (ii) periostitis of long bones; (iii) reactive CSF VDRL/RPR; (iv) CSF pleocytosis or raised CSF protein without other explanation; (v) reactive test for FTA-ABS 19S IgM antibody
From ref. [82].	

Table 17.4 Case definition for congenital syphilis

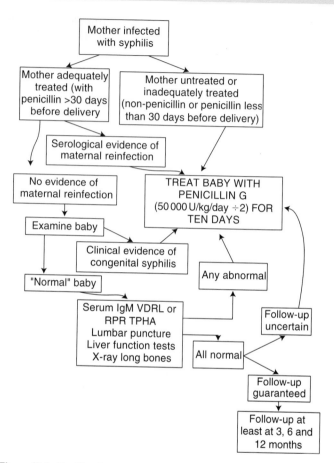

Figure 17.9 Algorithm for management of a baby born to a mother with syphilis

is certain; if follow-up is not certain, they should be treated as if 'definite' since infection cannot be excluded. This treatment is effective against neurosyphilis. There is no proven alternative antibiotic to penicillin.

Close follow-up of treated and untreated babies, at 3, 6 and 12 months at least, is essential, and serological tests should be repeated until they become negative. Persistently raised titres over several months are an indication for retreatment. Patients with neurosyphilis should also have serum and CSF serology repeated every 6 months for at least 3 years. Retreatment should be considered if clinical signs persist or recur, if there is a persistent fourfold rise in a non-specific antibody test, or if a high titre fails to decrease fourfold within 1 year [77].

WHICH SEROPOSITIVE BABIES SHOULD BE TREATED?

A flowchart for deciding which babies to treat is shown in Figure 17.9. In clinical practice, it may be extremely difficult to guarantee follow-up of babies born to women with syphilis, who are often from disadvantaged backgrounds. If there is any doubt about the completeness of follow-up, or the diagnosis is uncertain, it seems wise to treat the baby with parenteral penicillin G for a full 10 days. This pragmatic, but realistic, approach could be criticized as overtreating a number of normal babies, but we believe that the devastating effects of untreated congenital syphilis justify such pragmatism.

Case history 17.4

A 1-day-old baby boy was referred with suspected congenital herpes simplex virus infection. Mother was 21, single and had received no antenatal care. She reported no problems in pregnancy. The baby weighed 2080 g at birth at full term. He had desquamation over the trunk and limbs, and the skin peeled with pressure. Bullae containing mucopurulent fluid were present over the arms, ankles, wrists and abdomen (Colour plate 17.5a). The palms and soles were bright red and indurated (Colour plate 17.5b). The baby had hepatosplenomegaly. The VDRL test was positive on mother's and baby's serum. The baby's CSF contained 30 lymphocytes and was VDRL, TPHA and FTA positive, with specific IgM to *T. pallidum* detected. Radiographs of the long bones showed periostitis (Figure 17.10). The baby was successfully treated for neurosyphilis and the mother for syphilis. No contacts could be traced.

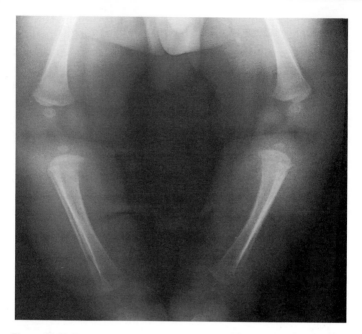

Figure 17.10 Periosteal elevation of femora plus bilateral erosions of medial tibial epiphyses (Wimberger's sign)

CONGENITAL MALARIA

Congenital malaria is rare in industrialized countries, with about one case per year reported in the United States since 1950 [79], while it occurs in the offspring of up to 3 per 1000 immune and 7.4% of non-immune mothers with mainly falciparum malaria in non-industrialized countries [80].

The clinical features can mimic other congenital infections, with hepatosplenomegaly, jaundice and anaemia as prominent features, but the presence of fever is almost invariable in congenital malaria (see Table 17.5). Babies with congenital malaria tend to present late, with a mean age of presentation of $5^1/_2$ weeks in 46 babies in Hulbert's series, of whom 96% developed signs or symptoms between 2 and 8 weeks after birth [79]. It is thought that fetal haemoglobin may provide some protection against infection. However, the symptoms of congenital malaria may occasionally be present in the first week of life or be delayed (as with congenital syphilis) until as late as 60 weeks of age.

Haematological features of congenital malaria include anaemia (in Hulbert's series, the mean Hb concentration was 8 g/dL, with a range from 4 to 16.5), normal or low neutrophil count, and thrombocytopenia (mean 72, range 27–257, 90% below 100).

Most cases of congenital malaria in an industrialized country occur in recent immigrants, although occasionally the mother has been away from a malarious area for up to 5–7 years. Transmission probably occurs around the time of delivery rather than transplacentally. A history of maternal fever at any time in pregnancy is obtained in only about 70% of mothers, and by the time the baby presents only about half the mothers have blood smears positive for malaria [79]. In non-industrialized countries, malaria may be acquired by blood transfusion.

Hulbert described that over 80% of cases were caused by *Plasmodium vivax*, but all species were represented and one baby had dual infection [79]. However, in a series of over 100 babies with congenital malaria reported in 1950, mostly from

Clinical feature	Proportion of affected babies with feature
Fever	100%
Splenomegaly	93%
Hepatomegaly	84%
Jaundice	79%
Anaemia	84%
Irritability	85%
Anorexia	>50%
Lethargy	>50%
From ref. [79].	

Table 17.5 Clinical features of congenital malaria

malarial areas, 64% were due to *P. falciparum* and 32% to *P. vivax* [81].

Diagnosis of congenital malaria is by microscopy of thick and thin blood films, and treatment is with antimalarials appropriate to the parasite identified and appropriate supportive therapy as necessary, such as blood transfusion.

References

1 Garland S, Gilbert GL, Ferson M *et al.* Investigation of congenital infection: the TORCH screen is not a legitimate test. *Med J Aust* 1993; **159**: 346–8.

2 Desmonts G, Couvreur J, Alison F *et al.* Étude épidémiologique sur la toxoplasmose: de l'influence de la cuisson des viandes de boucherie sur la fréquence de l'infection humaine. *Rev Fr Étude Clin Biol* 1965; **10**: 952–8.

3 Sabin AB. Toxoplasmosis: recently recognized disease of human beings. V. Clinical manifestations of toxoplasmosis in man. *Adv Pediatr* 1942; **1**: 1–56.

4 Alford CA, Stagno S & Reynolds DW. Congenital toxoplasmosis: clinical, laboratory and therapeutic considerations, with special reference to subclinical disease. *Bull NY Acad Med* 1974; **50**: 160–81.

5 Gilbert GL. Congenital fetal infections. *Semin Neonatal* 1996; **1**: 91–105.

6 Daffos F, Forestier F, Capella-Pavlovsky M *et al.* Prenatal management of 746 pregnancies at risk for congenital toxoplasmosis. *N Engl J Med* 1988; **318**: 271–5.

7 Hohlfeld P, Deffos F, Costa JM, Thulliez P, Forestier F & Vidaud M. Prenatal diagnosis of congenital toxoplasmosis with a polymerase chain reaction test on amniotic fluid. *N Engl J Med* 1994; **331**: 695–9.

8 McAuley J, Boyer KM, Patel D *et al.* Early and longitudinal evaluations of treated infants and children and untreated historical patients with congenital toxoplasmosis: the Chicago collaborative treatment trial. *Clin Infect Dis* 1994; **18**: 38–72.

9 Desmonts G, Daffos F, Forestier F *et al.* Prenatal diagnosis of congenital toxoplasmosis. *Lancet* 1985; **i**: 500–4.

10 Hohlfeld P, Daffos F, Thulliez P *et al.* Fetal toxoplasmosis: outcome of pregnancy and infant follow-up after *in utero* treatment. *J Pediatr* 1989; **115**: 765–9.

11 McCabe R & Remington JS. Toxoplasmosis: the time has come. *N Engl J Med* 1988; **318**: 313–15.

12 Jeannel D, Costagliola D, Niel G *et al.* What is known about the prevention of congenital toxoplasmosis. *Lancet* 1990; **336**: 359–61.

13 Guerina NG, Hsu H-W, Meissner HC *et al.* Neonatal serologic screening and early treatment for congenital *Toxoplasma gondii* infection. *N Engl J Med* 1994; **330**: 1858–63.

14 Strannegard O, Holm SE, Hermodsson S *et al.* Case of apparent reinfection with rubella. *Lancet* 1970; **i**: 240–1.

15 Haukenes G & Haram KO. Clinical rubella after reinfection. *N Engl J Med* 1972; **287**: 1204.

16 Northrop RL, Gardner WM & Geittmann WF. Rubella reinfection during early pregnancy: a case report. *Obstet Gynecol* 1972; **39**: 524–6.

17 Eilard T & Strannegard O. Rubella reinfection in pregnancy followed by transmission to the fetus. *J Infect Dis* 1974; **129**: 594–6.

18 Forsgren M, Carlstrom G & Strangert K. Congenital rubella after maternal reinfection. *Scand J Infect Dis* 1979; **11**: 81–3.

19 Best JE, Banatvala JE, Morgan-Capner P & Miller E. Fetal infection after maternal reinfection with rubella: criterion for defining reinfection. *BMJ* 1989; **299**: 773–5.

20 Miller E, Cradock-Watson JE & Pollock TM. Consequences of confirmed maternal rubella at successive stages of pregnancy. *Lancet* 1982; **ii**: 781–4.

21 Menser MA, Dods L & Marley JD. A twenty-five year follow-up of congenital rubella. *Lancet* 1967; **ii**: 1347–50.

22 McIntosh EDG & Menser MA. A fifty-year follow-up of congenital rubella. *Lancet* 1992; **340**: 414–15.

23 Daffos F, Forestier F, Grangeot-Keros L *et al.* Prenatal diagnosis of congenital rubella. *Lancet* 1984; **ii**: 1–3.

24 Robinson J, Lemay M & Vaudry WL. Congenital rubella after anticipated maternal immunity: two cases and a review of the literature. *Pediatr Infect Dis J* 1994; **13**: 812–15.

25 Burgess MA. Rubella reinfection – what risk to the fetus? *Med J Aust* 1992; **156**: 824–5.

26 Centers for Disease Control. Rubella and congenital rubella – United States, 1984–6. *MMWR* 1987; **36**: 457.

27 Wild NJ, Sheppard S & Smithells RW. The consequences of antenatal rubella testing. *Health Trends* 1986; **18**: 9–10.

28 Modlin JF, Hermann K, Brandling-Bennett AD *et al.* Risk of congenital abnormality after inadvertent rubella vaccination of pregnant women. *N Engl J Med* 1976; **294**: 972–4.

29 Preblud SR, Stetler HC, Frank JA *et al.* Fetal risk associated with rubella vaccine. *JAMA* 1981; **246**: 1413–17.

30 Vaheri A, Vesikari T, Oker-Blom N *et al.* Isolation of attenuated

rubella-vaccine virus from human products of conception. *N Engl J Med* 1972; **286**: 1071–4.

31 Fleet WF, Benz EW, Karzon DT *et al.* Fetal consequences of maternal rubella immunisation. *JAMA* 1974; **227**: 621–7.

32 Boppana SB, Pass RF & Britt WJ. Virus-specific antibody responses in mothers and their newborn infants with asymptomatic congenital cytomegalovirus infections. *J Infect Dis* 1993; **167**: 72–7.

33 Fowler KB, Stagno S, Pass RF, Britt WJ, Boll TJ & Alford CA. The outcome of congenital cytomegalovirus infection in relation to maternal antibody status. *N Engl J Med* 1992; **326**: 663–7.

34 Stagno S, Reynolds DW, Pass RF & Alford CA. Breast milk and the risk of cytomegalovirus infection. *N Engl J Med* 1980; **302**: 1073–6.

35 Yeager AS. Transfusion-acquired cytomegalovirus infections in newborn infants. *Am J Dis Child* 1974; **128**: 478–83.

36 Kumar ML, Nakervis GA, Cooper AR & Gold E. Postnatally acquired cytomegalovirus infections in infants of CMV-excreting mothers. *J Pediatr* 1984; **104**: 669–73.

37 Peckham CS, Coleman JC, Hurley R *et al.* Cytomegalovirus infection in pregnancy: preliminary findings from a prospective study. *Lancet* 1983; **i**: 1352–5.

38 Ahlfors K, Ivarsson SA, Johnsson T & Svanberg L. A prospective study on congenital and acquired cytomegalovirus infections in infants. *Scand J Infect Dis* 1979; **11**: 177–8.

39 Birnbaum G, Lynch JI, Margileth AM *et al.* Cytomegalovirus infections in newborn infants. *J Pediatr* 1969; **75**: 789–95.

40 Stagno S, Reynolds DW, Huang ES *et al.* Congenital cytomegalovirus infection. Occurrence in an immune population. *N Engl J Med* 1977; **296**: 1254–8.

41 Preece PM, Pearl KN & Peckham CS. Congenital cytomegalovirus infection. *Arch Dis Child* 1984; **59**: 1120–6.

42 Numazaki Y, Yano N, Morizuka T *et al.* Primary infection with cytomegalovirus: virus isolation from healthy infants and pregnant women. *Am J Epidemiol* 1970; **91**: 410–17.

43 Schopfer K, Lauber E & Krech U. Congenital cytomegalovirus infection in newborn infants of mothers infected before pregnancy. *Arch Dis Child* 1978; **53**: 536–9.

44 Griffiths PD, Campbell-Benzie A & Heath RB. A prospective study of cytomegalovirus infection in pregnancy. *Br J Obstet Gynaecol* 1980; **87**: 308–14.

45 Grant S, Edmond E & Syme J. A prospective study of primary cytomegalovirus infection during pregnancy. *J Infect* 1981; **3**: 24–31.

46 Stagno S, Pass RF, Dworsky ME *et al.* Congenital cytomegalovirus infection. The relative importance of primary and recurrent maternal infection. *N Engl J Med* 1982; **306**: 945–9.

47 Stagno S, Pass RF, Cloud G *et al.* Primary cytomegalovirus infection in pregnancy. *JAMA* 1986; **256**: 1904–8.

48 Ahlfors K, Ivarsson SA, Harris S *et al.* Congenital cytomegalovirus infection and disease in Sweden and the relative importance of primary and secondary maternal infections. *Scand J Infect Dis* 1984; **16**: 129–37.

49 Griffiths PD & Baboonian C. A prospective study of primary cytomegalovirus infection during pregnancy: final report. *Br J Obstet Gynaecol* 1984; **91**: 307–15.

50 Rutter D, Griffiths P & Trompeter RS. Cytomegalovirus inclusion disease after recurrent maternal infection. *Lancet* 1985; **ii**: 1182.

51 Nigro G, Clerico A & Mondaini C. Symptomatic congenital cytomegalovirus infection in two consecutive sisters. *Arch Dis Child* 1993; **69**: 527–8.

52 Preece PM, Tookey P, Ades A & Peckham CS. Congenital cytomegalovirus infection: predisposing maternal factors. *J Epidemiol Community Health* 1986; **40**: 205–9.

53 Reynolds DW, Stagno S, Stubbs KG *et al.* Inapparent congenital cytomegalovirus infection with elevated cord blood IgM levels: causal relation with auditory and mental deficiency. *N Engl J Med* 1974; **290**: 291–6.

54 Hanshaw JB, Scheiner AP, Moxley AW *et al.* School failure and deafness after 'silent' congenital cytomegalovirus infection. *N Engl J Med* 1976; **295**: 468–70.

55 Saigal S, Lunyk O, Larke RPB & Chernesky MA. The outcome in children with congenital cytomegalovirus infection. *Am J Dis Child* 1982; **136**: 896–901.

56 Kumar ML, Nakervis GA, Jacobs IB *et al.* Congenital and postnatally acquired cytomegalovirus infections: long-term follow-up. *J Pediatr* 1984; **104**: 674–9.

57 Davis LE, James CG, Fiber F & MacLaren LC. Cytomegalovirus isolation from a human ear. *Ann Otol Rhinol Laryngol* 1979; **88**: 424–6.

58 Yeager AS, Hafleigh MT, Arvin AM *et al.* Prevention of transfusion-acquired cytomegalovirus infection in newborn infants. *J Pediatr* 1981; **98**: 281–7.

59 Jones CA & Isaacs D. Predicting the outcome of symptomatic congenital cytomegalovirus infection. *J Paediatr Child Health* 1995; **31**: 70–1.

60 Nigro G, Scholz H & Bartmann U. Ganciclovir therapy for symptomatic congenital cytomegalovirus in infants: a two-regimen experience. *J Pediatr* 1994; **124**: 318–22.

61 Gilbert GL, Hayes K, Hudson IL *et al.* Prevention of transfusion-acquired cytomegalovirus infection in infants by blood filtration to remove leucocytes. *Lancet* 1989; **i**: 1228–31.

62 Ahlfors K, Ivarsson SA, Johnson T *et al.* Risk of cytomegalovirus infection in nurses and congenital infection in their offspring. *Acta Paediatr Scand* 1981; **70**: 819–23.

63 Dworsky M, Welch K, Cassady G *et al.* Occupational risk for primary cytomegalovirus infection among paediatric health-care workers. *N Engl J Med* 1983; **309**: 950–3.

64 Yeager AS. Longitudinal, serological study of cytomegalovirus infections in nurses and in personnel without patient contact. *J Clin Microbiol* 1975; **2**: 448–52.

65 Haneberg B, Bertnes E & Haukenes G. Antibodies to cytomegalovirus among personnel at a children's hospital. *Acta Paediatr Scand* 1980; **69**: 407–9.

66 Friedman HM, Lewis MR, Nemerofsky DM & Plotkin SA. Acquisition of cytomegalovirus infection among female employees at a pediatric hospital. *Pediatr Infect Dis J* 1984; **3**: 233–5.

67 Haldane EV, van Rooyan CE, Embil JA *et al.* A search for transmissible birth defects of virologic origin in members of the nursing profession. *Am J Obstet Gynecol* 1968; **105**: 1032–40.

68 Young AB, Reid D & Grist NR. Is cytomegalovirus a serious hazard to female staff? *Lancet* 1983; **i**: 975–6.

69 Abughali N, Van der Kuyp F, Annable W & Kumar ML. Congenital tuberculosis. *Pediatr Infect Dis J* 1994; **13**: 738–41.

70 Kendig EI. The place of BCG vaccine in the management of infants born to tuberculous mothers. *N Engl J Med* 1969; **281**: 520–3.

71 Dormer BA, Harrison I, Swart JA *et al.* Prophylactic isoniazid protection of infants in a tuberculosis hospital. *Lancet* 1959; **ii**: 902–3.

72 American Academy of Pediatrics. Revised guidelines for prevention of early-onset group B streptococcal. (GBS) infection. *Pediatrics* 1997; **99**: 489–96.

73 Smith MHD, Starke JR & Marquis JR. Tuberculosis and opportunistic mycobacterial infections. In: Feigin RD & Cherry JD (eds) *Textbook of Pediatric Infectious Diseases*, 3rd edn. Philadelphia: WB Saunders, 1992.

74 Colditz GA, Brewer TF, Berkey JD *et al.* Efficacy of BCG vaccine in the prevention of tuberculosis. *JAMA* 1994; **271**: 698–702.

75 Stray-Pederson B. Economic evaluation of maternal screening to prevent congenital syphilis. *Sex Transm Dis* 1983; **10**: 167–72.

76 Stoll BJ, Lee FK, Larsen S *et al.* Clinical and serologic evaluation of neonates for congenital syphilis: a continuing diagnostic dilemma. *J Infect Dis* 1993; **167**: 109.

77 Centers for Disease Control. Guidelines for the prevention and control of congenital syphilis. *MMWR* 1988; **37** (Suppl S-1): 1–13.

78 Sanchez PJ, Wendel GD Jr, Grimprel E *et al.* Re-evaluation of molecular methodologies and rabbit infectivity testing for the diagnosis of congenital syphilis and neonatal central nervous system invasion by *Treponema pallidum*. *J Infect Dis* 1993; **167**: 148–57.

79 Hulbert TV. Congenital malaria in the United States: report of a case and review. *Clin Infect Dis* 1992; **14**: 922–6.

80 McGregor IA. Epidemiology, malaria and pregnancy. *Am J Trop Med Hyg* 1984; **33**: 517–25.

81 Covell G. Congenital malaria. *Trop Dis Bull* 1950; **47**: 1147–67.

82 Zenker PN & Berman SM. Congenital syphilis: trends and recommendations for evaluation and management. *Pediatr Infect Dis J* 1991; **10**: 516–22.

18 | Surveillance and managing outbreaks

INTRODUCTION

'Surveillance' is a term frequently used in the neonatal unit. Resistant organisms are often selected by the extensive use of antibiotics and may be transmitted from baby to baby. Traditional practice has been to perform routine bacterial and fungal culture of various sites from most or all babies on the neonatal unit, so-called 'surveillance cultures'; these would be performed at least once a week.

The rationale for performing frequent surveillance cultures is really twofold. One intention is to know which organisms are colonizing an individual baby so that, if the baby develops systemic sepsis, appropriate antibiotic therapy based on the colonizing organisms can be started. The second aim of surveillance cultures is to identify resistant organisms that have spread from baby to baby, so that infection control measures can be introduced or reinforced to prevent spread and so that antibiotic policies can, if necessary, be changed if colonization is widespread.

In many neonatal units, a large number of surveillance cultures are performed at great expense in time and cost. The advisability of these cultures has been questioned [1].

DO SURVEILLANCE CULTURES PREDICT THE ORGANISMS CAUSING SYSTEMIC SEPSIS?

Early studies suggested that babies with abnormal pharyngeal colonization, defined as a heavy growth of Gram-negative bacilli, *Staphylococcus aureus*, *S. epidermidis* or other organisms (*Haemophilus*, enterococci, yeasts) from throat swabs, were the only babies who developed late-onset or nosocomial sepsis [2]. Babies with 'normal flora' (defined as no growth, a light growth, or α-haemolytic streptococci as the predominant organism) did not develop sepsis. Most of the babies who developed sepsis had required endotracheal intubation for hyaline membrane disease; we are not told what proportion of the controls required intubation, so the authors may merely have been describing an epiphenomenon in a high-risk group.

It is, perhaps, not surprising that intubated babies develop septicaemia. Storm showed that a transient bacteraemia lasting <10 min occurred in three of ten intubated babies during routine suctioning of the endotracheal tube [3]. Others have shown that most babies who develop late-onset sepsis are preterm babies receiving mechanical ventilation [4,5].

Harris *et al.* [6] and Sprunt *et al.* [2] found a close correlation between the organisms colonizing the oropharynx or endotracheal tube and the organisms causing subsequent sepsis. However, more recent papers have tended to show that surveillance cultures are poorly predictive of the organisms responsible for systemic sepsis. In the late 1980s Slagle and colleagues found that routine endotracheal cultures were poorly predictive of the organisms causing septicaemia and often misleading [7]. Evans and co-workers analysed over 24 000 cultures taken from 3000 babies over 3 years. They found that the maximum sensitivity of cultures from ear, nasopharynx, axilla, umbilicus, groin, rectum, stomach and endotracheal tube in predicting the organisms causing sepsis was only 56%, with a specificity of 82%; only 1 in 30 babies with suspected sepsis proved to have true sepsis [8]. Webber and colleagues found that endotracheal and nasopharyngeal cultures predicted the organism or organisms obtained from blood cultures in only one of seven babies with late-onset pneumonia and septicaemia [9].

It is not clear why there has been an apparent change in the value of surveillance cultures for predicting the organisms causing sepsis. It may be a facet of the increasingly invasive procedures needed to care for very preterm babies, including the use of central venous catheters, which have altered the possible routes of entry of organisms and increased the likelihood of catheter-associated organisms such as coagulase-negative staphylococci. Whatever the reason for the change, surveillance cultures have been described by Fulginiti and Ray as 'an exercise in futility, wastefulness and inappropriate practice' [1]. This would certainly appear true for predicting sepsis in an individual baby and we have argued already (Chapter 6) that the choice of antibiotics for a baby should be based on a unit antibiotic policy, itself based on episodes of sepsis, rather than on the organisms colonizing babies.

DO SURVEILLANCE CULTURES HELP IN MANAGING OUTBREAKS?

If cultures from surface and deep sites are not predictive of sepsis in an individual baby, it may be important to know what organisms are circulating on the neonatal unit, their sensitivity patterns and whether there is a lot of spread from baby to baby. Organisms may be colonizing the upper respiratory tract, skin or bowel and enter the bloodstream via the respiratory tract, for which endotracheal intubation is the most obvious risk factor; through the skin by means of local trauma or intravascular cannulas, particularly long-standing cannulas; or through the bowel wall, particularly where there has been necrosis as in necrotizing enterocolitis (NEC). Full surveillance cultures might then include cultures of nasopharyngeal or endotracheal secretions, skin and faeces. One of the main problems is that multiple organisms of varying sensitivities are usually present in each of these sites.

We have found that surveillance cultures do have a limited

value in telling us which organisms are prevalent. We would not change the unit antibiotic policy because of widespread colonization with resistant organisms without episodes of systemic sepsis (Chapter 6). We did, however, find at one time that six preterm babies requiring artificial ventilation were colonized with gentamicin-resistant *Klebsiella oxytoca*. It has been shown previously that babies who are artificially ventilated are the highest risk group for developing late sepsis [4]. When two of the six babies developed septicaemia with gentamicin-resistant *K. oxytoca*, we changed our antibiotic regimen for suspected late sepsis from flucloxacillin and gentamicin to flucloxacillin and netilmicin [10]. It was certainly helpful, when making the decision to change the antibiotic policy, to know the colonization status of the other high-risk babies. On the other hand, the same information could have been obtained rapidly by culturing endotracheal secretions from intubated babies for the first time only when there was an apparent outbreak of systemic sepsis, i.e. not performing regular surveillance cultures.

CULTURES FOR EARLY-ONSET SEPSIS

Although these are not strictly surveillance cultures, it has become routine to collect cultures from a number of different sites in babies with suspected early-onset sepsis. As the babies with systemic sepsis are usually those most heavily colonized, all these superficial and deep cultures tend to be positive when a baby has systemic sepsis [9]. Thus, it should be possible to cut down on the number of such cultures without increasing the risk of missing those babies with negative blood and CSF cultures who are colonized with a pathogen such as group B streptococcus or *Listeria* (Chapter 6).

CULTURES FOR NEW ADMISSIONS

In many neonatal units, it is standard practice to take multiple cultures from babies admitted to the unit. This may be confined to babies transferred from other hospitals or may include all inborn babies admitted to the neonatal unit.

We certainly perform selective cultures for methicillin-resistant *Staphylococcus aureus* (MRSA) from babies transferred to the unit from another hospital, because the baby may be colonized with MRSA, which is no longer prevalent on our unit. If this proves to be the case, the baby is isolated if possible, or at least the importance of handwashing after handling the baby is reinforced. On the other hand, cultures are not taken routinely from inborn babies unless they are suspected of being septic.

WHICH CULTURES ARE USEFUL?

After 4 years of carefully documented experience using multiple cultures for suspected early and late sepsis, and only moderately restricted surveillance cultures, we came to a similar, if slightly less extreme, conclusion to that of Fulginiti and Ray [1]. We decreased greatly the number of cultures for suspected early and late sepsis. Surveillance cultures were also decreased from thrice-weekly endotracheal and nasopharyngeal cultures from all preterm babies who were being or who had been artificially ventilated, to once-weekly endotracheal tube cultures from babies on mechanical ventilation. After 3 years, no increased problems were experienced in monitoring or treating sepsis, nor did any babies relapse after stopping antibiotics after 48 hours. We estimated the annual saving by reducing these cultures to be about £28 000 and there were savings in time and effort without adverse clinical outcome [11].

MANAGEMENT OF AN OUTBREAK

In managing an apparent outbreak of infection, the first question is whether it is truly an outbreak (Table 18.1). For example, it is not uncommon to have small clusters of necrotizing enterocolitis involving three or four babies. Almost always we

Questions:
Is it really an outbreak?
What is the organism?
What is the mode of spread?
Any possibility of a common source, e.g. intravenous fluids?
How can spread be prevented, e.g. improved handwashing?
Should the antibiotic policy be changed?

Possible actions:
Eradicate any common source
Improve handwashing: education of staff and visitors
Change the antibiotic policy
Cohorting of infected and colonized babies
Cohorting of staff

Table 18.1 Management of a possible outbreak

have found that all the babies had risk factors for NEC, and that there was no common organism identified. However, outbreaks of NEC have been associated with rotavirus, among other organisms, so the possibility of an outbreak should be investigated.

If an organism is identified as the cause of an outbreak, the mode of spread should be considered next. In the great majority of cases, the spread will be on the hands of staff, and the implication is that normal infection control procedures have lapsed, and that improved handwashing is the priority.

On the other hand, occasionally a common source is identified, so it is always worth considering possible sources (Table 18.2). Intravenous fluids can be contaminated in their preparation, and have caused outbreaks of infection due to *Enterobacter* species and coagulase-negative staphylococci. Outbreaks of conjunctivitis due to water-loving Gram-negative organisms have been associated with contaminated eyewash solutions. An outbreak of infection with *Candida parapsilosis* was attributed to the use of a common liquid suppository [12], while *Listeria monocytogenes* was transmitted from baby to baby by the use of a common rectal thermometer [13]. Other reported sources of outbreaks of infection with Gram-negative bacilli include

Organisms	Mode of spread
Gram-negative enteric bacilli	Hands of staff (exacerbated by increased workload) Resuscitation equipment Eyewash solutions Scrubbing brushes
Staphylococcus aureus	Hands of staff (exacerbated by increased workload) Nasal carriage by staff may be source
Coagulase-negative staphylococci	Hands of staff Contaminated intravenous fluids
Enterobacter species	Contaminated intravenous fluids
Listeria monocytogenes	Rectal thermometer In delivery suite Hands of mother
Respiratory syncytial virus	Hands of staff Staff infections
Enteroviruses	Hands of staff
Rhizopus	Surgical bandages Tongue depressor used as arm-splint
Candida parapsilosis	Liquid glycerin suppositories

Table 18.2 Modes of spread implicated in outbreaks of nosocomial infection

distilled water containers [14], resuscitation apparatus [15,16] and handwashing brushes [17].

We have argued that a response such as a change in antibiotic policy is justified only if there is an outbreak of systemic sepsis with a multiresistant organism (e.g. MRSA or an extended-spectrum β-lactamase-producing Gram-negative (ESBL) organism), not just widespread colonization. Indeed, we have argued that it is not worth performing routine surveillance cultures looking for colonization with resistant organisms.

When an outbreak of sepsis with the same organism does occur, it may be worth testing all babies on the unit to look for evidence of spread, as described in an outbreak of echovirus 11 infection [18]. It may, however, be unnecessary if a number of cases have occurred. Royle and co-workers assumed that all babies on the neonatal unit were colonized during an outbreak of ESBL *Klebsiella pneumoniae* infection, and aborted the outbreak by instituting measures to improve handwashing [19] as described in the Outbreak history below.

The theoretical situation during an outbreak, with some babies colonized and others not, is shown in Figure 18.1a. Performing surveillance cultures allows colonized babies and non-colonized babies to be 'cohorted', i.e. nursed separately (Figure 18.1b). However, if handwashing is performed assiduously, then cohorting should be unnecessary, since there should be no baby-to-baby spread on hands (Figure 18.1c).

Outbreak history [19]

A baby with bladder extrophy, known to be colonized with an extended-spectrum β-lactamase-producing *Klebsiella pneumoniae* (ESBLKp), became septic on day 25. Blood and urine grew ESBLKp and the baby recovered on amikacin, to which the organism was sensitive. No other babies were known to be colonized and policy was not changed.

Three months later, a second case occurred in a baby previously treated for NEC. Again the baby recovered on amikacin.

Cases 3 and 4 occurred 10 weeks later, in a baby with malrotation, volvulus and NEC, and in a baby with gastroschisis. The latter baby died. At this time, alterations in policy were considered, but not adopted.

Six weeks later a further two cases occurred and a second baby died. The infection control team elected:

1. to change empirical antibiotic policy for suspected late-onset sepsis from vancomycin and gentamicin to vancomycin and imipenem;

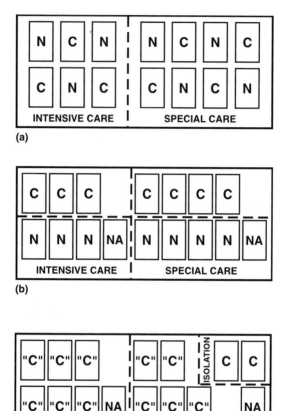

Figure 18.1 (a) Theoretical situation during outbreak of infection with multiresistant organism. About half the babies in intensive care are colonized (C), half not (N). (b) Surveillance cultures and cohorting. Colonized babies (C) are identified by surveillance cultures and cohorted apart from non-colonized (N) babies. New admissions (NA) are nursed with N babies. Regular surveillance cultures are necessary. (c) Low-cost approach. All babies are assumed to be colonized ('C'). Proven colonized or infected babies (C) are nursed in isolation. New admissions (NA) are nursed alongside 'C' babies, but protected by improved handwashing

2. to assume all babies on the unit were colonized, so not to perform immediate surveillance cultures;

3. to improve handwashing by conducting education sessions with the nursing staff, exhorting them to act as advocates for the babies and to get others to handwash.

A seventh case occurred 1 week after cases 5 and 6, but no further cases of systemic sepsis with ESBLKp. Ten weeks after the last case, it was elected to perform faecal cultures on all babies in the unit, to see how many colonized babies remained. At this point, there were only two colonized babies, so these were isolated in a sideroom and the antibiotic policy was changed back to vancomycin (subsequently flucloxacillin) and gentamicin for all other babies. Thus the outbreak was contained by cheap, simple methods, although in retrospect these might have been instituted after cases 3 and 4.

SURVEILLANCE OF SYSTEMIC SEPSIS AND ANTIBIOTIC USE

Although we have found surveillance cultures to be of limited use in managing infections, on the other hand we have found it extremely helpful to monitor episodes of systemic sepsis and antibiotic use.

The system devised in the John Radcliffe Hospital, Oxford, in conjunction with Prof. Andrew Wilkinson, the senior neonatologist, is for one infectious disease specialist to perform a weekly ward round, lasting about 2 hours, with the neonatal junior staff. All microbiology reports are seen by a junior doctor, signed and filed in alphabetical order of the baby's name in a box file. They are not filed in the babies' case notes until they have been seen and signed by the infectious disease specialist on the weekly ward round, who therefore has immediate access to the whole week's results, as do the neonatal junior staff who can look them up in the box file. The box file is a very cheap, but effective, way for the infectious disease specialist to have access to results without having to search through each baby's case notes. Computerized results are tending to replace report forms on paper, so the box file may sadly become obsolete.

On the weekly ward round, and by reviewing after the ward round the case notes of babies discharged from the unit during the week, the infectious disease doctor records episodes of systemic sepsis and other infections, contaminants of blood or CSF, and antibiotic use on a standard proforma (Figure 18.2). Infections and contaminants are defined as in Appendix 1. The number of baby-days are recorded, as well as the level of intensive care, as defined by the British Paediatric Association [20]; this has been used as a marker of workload and found to correlate with the spread of organisms [10].

The ward round acts as a teaching round on neonatal infections and as an opportunity to collect data. It also reminds junior staff to consider stopping antibiotics after 2–3 days when cultures are negative. When the ward rounds were started in April 1984, the unit antibiotic policy was, as it is now, to stop antibiotics if systemic cultures were negative unless there was either pneumonia or suspected early sepsis associated with heavy colonization with group B streptococcus, *Listeria* or another likely pathogen. In practice, however, antibiotics were often continued and at the start of surveillance the median duration of antibiotic courses was 5 days and, on average, a baby spent 1 in 4 days on antibiotics (Figure 18.3). The same average antibiotic use had occurred in the previous year. Within 2 years of starting infectious disease ward rounds, the median duration of antibiotic courses was 2 days, as it has remained [21]. The proportion of baby-days spent on antibiotics had fallen from the previous level of 25% and, although there was great fluctuation in antibiotic use from month to month (●), when examined over 6-month intervals (▲) antibiotic use remained constant at 15–20% of baby-days (Figure 18.3). This represents a substantial saving in antibiotic costs and in not having to perform serum aminoglycoside assays, which are generally done only if antibiotics are continued for longer than 3 days. The infectious disease doctor maintains a close liaison with the

NEONATAL INFECTION SURVEILLANCE

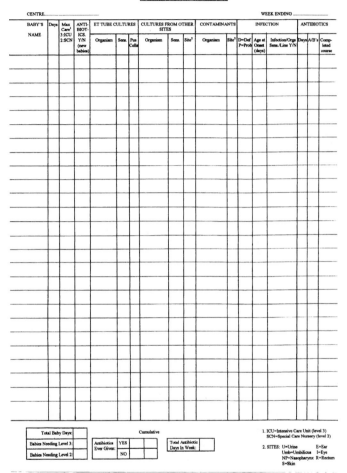

Figure 18.2 Standard proforma for recording information once weekly on infections, colonization, contaminants and antibiotic use

microbiology department on the significance of blood culture isolates, antibiotic treatment and general policy.

The organism is reviewed regularly using sepsis and the outcome of episodes of sepsis at a 6-monthly meeting. This

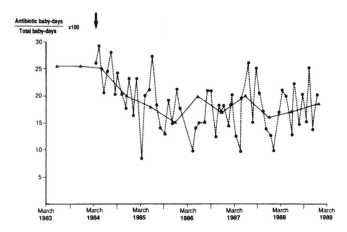

Figure 18.3 Antibiotic use expressed as the proportion of baby-days spent on antibiotics, e.g. 25% represents an average of 1 in 4 days spent on antibiotics. ▲, 6-monthly means; ●, 1-monthly means; arrow indicates start of regular surveillance of antibiotic use

allows staff to be aware rapidly of changing patterns of sepsis (Chapter 1) and of whether the unit's antibiotic policy is appropriate or is resulting in increased morbidity or mortality.

We would recommend this system of monitoring or 'surveillance' of infections and antibiotic use as being simple, cheap, economical of time and highly educational for the infectious disease doctors as well, it is hoped, as for the junior staff.

SURVEILLANCE OF NOSOCOMIAL INFECTIONS

Nosocomial infections prolong hospital stay and are expensive: Gray and colleagues estimated that each episode of coagulase-negative staphylococcal bacteraemia prolonged hospital stay by 14 days, at a cost of US$25 000 per patient [22].

What is an acceptable rate of nosocomial infection? A neonatal unit can compare its own nosocomial infection rate from year to year, but this will identify internal fluctuations and not whether the overall rate is satisfactory. Trying to compare rates between different hospitals suffers from variations in the populations of babies: some hospitals will be caring for much smaller, sicker babies than others. Gaynes and co-workers compared rates of nosocomial infection in neonatal units in the United States using National Nosocomial Infection Survey (NNIS) definitions [23]. These definitions were not developed for neonates, and the data are difficult to collect, but they do allow comparisons between hospitals while taking into account different severities of patient populations. Gaynes *et al.* found duration of stay and 'device utilization' (e.g. endotracheal tube, central venous catheter) to have the strongest correlation with rates of nosocomial infection [23].

Scores of severity of illness such as the SNAP (Score of Neonatal Acute Physiology) and CRIB (Clinical Risk Index for Babies) scores make allowances for patient populations. Both were designed to compare mortality rates. Higher SNAP [22] or CRIB [24] scores do correlate with greater risk of nosocomial infection, which is hardly surprisingly since smaller, sicker babies needing more intervention are the babies at highest risk of nosocomial infection. The lowest birthweight babies have the highest rate of infection [25]. However, there are other factors, e.g. bowel surgery, urinary tract abnormality, which increase the risk of nosocomial infection without necessarily increasing mortality. New risk of nosocomial infection scores are needed for comparing neonatal units.

SUMMARY

- Surveillance cultures for colonization should generally be kept to a minimum.
- During an outbreak of systemic sepsis due to a common organism:
  (a) eradicate any common source,
  (b) improve handwashing,
  (c) change the unit antibiotic policy, if appropriate, and
  (d) consider cohorting of colonized babies.

> • Surveillance and regular review of systemic sepsis on a neonatal unit is useful.

References

1 Fulginiti VA & Ray CG. Body surface cultures in the newborn infant. An exercise in futility, wastefulness and inappropriate practice. *Am J Dis Child* 1988; **142**: 19–20.

2 Sprunt K, Leidy G & Redman W. Abnormal colonization of neonates in an intensive care unit: means of identifying neonates at risk of infection. *Pediatr Res* 1978; **12**: 998–1002.

3 Storm W. Transient bacteremia following endotracheal suctioning in ventilated newborns. *Pediatrics* 1980; **65**: 487–90.

4 Isaacs D, Wilkinson AR & Moxon ER. Surveillance of colonisation and late-onset septicaemia in neonates. *J Hosp Infect* 1987; **10**: 114–19.

5 Stoll BJ, Gordon T, Korones SB *et al.* Late-onset sepsis in very low birth weight neonates: a report from the National Institute of Child Health and Human Development Neonatal Research Network. *J Pediatr* 1996; **129**: 63–71.

6 Harris H, Wirtshaffer D & Cassady G. Endotracheal intubation and its relationship to bacterial colonization and systemic infection of newborn infants. *Pediatrics* 1976; **58**: 816–23.

7 Slagle TA, Bifano EM, Wolf JW & Gross SJ. Routine endotracheal cultures for the prediction of sepsis in ventilated babies. *Arch Dis Child* 1989; **64**: 34–8.

8 Evans ME, Schaffner W, Federspiel CF *et al.* Sensitivity, specificity and predictive value of body surface cultures in a neonatal intensive care unit. *JAMA* 1988; **259**: 248–52.

9 Webber S, Lindsell D, Wilkinson AR *et al.* Neonatal pneumonia. *Arch Dis Child* 1990; **65**: 207–11.

10 Isaacs D, Catterson J, Hope PL *et al.* Factors influencing colonisation with gentamicin resistant Gram negative organisms in the neonatal unit. *Arch Dis Child* 1988; **63**: 533–5.

11 Dobson S, Isaacs D, Wilkinson A *et al.* Reduced use of surface cultures for suspected neonatal sepsis and surveillance is safe. *Arch Dis Child* 1992; **67**: 44–7.

12 Welbel SF, McNeil MM, Kuykendall RJ *et al. Candida parapsilosis* bloodstream infections in neonatal intensive care unit patients: epidemiologic and laboratory confirmation of a common source outbreak. *Pediatr Infect Dis J* 1996; **15**: 998–1002.

13 Larsson S, Cederberg A, Ivarsson S, Svanberg L & Cronberg S. *Listeria monocytogenes* causing hospital-acquired enterocolitis and meningitis in newborn infants. *BMJ* 1978; **ii**: 473–4.

14 Rapkin RH. *Pseudomonas cepacia* in an intensive care nursery. *Pediatrics* 1976; **57**: 239–43.

15 Drewitt SE, Payne DJH, Tuke W *et al.* Eradication of *Pseudomonas aeruginosa* infection from a special care nursery. *Lancet* 1972; **i**: 946–8.

16 Stone JW & Das BC. Investigation of an outbreak of infection with *Acinetobacter calcoaceticus* in a special care baby unit. *J Hosp Infect* 1985; **6**: 42–8.

17 Anagnostakis D, Fitsialos J, Koutsia C *et al.* A nursery outbreak of *Serratia marcescens* infection. Evidence of a single source of contamination. *Am J Dis Child* 1981; **135**: 413–15.

18 Isaacs D, Dobson SRM, Wilkinson AR *et al.* Conservative management of an echovirus 11 outbreak in a neonatal unit. *Lancet* 1989; **i**: 543–5.

19 Royle J, Halasz S, Eagles G *et al.* An outbreak of extended spectrum beta-lactamase producing *Klebsiella pneumoniae* in a neonatal unit. *Arch Dis Child* 1998 (in press).

20 British Paediatric Association. *Categories of Babies Receiving Neonatal Care*. London: British Paediatric Association, 1984.

21 Isaacs D, Bangham CRM & McMichael AJ. Cell-mediated cytotoxic response to respiratory syncytial virus in infants with bronchiolitis. *Lancet* 1987; **ii**: 769–71.

22 Gray JE, Richardson DK, McCormick MC & Goldmann DA. Coagulase-negative staphylococcal bacteremia among very low birthweight infants: relation to admission illness severity, resource use and outcome. *Pediatrics* 1995; **95**: 225–30.

23 Gaynes RP, Martone WJ, Culver DH *et al.* Comparison of rates of nosocomial infection in neonatal intensive care units in the United States. *Am J Med* 1991; **91**: 192–5.

24 Fowlie PW, Gould CR, Parry GJ, Phillips G, Tarnow-Mordi WO. CRIB. Clinical Risk Index for Babies; in relation to nosocomial bacteraemia in very low birthweight or preterm infants. *Arch Dis Child* 1996; **75**: F49–F52.

25 Isaacs D, Barfield C, Clothier T *et al.* Late onset infections of infants in neonatal units. *J Paediatr Child Health* 1996; **32**: 158–61.

19 | **Prevention**

INTRODUCTION

In view of the high mortality and morbidity of neonatal infections, prevention of such infections should have a high priority. Reference to this has been made in many of the chapters on specific infections, but this chapter examines more general aspects of prevention.

CONGENITAL INTRAUTERINE INFECTIONS

Immunization is arguably the single most effective preventive measure available to doctors. Immunization of mothers against rubella has the potential to eliminate congenital rubella syndrome, while maternal immunization against tetanus prevents neonatal tetanus. When immunizations are not available, as for toxoplasmosis and cytomegalovirus (CMV) infection, other strategies of prevention need to be considered. Serological screening programmes of pregnant women for toxoplasmosis have been introduced in France and their possible use in other countries may be considered in future.

Any maternal illness in the first trimester of pregnancy should be taken seriously, and serological tests for toxoplasma, rubella and CMV, if clinically indicated, may help to identify at-risk pregnancies. Antenatal diagnosis of fetal infections using fetal blood samples or cordocentesis is increasingly possible, and counselling based on the state of knowledge can then be offered.

EARLY-ONSET INFECTIONS

The prevention of infections due to group B streptococci (GBS) and *Listeria* has been discussed in Chapter 14. Screening of pregnant women for GBS carriage, by culturing either cervical secretions or urine, can identify high-risk pregnancies. Maternal *Listeria* infection is often undiagnosed clinically, but dietary advice may allow women to reduce their risk of contracting *Listeria* infection during pregnancy.

When women in labour have risk factors for neonatal infection (fever, prolonged membrane rupture, premature onset of labour), it may be decided to start them on antibiotic therapy. Although this is the obstetrician's decision, paediatricians should not be slow in pointing out that there is sound evidence that intrapartum ampicillin (2 g i.v. at once and 1 g i.v. 4-hourly until delivery) reduces maternal and neonatal GBS infection [1] and it may also reduce the severity of neonatal listeriosis. Ampicillin is probably effective cover against *Haemophilus influenzae* and pneumococcus, as well as some Gram-negative organisms, so it seems the antibiotic of choice for intrapartum therapy. Alternatives are penicillin G and erythromycin.

Women who have had a baby with congenital listeriosis are at low risk for their subsequent babies to be infected. This is not true for women who have had a baby with early-onset GBS sepsis, and they should be given intrapartum ampicillin at the above dose from the onset of labour in all subsequent pregnancies.

LATE-ONSET INFECTIONS

BREASTFEEDING

Human breast milk is protective against gastroenteritis, many respiratory infections including RSV infection, gastroenteritis and necrotizing enterocolitis. There is surprisingly little evidence on breast milk and nosocomial infections (see Chapter 22)[2], but the limited evidence certainly suggests it protects against nosocomial infections, diarrhoea and NEC. Women should be strongly encouraged to breastfeed their babies. If the baby is preterm and not sucking, the mother should be given encouragement and assistance in expressing her milk.

EARLY ENTERAL FEEDING

In the unit at Oxford, enteral feeding has traditionally been introduced very early, even for very preterm babies requiring ventilatory support, because of its importance in stimulating gut hormonal development. This has meant that it has often been possible to maintain babies' nutritional status without resort to central venous catheters and parenteral nutrition, both of which carry an inherent risk of sepsis.

SKIN CARE

Hexachlorophene baths halve the incidence of *Staphylococcus aureus* skin colonization compared with water, with or without soap or detergent [3]. However, there have been worries about systemic absorption of disinfectants, such as hexachlorophene, leading to neurotoxicity. Babies are now cleaned at birth by washing with soap and water, although the use of dilute 3% hexachlorophene, followed by thorough rinsing is used, with caution, in the face of epidemics of *S. aureus*. Chlorhexidine baths seem to be safer than hexachlorophene and at least as effective in reducing colonization [3].

UMBILICAL CORD CARE

There is little doubt that attention to umbilical cord care was highly important in reducing the incidence of local and systemic staphylococcal infections in the 1950s and 1960s. There is some debate as to the relative merits of various topical antibiotics and antimicrobials, including triple dye (brilliant green, proflavin hemisulphate and gentian violet), gentian violet alone and bacitracin ointment or powder, to sterilize the cord.

Triple dye application to the umbilicus reduces umbilical and nasal colonization with *S. aureus* by over 50%, compared with soap and water, although it has no effect on colonization with Gram-negative organisms. It also reduces group B streptococcal colonization by 20%, which approaches statistical significance [3]. Silver sulphadiazine is almost as effective as triple dye for *S. aureus* and significantly reduces group B streptococcal or Gram-negative bacillary colonization. Chlorhexidine is not absorbed through the skin of newborns, and chlorhexidine baths reduce *S. aureus* colonization at least as much as hexachlorophene, although chlorhexidine application only to the cord is ineffective [3].

What is clear is that, if no cord care is given, we can expect to see a return of serious infection due to *S. aureus* and, in the neonatal unit, omphalitis due to Gram-positive and Gram-negative organisms [4].

EYE CARE

The use of prophylactic antibiotics to prevent gonococcal and chlamydial conjunctivitis is discussed in Chapter 12. In the UK and Australia, prophylactic antibiotics are not given, the occurrence of gonococcal conjunctivitis being used as a marker to treat the baby, the mother and her sexual contacts. Chlamydial conjunctivitis is underdiagnosed, but it may be important to attempt to diagnose it rather than to prevent it, because without systemic erythromycin about one-half of the babies with chlamydial conjunctivitis will develop chlamydial pneumonitis. As the latter presumably follows nasopharyngeal colonization, eye prophylaxis would not prevent pneumonitis, but would prevent recognition of at-risk babies.

INVASIVE PROCEDURES

Invasive procedures for monitoring and treating the fetus and newborn baby have become an integral part of obstetric and neonatal care. To a large extent these have been inextricably linked with falling perinatal mortality rate, but they carry a price in terms of infection.

Fetal scalp monitors should be used with circumspection and care because they may result in scalp abscesses and, very occasionally, osteomyelitis of the skull. They should not be used when there is active herpes simplex virus infection of the cervix or a history of maternal HSV, because neonatal HSV infection has been introduced through fetal scalp monitors.

Umbilical vessel catheterization carries a modest risk of infection, but this is far higher for umbilical venous than for arterial catheters. If umbilical venous catheters are to be used it should be for as short a time as possible. Although infection of umbilical artery catheters is fairly uncommon, infection of peripheral artery catheters is even rarer [5] and they may be safer as regards infection.

Bacteraemia or fungaemia complicate the use of cental venous catheters in about 10% of patients [6].

Indwelling peripheral venous polyethylene catheters used for prolonged intravenous therapy may become infected in up to 8% of cases [6]. The use of topical antibiotics at the site of catheter entry and the use of prophylactic parenteral antibiotics have no effect on the incidence of bacteraemia [6].

Heat is generally a more effective disinfectant than solutions, and, whenever possible, equipment should be autoclaved rather than using liquid disinfectants. This applies particularly to ventilator tubing, humidifiers and suction equipment, which should be changed and autoclaved regularly. Nebulizer equipment and humidifiers are particularly prone to contamination with water-loving organisms. Closed incubators must be cleaned with disinfectant if they cannot be autoclaved, and an iodophor or quaternary disinfectant is preferable.

STAFFING ARRANGEMENTS

Understaffing and overcrowding (Figure 19.1) have been associated with an increased risk of all nosocomial infections [7], with spread of gentamicin-resistant Gram-negative bacilli [8] and with outbreaks of staphylococcal infection [9]. The most likely explanation for this is that normal infection control measures such as handwashing are compromised by increased workload, but whether this is because staff are busy and forget to wash their hands between handling different babies, or whether they do wash their hands, but are looking after more babies, is not clear. It seems unlikely that droplet spread is a major mechanism of baby-to-baby transmission.

Spread from sinks seems to be less important than was once thought. Although swabbing sinks will often yield water-loving organisms such as *Pseudomonas* species, in outbreaks of *Pseudomonas* species infection in adult intensive care units, the patients are usually infected with different strains from those found in the sink [10].

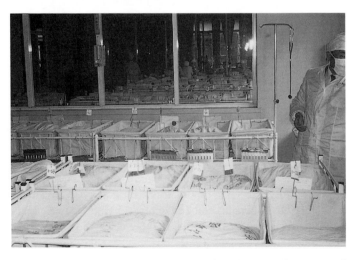

Figure 19.1 Overcrowding in a neonatal unit in China (photography courtesy of Professor Peter Rolfe). There was an exceptionally high incidence of staphylococcal skin infections

HANDWASHING

Handwashing is the single most effective infection-control measure available in the neonatal intensive care unit. Despite this, countless studies have shown that medical staff are extremely poor at washing their hands before handling babies, and that doctors are consistently the worst offenders. Semmelweis, working in Vienna in 1861, noted that women delivered by doctors had an incidence of puerperal fever three times greater than that in women delivered by midwives. When a colleague died from sepsis after cutting his hand performing an autopsy, Semmelweis realized that the doctors were probably transmitting organisms acquired when performing autopsies. He introduced strict handwashing with chlorine water, and the maternal mortality rate dropped from 12% to 3% within weeks. Almost simultaneously, Florence Nightingale was stressing the importance of handwashing while nursing in the Crimean War.

Larson reviewed over 400 articles on handwashing published from 1879 to 1986 and concluded that there was strong evidence that handwashing prevents infection [11]. The use of soap and water for 15 seconds removes most superficial bacteria from hands, while chlorhexidine or iodine-based soaps increase the effectiveness [12]. Alcohol rubs are very effective in preventing spread of viruses [13]. Constant reminders on ward rounds about not leaning on incubators and about washing hands before and after handling babies can help to reduce the spread of organisms.

MANAGEMENT OF OUTBREAKS

There are many reports of outbreaks of neonatal infection, often with resistant Gram-negative bacilli, other bacteria, fungi or enteroviruses. In some reports it is clear that a new organism has entered the neonatal unit and spread to many babies, colonizing many and infecting some. In other cases the evidence of a true outbreak is less clear-cut.

We have reported previously [14] that when we started surveillance of infections in Oxford about 30% of all babies cultured were colonized with *Pseudomonas aeruginosa*, which was the commonest cause of late-onset sepsis. Nine months later, and without introducing any special infection control measures, it was rarely possible to culture *Pseudomonas* from any of the babies (Figure 19.2). In our opinion, this casts doubt on the validity of expensive infection-control measures, such as bacterial surveillance cultures on all babies and swabbing possible environmental sources such as sinks, unless there is clear evidence of a true outbreak. Babies will inevitably become colonized with one or more organisms, and systemic sepsis with those organisms is likely to occur in babies with multiple risk factors for infection. Our observations (Figure 1.3) suggest that approximately the same total number of late-onset infections occur each year, but with different organisms, depending on which are colonizing babies. Thus, the particular virulence of organisms does not appear to be a major factor in determining the incidence of late-onset infection.

We have found a low mortality rate from late-onset infections. Unless an organism colonizing babies was causing particularly frequent, severe infections, we would argue that infection-control measures, other than to reinforce the importance of handwashing, are of unconfirmed benefit, often expensive and probably unnecessary. Outbreak control is considered in more detail in Chapter 18.

COHORTING

'Cohorting' of staff and babies may be an effective measure if there is documented spread of an organism. Babies known to be colonized or infected are segregated from non-infected babies and cared for only by the same staff, who do not handle non-infected babies, including new admissions. If the staff are ill but still working, they handle only infected babies. In busy neonatal units, where infected babies require varying levels of intensive care, this is rarely a practical proposition.

ISOLATION

Isolation of babies who are colonized or infected is rarely necessary. The indications for isolation include suspected or

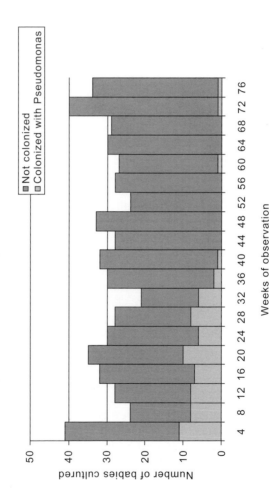

Figure 19.2 Sequential observations on colonization of babies with *Pseudomonas aeruginosa*. Neonatal unit, John Radcliffe Hospital, Oxford, starting May 1984. Shaded areas represent babies colonized with *P. aeruginosa*

confirmed infections with diarrhoeal organisms, rubella, chickenpox, herpes simplex virus, enteroviruses (particularly coxsackievirus), syphilis and gonorrhoea. *Listeria* has occasionally caused serious nosocomial infections and we routinely isolate mother and baby. Group B streptococci occasionally cause outbreaks, but this is rare and, as most colonized babies are not detected because they are never swabbed, we do not isolate babies with GBS colonization or sepsis.

GLOVES, GOWNS AND MASKS

Gloves, gowns and masks need be worn by staff to prevent neonatal infections only during surgical procedures. We do recommend that staff with colds wear masks. Baley and Fanaroff reviewed studies on the effects of gowning or of eliminating gowning in the newborn nursery [3]. They consistently found that eliminating gowning did not result in increased colonization, nor in increased sepsis.

VISITORS

There are many reasons for allowing free access to relatives and friends to visit babies on the neonatal unit and, fortunately, nosocomial viral infections are fairly uncommon, even in winter [15]. We ask visitors to wash their hands to the elbow and to handle their own baby only. We ask family and friends not to visit if they have a respiratory or gastrointestinal infection.

ANTIBIOTIC USE

In Chapter 6 it was argued in detail that antibiotic use can be, and should be, kept to a minimum. Prolonged use of antibiotics creates 'antibiotic pressure' which selects for resistant organisms and is associated with an increased risk of systemic candidiasis [16]. Antibiotics should not be continued for longer than 2–3 days just because the baby is 'still sick' or has 'lots of lines'. It has been shown that, in most instances, antibiotics can safely be stopped after 48–72 hours without risk of missing occult infection [17].

BLOOD PRODUCTS

All human blood products used in the neonatal unit should come from donors who have been screened for antibodies to HIV, hepatitis B virus, and hepatitis C virus. Furthermore, the risk of transmitting CMV to babies should be minimized, either by using only blood products from known CMV-seronegative donors [18] or by using filtered blood [19].

IMMUNOGLOBULINS

The potential ability of oral immunoglobulin preparations rich in IgG and IgA to prevent necrotizing enterocolitis is discussed in Chapter 13.

It has been proved that i.m. immunoglobulin preparations rich in specific antibody are effective in decreasing the severity of neonatal chickenpox (Chapter 16) and normal human immunoglobulin can protect against severe measles in older immune-compromised children. Specific immunoglobulin preparations have also been used successfully to prevent infections with RSV in high-risk infants [20].

Intravenous immunoglobulin (IVIG) preparations have been given prophylactically to low-birthweight preterm babies who are at high risk of late infection and have relatively low levels of transplacental antibodies. The consensus view, summarized in Chapter 7, is that IVIG preparations are of at best marginal benefit in preventing late-onset infections in industrialized countries, and that other measures are more effective. In developing countries, some benefit has been shown, but IVIG may be being used instead of handwashing, and there would be little doubt of the outcome of a cost–benefit analysis of the two interventions.

NON-INDUSTRIALIZED COUNTRIES

Prevention of infections in non-industrialized countries is considered in Chapter 22.

SUMMARY

- Handwashing is the single most important and most cost-effective means to reduce nosocomial infections.
- Breast milk is preferable to formula, and mothers should be encouraged and helped to express or to breastfeed.
- Chlorhexidine baths reduce colonization with *Staphylococcus aureus*.
- Umbilical cord care with antiseptics like triple dye significantly reduces umbilical and nasal *S. aureus* colonization.
- Understaffing and overcrowding increase the risk of nosocomial infection.
- Wearing gowns does not reduce nosocomial infections.

References

1 Boyer KM & Gotoff SP. Prevention of early-onset neonatal group B streptococcal disease with selective intrapartum chemoprophylaxis. *N Engl J Med* 1986; **314**: 1665–9.

2 Relucio-Clavano N. The results of a change in hospital practices. A paediatrician's campaign for breast-feeding in the Philippines. *Assignment Children* 1981; **55/56**: 139–61.

3 Baley JE & Fanaroff AA. Neonatal infections, Part 1: Infection related to nursery care practices. In: Sinclair JC & Bracken MB (eds) *Effective Care of the Newborn Infant*. Oxford: Oxford University Press, 1992: 454–75.

4 Mason WH, Andrews R, Ross LA & Wright HT. Omphalitis in the newborn infant. *Pediatr Infect Dis J* 1989; **8**: 521–5.

5 Adams JM, Speer ME & Rudolph AJ. Bacterial colonization of radial artery catheters. *Pediatrics* 1980; **65**: 94–7.

6 Nelson JD. Control of infection acquired in the nursery. In: Remington JS & Klein JO (eds) *Infectious Diseases of the Fetus and Newborn Infant*, 2nd edn. Philadelphia: WB Saunders, 1983: 1035–52.

7 Goldmann DA, Durbin WA & Freeman, J. Nosocomial infections in a neonatal intensive care unit. *J Infect Dis* 1981; **144**: 449–59.

8 Isaacs D, Catterson J, Hope PL *et al.* Factors influencing colonisation with gentamicin resistant Gram negative organisms in the neonatal unit. *Arch Dis Child* 1988; **63**: 533–5.

9 Haley RW & Bregman DA. The role of understaffing and over-crowding in recurrent outbreaks of staphylococcal infection in a neonatal intensive care unit. *J Infect Dis* 1982; **145**: 875–85.

10 Morrison AJ & Wenzel RP. Epidemiology of infections due to *Pseudomonas aeruginosa. Rev Infect Dis* 1984; **6** (Suppl): 627–42.

11 Larson E. A causal link between handwashing and risk of infection? Examination of the evidence. *Infect Control Hosp Epidemiol* 1988; **9**: 28–36.

12 Sprunt K, Redman W & Leidy G. Antibacterial effectiveness of routine hand-washing. *Pediatrics* 1973; **52**: 264–7.

13 Isaacs D, Dobson SRM, Wilkinson AR *et al.* Conservative management of an echovirus 11 outbreak in a neonatal unit. *Lancet* 1989; **i**: 543–5.

14 Isaacs D, Wilkinson AR & Moxon ER. Surveillance of colonisation and late-onset septicaemia in neonates. *J Hosp Infect* 1987; **10**: 114–19.

15 Rudd PT & Carrington D. A prospective study of chlamydial, mycoplasmal and viral infections in a neonatal intensive care unit. *Arch Dis Child* 1984; **59**: 120–5.

16 Weese-Mayer DE, Fondriest DW, Brouillette RT & Shulman ST. Risk factors associated with candidemia in the neonatal intensive care unit: a case–control study. *Pediatr Infect Dis J* 1987; **6**: 190–6.

17 Isaacs D, Wilkinson AR & Moxon ER. Duration of antibiotic courses for neonates. *Arch Dis Child* 1987; **62**: 727–8.

18 Yeager AS, Hafleigh MT, Arvin AM *et al.* Prevention of transfusion-acquired cytomegalovirus infection in newborn infants. *J Pediatr* 1981; **98**: 281–7.

19 Gilbert GL, Hayes K, Hudson IL *et al.* Prevention of transfusion-acquired cytomegalovirus infection in infants by blood filtration to remove leucocytes. *Lancet* 1989; **i**: 1228–31.

20 Groothuis JR, Simoes EAF, Levin MJ *et al.* Prophylactic administration of respiratory syncytial virus immune globulin to high-risk infants and young children. *N Engl J Med* 1993; **329**: 1524–30.

20 | The mother: obstetric aspects

Early-onset neonatal infection results from organisms acquired from the mother at the time of delivery. However, the organisms colonizing the mother's genital tract are important in neonatal sepsis in another way. There is increasing evidence that heavy or 'abnormal' colonization of the maternal genital tract may predispose to preterm labour, and this greatly increases the risk of neonatal sepsis.

In this chapter, we will consider:

- Bacterial vaginosis
- Bacteriuria
- Preterm prolonged ruptured membranes
- Chorioamnionitis (symptomatic and asymptomatic)
- Peripartum maternal risk factors for neonatal sepsis
- Prevention of early-onset group B streptococcal infection.

BACTERIAL VAGINOSIS

Bacterial vaginosis is not truly an infection, but an imbalance in the vaginal microflora, with reduced lactobacilli and an increase in various endogenous organisms [1].

Gilbert [2] defined bacterial vaginosis as a common condition characterized by:

- an offensive, non-irritant vaginal discharge,
- high vaginal pH >4.5,
- clue cells (epithelial cells covered with Gram-variable coccobacilli), but no or few pus cells in the vaginal discharge, and

- altered bacterial flora with virtually no lactobacilli, but over-growth of organisms such as *Gardnerella vaginalis*, genital mycoplasmas and anaerobes.

Bacterial vaginosis has been shown in studies in the UK [3], in the USA [4] and Australian Aborigines [5] to increase the risk of preterm labour or preterm delivery about threefold, and also to cause late miscarriages. In addition, tocolytics are less effective in aborting preterm labour in women with bacterial vaginosis.

McGregor and colleagues screened women at their first booking antenatal visit to Denver Hospital for bacterial vaginosis [4]. If bacterial vaginosis was present, the women were treated with the antibiotic appropriate to their predominant organism (ceftriaxone for *Neisseria gonorrhoeae*, erythromycin for *Chlamydia trachomatis*, metronidazole for *Trichomonas vaginalis*, clindamycin for bacterial vaginosis). Outcome was compared with a previous period of observation without treatment. Treatment of bacterial vaginosis was associated with a halving of the incidence of preterm birth and of preterm premature ruptured membranes.

Screening women for bacterial vaginosis, by obtaining a vaginal swab for Gram stain and culture at booking, and treating affected women with oral clindamycin 300 mg 12-hourly for 7 days, could significantly reduce the incidence of preterm birth and hence of neonatal infection.

BACTERIURIA

Bacteriuria is a reflection of heavy colonization. As such, it is relatively uncommon, only 1–2% of women having group B streptococcal (GBS) bacteriuria [6,7], but is strongly associated with preterm labour [7,8]. In Denmark, 69 (1.7%) of 4122 women screened at 27–31 weeks' gestation had GBS bacteriuria. Oral penicillin (1 million units 8-hourly for 3 days, repeated if colonization recurred) significantly reduced the incidence of preterm delivery from 12 (38%) of 32 in the placebo group to 2 (5%) of 37, and increased the mean gestational age at delivery from 36.2 to 39.6 weeks. Thus, 10 preterm deliveries were prevented in 4000 deliveries.

Screening by urine culture for GBS bacteriuria is relatively insensitive, but has the power to prevent some preterm deliveries.

PRETERM PROLONGED RUPTURED MEMBRANES

Sometimes, the mother's membranes may rupture before term (preterm), and also before labour ('prematurely'). This condition of preterm premature rupture of membranes (pPROM) increases the morbidity of both baby and mother. The baby is at risk from sepsis and from effects of prematurity such as intraventricular haemorrhage (IVH). The cause of pPROM is multifactorial, but infection plays an important role [9].

Mercer and Arheart performed a meta-analysis of the controlled trials of antibiotic therapy for pPROM [10]. They found that antimicrobials, usually ampicillin or erythromycin, reduced neonatal sepsis by half, neonatal pneumonia by two-thirds, and also reduced maternal chorioamnionitis by just over half.

French and McGregor argue for the use of a 7-day course of an oral macrolide, erythromycin or clindamycin, although more on theoretical grounds than any proven advantage over ampicillin [11]. However, in a controlled trial, ampicillin–sulbactam, which has improved anaerobic cover, was significantly better than ampicillin in terms of the latency period from pPROM to delivery, and in the incidence of sepsis, pneumonia and other neonatal complications [12].

CHORIOAMNIONITIS

Chorioamnionitis is inflammation of the fetal membranes and placenta, usually with associated infection of the amniotic fluid. Other names used for this condition are intra-amniotic infection or amniotic fluid infection, although, strictly speaking, chorioamnionitis is a histopathological diagnosis, rather than a microbiological one. When careful cultures are taken, bacteria or mycoplasmas can be grown from about 75% of placentas with histological chorioamnionitis [13].

Chorioamnionitis is common, and histological evidence can be found in up to 40% of unselected placentas [2]. Most women with histological chorioamnionitis are asymptomatic, fewer than 10% being febrile. When clinical chorioamnionitis occurs, the features are fever, tachycardia, uterine tenderness and foul-smelling liquor.

The pathogenesis of chorioamnionitis is primarily ascending infection from the maternal genital tract, although *Listeria* and group A streptococci are organisms that can also spread haematogenously. Most cases of chorioamnionitis are polymicrobial, with low-grade pathogens, such as facultative Gram-negative and Gram-positive bacteria, anaerobes and mycoplasma (*Ureaplasma urealyticum* and *Mycoplasma hominis*) being isolated more often than from controls [9]. However, group B streptococcus and *Escherichia coli* are major causes of chorioamnionitis, together causing 45% of isolates in one study [14].

Chorioamnionitis is associated with preterm labour, and as such puts babies at risk of sepsis, although only around 5–6% of babies born to women with chorioamnionitis develop proven sepsis. Does chorioamnionitis *cause* preterm labour or *result* from it? This is a traditional chicken-and-egg question. Gibbs favours the idea that low-grade sepsis causes chorioamnionitis and initiates preterm labour [9]. There is a plausible mechanism for this: genital tract bacteria elaborate phospholipase A_2 which is involved in prostaglandin synthesis. Prostaglandins are produced by amniotic cells and increased levels of prostaglandins, as well as metabolites of arachidonic acid, are found in the amniotic fluid of women with chorioamnionitis in preterm labour [9].

Two approaches might be considered to antibiotic therapy of chorioamnionitis. One is to identify and treat likely causative organisms in advance, to try to prevent later chorioamnionitis. Retrospective studies suggested that erythromycin treatment of women with genital mycoplasmas might reduce preterm labour. However, Eschenbach and colleagues randomized over 900 women colonized with *Ureaplasma urealyticum* to erythromycin or placebo for at least 7 weeks from 26–38 weeks' gestation [15]. They found no improvement in the rate of preterm labour.

A second approach would be to treat women in preterm labour with antibiotics, as well as tocolytics, to try to prolong the pregnancy. Such studies have shown statistically significant prolongation of pregnancy in antibiotic-treated groups, compared with controls. However, none has shown a decrease in perinatal mortality [9].

The situation with chorioamnionitis in association with group B streptococci is totally different: here, antibiotic therapy in labour is of proven benefit. This situation will be covered in the section below on Prevention of early-onset group B streptococcal sepsis.

PERIPARTUM MATERNAL RISK FACTORS FOR NEONATAL SEPSIS

There are certain common maternal risk factors for early-onset neonatal sepsis which may occur during labour. These have been carefully established and validated as increasing the risk of early-onset group B streptococcal infection [16], but probably apply to other early-onset pathogens, such as *Streptococcus pneumoniae*. The risk factors are shown in Table 20.1. As discussed in Chapter 6, the maternal risk factor most frequently overlooked by junior doctors and nurses is spontaneous preterm onset of labour.

The presence of one or more of these risk factors should lead to two considerations:

1. To treat the mother with intrapartum antibiotics, which has been shown to reduce maternal and neonatal sepsis from GBS.

Proven	Maternal fever	>37.5°C
	Prolonged rupture of membranes	>18 hours
	Spontaneous preterm onset of labour or rupture of membranes	<37 weeks' gestation
	Previous baby with GBS sepsis	Specifically for risk of GBS
Probable	Offensive liquor	

Table 20.1 Maternal risk factors for neonatal sepsis

2. To treat the baby with antibiotics if appropriate or to take cultures and observe closely.

PREVENTION OF EARLY-ONSET GROUP B STREPTOCOCCAL INFECTION

Various approaches to the prevention of early-onset GBS infections have been proposed (see Table 20.2). Intrapartum antibiotics have been shown to reduce the incidence of early-onset neonatal GBS sepsis and of maternal GBS infection in the babies of colonized women with risk factors [17]. However, screening for maternal recto-vaginal carriage at 26–28 weeks and intrapartum antibiotics for women with risk factors will only prevent about 50% of cases, although as few as 3.4% of women will need intrapartum antibiotics [18].

A second approach is to screen for carriage at 26–28 weeks' gestation and treat all GBS colonized women with intrapartum antibiotics: screening and non-selective chemoprophylaxis [19]. This will prevent about 60–70% of GBS cases, but about 15–25% of women will receive antibiotics. A third 'combination' approach, again using screening, is to treat all women with risk factors, such as spontaneous onset of preterm labour, but also to screen for GBS carriage at 35–37 weeks' gestation and treat all carriers with intrapartum antibiotics [20,21]. This will prevent around 85% of cases of early-onset GBS sepsis, but over 25% of women will receive antibiotics [21]. These three approaches are all costly and involve screening. A fourth approach is not to screen for carriage, but to treat

Prevention strategy	Proportion of early-onset GBS cases prevented	Proportion of mothers treated with antibiotics	Cost
Selective chemoprophylaxis Screen at 26–28 weeks for GBS carriage Treat colonized women with risk factors with IPA	} 50%	3–5%	+++
Non-selective chemoprophylaxis Screen at 26–28 weeks Treat all colonized mothers with IPA	} 60–70%	15–25%	+++
Combination approach Treat all women with risk factors with IPA, whether or not colonized Screen at 35–37 weeks and treat all GBS carriers with IPA	} 85%	25–30%	+++
Empirical strategy Do not screen Treat all women with risk factors with IPA	} 60–70%	15–20%	+

Table 20.2 Prevention strategies for early-onset group B streptococcal neonatal infection

IPA, intrapartum antibiotics.

all women with risk factors for neonatal sepsis, as described in the previous section, with intrapartum antibiotics. This will prevent 70% of cases and 18% of women will receive antibiotics and has the advantage of being far cheaper than the other strategies. The last two strategies will also prevent sepsis due to some organisms other than GBS. The two antibiotics that have been proven to be successful in preventing neonatal GBS sepsis are ampicillin and penicillin G [18]. Erythromycin has been recommended for women who are allergic to penicillin. The rate of fatal anaphylaxis to penicillin has been estimated at 0.001% or 1 in 100 000 women, while babies may die or have severe sequelae to non-fatal maternal anaphylaxis.

The high morbidity and mortality rates of neonatal early-onset GBS disease and the fact that maternal morbidity and even mortality due to GBS can occur argues heavily for the use of some form of preventive strategy. Cost–benefit analyses favour intrapartum antibiotic use whenever the rate of early-onset GBS sepsis is about 0.5 per 1000 live births [22], although in the long term effective vaccination of women of child-bearing age against GBS is likely to be the most cost-effective preventive strategy [23].

SUMMARY

- Bacterial vaginosis can be diagnosed at booking and treatment with clindamycin or erythromycin halves the rate of preterm birth.
- Group B streptococcal bacteriuria is rare, but associated with preterm labour; screening at 27–31 weeks' gestation and administration of oral penicillin reduce the incidence of preterm labour.
- Treatment of women with preterm prolonged rupture of membranes with antibiotics reduces neonatal sepsis.
- Chorioamnionitis is usually asymptomatic and is associated with preterm labour; treatment with antibiotics has been shown to prolong pregnancy.

- Peripartum maternal risk factors for early-onset neonatal sepsis are maternal fever, prolonged rupture of membranes, spontaneous preterm onset of labour, or a previous baby with GBS sepsis.
- Early-onset neonatal group B streptococcal sepsis can be prevented by intrapartum antibiotics; strategies include maternal screening for GBS carriage with selective or non-selective antibiotics, or empirical therapy of women with risk factors.

References

1 Hay PE & Taylor-Robinson D. Defining bacterial vaginosis: to BV or not to BV, that is the question. *Int J STD AIDS* 1996; **7**: 233–5.

2 Gilbert GL. *Infectious Disease in Pregnancy and the Newborn Infant.* Harwood: Chur, 1991.

3 Hay PE, Lamont RF, Taylor-Robinson D *et al.* Abnormal bacterial colonisation of the genital tract and subsequent preterm delivery and late miscarriage. *BMJ* 1994; **308**: 295–8.

4 McGregor JA, French JI, Parker R *et al.* Prevention of premature birth by screening and treatment for common genital infections: results of a prospective, controlled evaluation. *Am J Obstet Gynecol* 1995; **173**: 157–67.

5 Schultz R, Read AW, Straton JAY *et al.* Genito-urinary tract infections in pregnancy and low birthweight: case control study in Australian Aboriginal women. *BMJ* 1991; **303**: 1369–73.

6 Wood EG & Dillon HC. A prospective study of group B streptococcal bacteriuria in pregnancy. *Am J Obstet Gynecol* 1981; **140**: 515–20.

7 Thomsen AC, Morup L & Hansen KB. Antibiotic elimination of group-B streptococci in urine in prevention of preterm labour. *Lancet* 1987; **i**: 591–3.

8 Moller M, Thomsen AC, Borch K, Dinesen K & Zdravkovic M. Rupture of fetal membranes and premature delivery associated with group B streptococci in urine of pregnant women. *Lancet* 1984; **ii**: 69–70.

9 Gibbs RS. Obstetric factors associated with infections of the fetus and newborn infant. In: Remington JS & Klein JO (eds) *Infectious Diseases of the Fetus and Newborn Infant*, 4th edn. Philadelphia: WB Saunders, 1995: 1241–63.

10 Mercer BM & Arheart KL. Antimicrobial therapy in expectant management of preterm premature of the membranes. *Lancet* 1995; **346**: 1271–9.

11 French JI & McGregor JA. The pathobiology of premature rupture of membranes. *Semin Perinatol* 1996; **20**: 344–68.

12 Lewis DF, Fontenot MT, Brooks GG, Wise R, Perkins MB & Heymann AR. Latency period after preterm premature rupture of membranes: a comparison of ampicillin with and without sulbactam. *Obstet Gynecol* 1995; **86**: 392–5.

13 Pankuch GA, Appelbaum PC, Lorenz RP *et al.* Placental microbiology and histology and the pathogenesis of chorioamnionitis. *Obstet Gynecol* 1984; **64**: 802–6.

14 Sperling RS, Newton E & Gibbs RS. Intraamniotic infection in low-birth-weight infants. *J Infect Dis* 1988; **157**: 113.

15 Eschenbach DA, Nugent RP, Rao AV *et al.* A randomized placebo-controlled trial of erythromycin for the treatment of *Ureaplasma urealyticum* to prevent premature delivery. *Am J Obstet Gynecol* 1991; **164**: 734.

16 Boyer KM, Gadzala CA, Burd LI *et al.* Selective intrapartum chemoprophylaxis of group B streptococcal early-onset disease. I. Epidemiologic rationale. *J Infect Dis* 1983; **148**: 795–801.

17 Boyer KM & Gotoff SP. Prevention of early-onset neonatal group B streptococcal disease with selective intrapartum chemoprophylaxis. *N Engl J Med* 1986; **314**: 1665–9.

18 Schuchat A, Whitney C & Zangwill K. Prevention of perinatal group B streptococcal disease: a public health perspective. *MMWR* 1996; **45**: 1.

19 Jeffery HE & McIntosh EDG. Antenatal screening and non-selective intrapartum chemoprophylaxis for group B streptococcus. *Aust NZ J Obstet Gynaecol* 1994; **34**: 14–19.

20 Gilbert GL, Isaacs D, Burgess MA *et al.* Prevention of neonatal group B streptococcal sepsis: is routine antenatal screening appropriate? *Aust NZ J Obstet Gynaecol* 1995; **35**: 120–6.

21 CDC (Centers for Disease Control). Prevention of perinatal group B streptococcal disease: a public health perspective. *MMWR* 1996; **45** (RR-7): 1–24.

22 Mohle-Boetani JC, Schuchat A, Plikyatis BD, Smith JD & Broome CV. Comparison of prevention strategies for neonatal group B streptococcal infection. A population-based economic analysis. *JAMA* 1993; **270**: 1442–8.

23 Jeffery HE. Group B streptococcus infections. *Semin Perinatol* 1996; **1**: 77–89.

21 | **Immunizations**

Prevention of infections through vaccination or immunization is one of the most important medical advances ever made. Neonates are at high risk of infection and survivors of neonatal intensive care, especially those with chronic lung disease, are at particular risk of severe disease from respiratory pathogens such as *Bordetella pertussis*. Thus, expedient immunization of preterm babies, including immunization prior to discharge from the neonatal unit whenever possible, is a high priority.

PRETERM VERSUS TERM

As already emphasized in Chapter 2, the immune response of preterm newborns is dependent on postnatal antigen exposure, and hence depends more on postnatal age than on postgestational age. In other words, preterm neonates can respond immunologically to many antigens at about the same age after birth as full-term neonates.

This is an oversimplification, of course, since the term 'immune response' begs the question 'to what?' The response to BCG vaccine is almost exclusively a T cell-mediated, memory T cell response. In contrast, the response to tetanus toxoid protein depends on T cell processing of the protein antigen followed by B cell recognition and function. As a general rule, preterm infants respond well to vaccines and can be immunized at the same postnatal age as term infants.

WHY NOT IMMUNIZE AT BIRTH?

Some vaccines can be given at birth, and will induce a good immune response. BCG vaccine given at birth is as effective as if it is given later in infancy [1]. Here a T cell memory response is produced, and antibodies are not involved.

For viral vaccines, the response of babies immunized at birth is variable. Live, attenuated poliovirus (oral poliovirus, OPV, Sabin) induces antibodies when given at birth, and maternal antibodies do not interfere, perhaps because the vaccine is given orally. In contrast, passively acquired maternal antibodies to measles virus interfere with the baby's immune response to measles vaccine, which is suboptimal under 6 months of age. It is thought that the mechanism is maternal antibodies neutralizing the vaccine strain and rendering the vaccine virus non-immunogenic.

Protein antigens given at birth may induce a poor response compared with the same antigen given at 2 months of age. The major example is whole-cell pertussis vaccine [2–4] but the same phenomenon has been seen with diphtheria toxoid [5]. If a dose of vaccine is given at birth, not only is the initial response poor, but when further doses are given, the antibody response may continue to be suboptimal, compared with starting at 2 months old. This is the phenomenon of tolerance. The newborn baby needs to distinguish 'self' and 'non-self' antigens. It appears that some vaccines, if given at birth, may be seen as 'self' antigens. When these vaccines are given again later they will induce at best a low level antibody response. It is for this reason that triple vaccine (diphtheria–tetanus–pertussis) is given no sooner than 2 months after birth. In contrast, hepatitis B surface antigen (a viral protein) is extremely immunogenic at birth, indeed more so than in older children and adults.

BCG VACCINE

Full-term neonates can respond well to BCG vaccine. Indeed, a meta-analysis found that neonatal BCG was as effective as

BCG given later in infancy [1]. BCG vaccine is a live, attenuated strain of *Mycobacterium bovis*. It is only moderately protective against tuberculosis with an efficacy of 50%. However, it has a 64% efficacy against meningeal TB, and a 71% efficacy against dying from TB [1], so is well worth giving.

Neonatal BCG vaccine is one of the vaccines recommended for all babies in non-industrialized countries, as part of the Expanded Programme of Immunization (EPI) of the World Health Organization. In industrialized countries, neonatal BCG immunization is recommended for babies at high risk for TB. The exact recommendations vary and are shown in Table 21.1. There are no data on the response of preterm babies to BCG vaccine.

PROTEIN ANTIGENS (DIPHTHERIA, TETANUS)

Diphtheria and tetanus toxoids are protein antigens. They are not given at birth because of concern about inducing tolerance to later doses. Most countries use a 2, 4, 6 month regimen for

	Aus	UK	US	NZ
Babies who will be living in a household which includes immigrants or visitors from countries of high prevalence	✓	✓	✓	✓
Babies who are born into a household where they will continue to be exposed to a person with active tuberculosis (or where there is a person with past TB – NZ)	✓	✓	✓	✓
High incidence area or population, e.g. Australian Aborigine, Maori	✓			✓
Neonate whose family is emigrating to a high-risk country	✓	✓		✓
Babies born to patients with leprosy	✓			
Where the parents request neonatal BCG		✓		✓
Data from refs [12–15].				

Table 21.1 Indications for neonatal BCG vaccine in Australia, the UK, the USA and New Zealand

triple antigen, diphtheria–tetanus–pertussis (DTP), but the UK uses 2, 3, 4 months without any drop in immunogenicity [6].

DTP is immunogenic when given at 2 months of postnatal age, even to extremely premature infants. In the study by D'Angio and colleagues, all 16 babies born before 29 weeks' gestation and with birthweight <1000 g seroconverted to three doses of tetanus toxoid [7]. Studies of babies of 28–36 weeks' gestation show serological responses to diphtheria, tetanus and pertussis equivalent to full-term babies [8–10].

The dose of DTP vaccine is the same for preterm as for full-term babies. Half doses of vaccine should never be given. They are poorly immunogenic in preterm babies [11].

CARBOHYDRATE ANTIGENS

Bacterial polysaccharide carbohydrate antigens form the capsules of capsulated organisms such as *Haemophilus influenzae* type b (Hib), *Streptococcus pneumoniae*, *Neisseria meningitidis* and group B streptococcus. Although immunogenic to older children and adults, these polysaccharide (sugar) antigens are poor immunogens to children under 18–24 months old and particularly to babies. This largely explains the increased susceptibility of babies and infants to severe infections with capsulated organisms.

The reason for the poor response is that these are so-called T cell-independent antigens. The pioneering work of Porter Anderson from Rochester showed that conjugation of a carbohydrate antigen (the type b capsule or polyribosyl ribitol phosphate (PRP) of *H. influenzae* type b) to an immunogenic protein (diphtheria toxoid) converted the response into a T cell-dependent one. The conjugate vaccines stimulated antibody production to both PRP and diphtheria toxoid in babies as young as 2 months. Subsequently, other protein antigens, such as tetanus toxoid, have also been conjugated to PRP (PRP-T) and proved effective.

In most current immunization schedules in industrialized countries, Hib conjugate vaccines are routinely commenced at

2 months of age. There is an immediate antibody response to the first dose of PRP-outer membrane protein (PRP-OMP) vaccine, which is consequently preferred for groups at risk for early Hib disease, such as native Americans and Australian Aborigines. PRP-T and HbOC vaccines do not produce an antibody rise until after the second dose of vaccine.

Two doses of PRP-OMP vaccine at 2 and 4 months produced a reduced antibody response in preterm babies (median 28 weeks' gestation at birth) with chronic lung disease compared with well full-term babies [16] and in low birthweight babies [17]. However, even sick preterm babies still produced an antibody response sufficient to give short-term protection. Well preterm babies under 1000 g and under 29 weeks' gestation at birth produced a comparable response to full-term babies to a three-dose regimen of HbOC vaccine [7]. Preterm babies (27–36 weeks) had a reduced response after two doses but normal response after three doses of PRP-T vaccine [18].

It appears that the immune response of preterm babies is poor to PRP-OMP but is good to HbOC and PRP-T vaccines, and either of the latter two vaccines should be preferred.

If PRP-OMP Hib vaccine (Pedvax HIB) is used in a preterm baby, an additional dose of vaccine should be given at 6 months of age (i.e. doses should be given at 2, 4, 6 and 12 months of age) [13].

VIRAL VACCINES

POLIOVIRUS

Full-term neonates respond well to oral live attenuated poliovirus vaccine (OPV) given at birth, and indeed administration of OPV to newborns is recommended in non-industrialized countries. OPV stimulates both systemic and local gut mucosal immunity. Preterm babies respond normally to OPV commenced at 2 months' postnatal age [19].

OPV causes paralytic poliomyelitis in about 1 in 1 000 000 recipients and in occasional contacts. For this reason the USA has changed to giving killed vaccine (enhanced potency injectable polio vaccine or eIPV) for the first two doses followed by OPV for subsequent doses.

The incidence of vaccine-associated paralysis is increased about tenfold in hypogammaglobulinaemic subjects, and OPV is contraindicated for babies with possible or proven immune deficiency or who will be in close contact with immune deficient subjects; eIPV is given instead.

OPV spreads readily and is not recommended to be given to babies on neonatal units until after discharge. The rationale is a theoretical one: preterm babies have lower levels of maternal antibody and are immunologically immature, so might be at greater risk of vaccine-associated poliomyelitis. However, no cases of vaccine-induced disease in conjunction with nursery spread have ever been reported.

Well preterm babies respond normally to eIPV [20], although very low birthweight babies have a poor response to serotype 2 [7]. In contrast, sick preterm babies respond poorly to all three serotypes [21].

HEPATITIS B VACCINE

Full-term babies have an excellent response to hepatitis B vaccine, which is purified hepatitis B surface antigen (HBsAg). Indeed, the seroconversion rate for newborns given three doses at 0, 1 and 6 months is 95–99%, compared with about 90% for adults immunized with the same schedule [22].

Lau and co-workers found that babies with birthweight under 1750 g had a lower seroconversion rate and lower antibody response to hepatitis B vaccine than full-term babies [23]. The response of the preterm babies was improved if vaccine was delayed until they reached a weight of 2000 g (at about 30 days old) compared with immunization at birth or at a weight of 1000 g. Babies born to HBsAg-positive mothers were given hepatitis B immunoglobulin at birth as well as being immunized, and no baby became a chronic carrier [23].

For immunization of preterm babies against hepatitis B there are two options:

1. to give the first dose at birth, with additional doses at 1 month, 6 months and 12 months, preferably with measurement of antibody levels 1 month after the last dose; or
2. to delay vaccinating babies with birthweight less than 2000 g until 2 months of age, using a three-dose schedule (2, 3 and 8 months of age) and preferably measuring antibody levels after the third dose.

Preterm babies whose mothers are hepatitis B positive should be vaccinated according to option 1 and should also be given hepatitis B immunoglobulin. Option 2 may be preferred for low-risk babies, but there are no specific data in favour of this option.

HALF DOSES

Some carers have given half doses of vaccine to reduce the risk of side-effects or because preterm babies are so much smaller. Half doses of vaccines may not be immunogenic for preterm babies [11] and should never be given.

TEST DOSES

Test doses of vaccine to exclude allergy are never recommended and should not be given.

ADVERSE EVENTS

Preterm babies who have been discharged home do not have an increased rate of minor or serious adverse events following immunization [6]. However, about 20% of preterm babies on the neonatal unit will have apnoea or bradycardia within 24 hours of immunization, and although most episodes are minor and self-limiting, they may occasionally be more worrying [24]. The more premature babies with chronic lung disease are particularly likely to have apnoea or bradycardia.

This does not mean that immunization should be avoided in preterm babies. On the contrary, no babies came to harm, so immunization should be given to preterm hospitalized babies at 2 months' postnatal age, but they should have cardiorespiratory monitoring for 24–48 hours after each immunization [24]. Preterm babies who have been discharged home can safely be immunized.

SCHEDULE

A suggested immunization schedule is shown in Table 21.2. This is only a guide, and may need modifying depending on local immunization recommendations (most countries publish a book of immunization procedures via their Health Department or a specialist advisory body) and vaccine availability.

Age	BCG[a]	DTP	OPV	Hib conjugate (HbOC or PRP-T)	HepB[a] (see text)
Birth	T W S				T W
1 month					T W
2 months		T W S		T W S	S (2,3,8)
4 months		T W S		T W S	
6 months		T W S		T W S	T W
Delay until discharge			T W S		

T, Term baby; W, preterm well baby; S, preterm sick baby.
[a]If vaccine indicated.
NB: If mother is hepatitis B positive, then even preterm babies should be given hepatitis B vaccine as well as immunoglobulin at birth.

Table 21.2 Suggested immunization schedule for babies admitted to neonatal units

SUMMARY

- The immune response of neonates, including preterm babies, generally depends on postnatal antigen exposure and hence postnatal age.
- Preterm infants respond well to vaccines and well preterm babies can be immunized at the same postnatal age as full-term babies.

- Sick preterm babies respond less well to vaccines and may require a modified schedule.

- Half doses of vaccine should never be given; the dose for preterm babies is the same as for full-term babies.

- Some vaccines cannot be given at birth because they induce tolerance: the baby considers them to be 'self' antigens so the later immune response is impaired.

References

1 Colditz GA, Brewer TF, Berkey JES *et al.* Efficacy of BCG vaccine in the prevention of tuberculosis. *JAMA* 1994; **271**: 698–702.

2 Peterson JC & Peterson JC. Immunization in the young infant. Response to combined vaccines: I–IV. *Am J Dis Child* 1951; **81**: 484–91.

3 Provenzano RW, Wetterlow LH & Sullivan CL. Immunization and antibody response in the newborn infant. *N Engl J Med* 1965; **273**: 959–65.

4 Baraff LJ, Leake RD, Burstyn DG *et al.* Immunologic response to early and routine DTP immunization in infants. *Pediatrics* 1984; **73**: 37–42.

5 Lieberman JM, Greenberg DP, Wong VK *et al.* Effect of neonatal immunization with diphtheria and tetanus toxoids on antibody responses to *Haemophilus influenzae* type and conjugate vaccines. *J Pediatr* 1995; **126**: 198–205.

6 Ramsay ME, Miller E, Ashworth LAE, Coleman TJ, Rush M & Waight PA. Adverse events and antibody response to accelerated immunization in term and preterm infants. *Arch Dis Child* 1995; **72**: 230–2.

7 D'Angio CT, Maniscalco WM & Pichichero ME. Immunologic response of extremely premature infants to tetanus, *Haemophilus infleuzae* and polio immunizations. *Pediatrics* 1995; **96**: 18–22.

8 Bernbaum JC, Daft A, Anolik R *et al.* Response of preterm infants to diphtheria–tetanus–pertussis immunizations. *J Pediatr* 1985; **107**: 184–8.

9 Koblin BA, Townsend TR, Munoz A, Onorato I, Wilson M & Polk BF. Response of preterm infants to diphtheria–tetanus–pertussis vaccine. *Pediatr Infect Dis J* 1988; **7**: 704–11.

10 Pullan CR & Hull D. Routine immunization of preterm infants. *Arch Dis Child* 1989; **64**: 1438–41.

11 Bernbaum JC, Daft A, Samuelson J & Polin RA. Half-dose immunization for diphtheria, tetanus, pertussis: Response of preterm infants. *Pediatrics* 1989; **83**: 471–6.

12 Department of Health. *Immunisation Against Infectious Disease*. London: HMSO, 1996.

13 *The Australian Immunisation Procedures Handbook*, 6th edn. Canberra: NHMRC, 1997.

14 American Academy of Pediatrics. *Red Book: Report of the Committee on Infectious Diseases*, 24th edn. Elk Grove Village, IL: AAP, 1997.

15 Ministry of Health. *New Zealand Immunisation Guidelines*. Wellington: Ministry of Health, 1996.

16 Washburn LK, O'Shea M, Gillis DC, Block SM & Abramson JS. Response to *Haemophilus influenzae* type to conjugate vaccine in chronically ill premature infants. *J Pediatr* 1993; **123**: 791–4.

17 Munoz A, Salvador A, Brodsley NL, Arbeter AM & Porat R. Antibody response of low birth weight infants to *Haemophilus influenzae* type b polyribosylribitol phosphate outer membrane protein congugate vaccine. *Pediatrics* 1995; **96**: 216–19.

18 Kristensen K, Gyhrs A, Lausen B, Barington T & Heilmana C. Antibody response to *Haemophilus influenzae* type b capsular polysaccharide conjugated to tetanus toxoid in preterm infants. *Pediatr Infect Dis J* 1996; **15**: 525–9.

19 Smolen P, Bland R, Heiliejenstein E, Lawless MR, Dillard R & Abramson J. Antibody response to oral polio vaccine in premature infants. *J Pediatr* 1983; **103**: 917–19.

20 Adenyi-Jones SC, Faden H, Ferdon MB, Kwong MS & Ogra PL. Systemic and local immune responses to enhanced-potency inactivated poliovirus vaccine in premature and term infants. *J Pediatr* 1992; **120**: 686–9.

21 O'Shea TM, Dillard RG, Gillis DC & Abramson JS. Low rate of response to enhanced inactivated polio vaccine in preterm infants with chronic illness. *Clin Res Reg Affairs* 1993; **10**: 49–57.

22 McIntosh EDG. Immunization: hepatitis A and hepatitis B vaccines. In: Isaacs D & Moxon ER (eds) *A Practical Approach to Pediatric Infectious Diseases*. London: Churchill Livingstone, 1996: 571–7.

23 Lau Y-L, Tam AYC, Ng KW, Tsoi NS, Lam B, Lam P & Yeung CY. Response of preterm infants to hepatitis B vaccine. *J Pediatr* 1992; **121**: 962–5.

24 Botham SJ & Isaacs D. Incidence of apnoea and bradycardia in preterm infants following triple antigen immunization. *J Paediatr Child Health* 1994; **30**: 533–5.

22 | Neonatal care in non-industrialized countries

In non-industrialized countries, neonatal care is invariably compromised by lack of resources. The degree of compromise varies: in most such countries electricity supply cannot be guaranteed, oxygen is a luxury, and many antibiotics are unobtainable or only intermittently so. Under such conditions, babies cannot and probably should not be ventilated artificially.

Other aspects of neonatal care, notably prevention of infection, need an extremely high priority since optimal treatment of infection may not be possible.

ANTENATAL CARE

The first antenatal visit is an ideal time to examine the mother clinically, including for evidence of infection which will affect the baby, such as tuberculosis or sexually transmitted diseases. Ideally, blood should be taken for syphilis serology (see Chapter 14), a vaginal swab to look for bacterial vaginosis (Chapter 20) and a urine culture for bacteriuria (Chapter 20). One or more of these tests may not be available, but all of them identify conditions that can precipitate preterm labour and that are readily treatable with simple antibiotic regimens.

At this antenatal visit, women who are not up-to-date with their tetanus immunization should be commenced or continued on tetanus toxoid (with or without diphtheria toxoid) to try to prevent neonatal tetanus.

Follow-up antenatal visits are an opportunity to continue to check by history and examination for infectious diseases, which may be acquired later in the pregnancy. Antenatal attendance is improved by making clinics more accessible and by catering for the needs and wishes of pregnant women, rather than those of staff.

INTRAPARTUM ANTIBIOTICS

The use of parenteral antibiotics during labour has been shown to be effective in preventing neonatal sepsis and maternal morbidity from group B streptococcal (GBS) infection when used for colonized women with risk factors for sepsis [1]. GBS has traditionally been considered to be a rare cause of neonatal sepsis in non-industrialized countries, but has been described as the major early-onset pathogen in South Africa and parts of the West Indies, and of increasing importance in Malaysia (Chapters 1 and 8). It is too expensive and too impractical to screen for maternal GBS carriage in non-industrialized countries.

The use of intrapartum antibiotics (e.g. ampicillin 2 g i.v. stat, then 1 g 4-hourly, or penicillin G 5 mU stat, then 2.5 mU 4-hourly until delivery) should be strongly advocated for women with maternal risk factors (spontaneous preterm labour or preterm ruptured membranes <37 weeks' gestation, fever >37.5°C or prolonged rupture of the membranes >18 hours) in countries where GBS is known to be a major early-onset pathogen. The use of oral rather than parenteral antibiotics has not been studied.

If GBS is known from studies not to be a major pathogen in a country, there is no evidence that intrapartum antibiotics are helpful or harmful, and their use should be discretionary. If the local organisms are unknown, a similar situation prevails: a lack of data on which to base decisions. Nevertheless, extrapolation from GBS data would favour the use of intrapartum antibiotics (ampicillin, penicillin G or erythromycin) for women with risk factors for neonatal sepsis, if antibiotics can safely be given and are available.

HANDWASHING

There is no doubt that handwashing prevents nosocomial infections: Larson found 423 articles supporting the efficacy of handwashing [2]. It is the cheapest of interventions, since soap is virtually as effective as expensive proprietary antimicrobial solutions. Neonatal staff in industrialized countries are fair at washing their hands, but lapse when the workload increases [3]. Staff on paediatric wards or in paediatric intensive care units for older children are extremely poor at handwashing [4].

In non-industrialized countries, water is not always available. Sinks are scarce, and functioning sinks with functioning taps are scarcer still. Soap is often homemade and greasy. Towels are often dirty. Frequently, the distance from a patient's bed to the nearest sink is several hundred metres. When the wards are overflowing with patients, it is hardly surprising that handwashing is rarely practised at all, let alone well. Yet, if outbreaks of gastroenteritis and spread of resistant organisms are to be prevented, handwashing is essential.

What are the possible answers? Old-style physicians used to take a bowl of water, containing a disinfectant such as Dettol, with them on the ward trolley when doing ward rounds. This is a simple, cheap alternative. Although it is best suited to the ward round, bowls of disinfected water could be placed on wards at strategic points, such as non-functioning sinks, so that hands could be washed at other times.

Dirty towels negate handwashing. It is better to shake hands dry than to recontaminate them. In Port Moresby General Hospital, electric hand dryers have been installed, like those used in public washrooms. However, these depend on having electricity.

Where resources are limited, the importance of simple hygienic measures like handwashing to prevent infection cannot be overemphasized. A doctor working on a busy neonatal unit in a developing country asked us for advice on how to cope with their very high rate of nosocomial septicaemia with different Gram-negative organisms. After a period of observation and discussion with the staff, we pointed out that no-one washed their hands. 'We're too busy to wash our hands', we were told. Too busy doing septic screens on infected babies we thought, but were too polite to say. When handwashing improved on this unit, the incidence of infection fell sharply, and the staff became less busy.

BREASTFEEDING

There is little need to emphasize the advantages of breastfeeding in most non-industrialized countries. Breast milk is cheaper and cleaner than formula milk and gives much better protection against nosocomial infections, particularly those due to enteric organisms, and against necrotizing enterocolitis. Early administration of breast milk by breastfeeding or by gavage (tube) feeds saves lives.

There is surprisingly little objective evidence of the advantages of using breast milk to feed neonates in non-industrialized countries [5]. Relucio-Clavano described a dramatic reduction in the incidence of episodes of clinical sepsis and mortality from such episodes (Figure 22.1) and reduction in episodes of diarrhoea (Figure 22.2) after a programme to encourage use of breast milk by breastfeeding or gavage

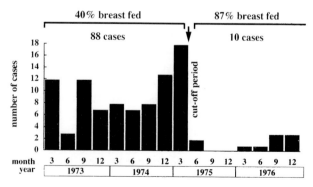

Figure 22.1 Effect of the introduction of a programme promoting breastfeeding on the incidence of clinical sepsis. There were 9886 infants in the study [6]

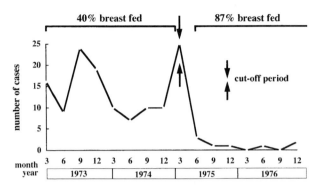

Figure 22.2 Effect of the introduction of programme promoting breastfeeding on the incidence of diarrhoea. There were 9886 infants in the study [6]

feeds was introduced [6]. There have been no controlled trials comparing breast milk and formula feeds in a neonatal unit in a non-industrialized country, and such a study might not be ethical.

Encouragement of the use of breast milk is a cheap, simple and probably highly effective means of reducing or preventing infections in neonatal units in non-industrialized countries.

RATIONAL ANTIBIOTIC USE

Antibiotics can be expensive and toxic. Simple cheap regimens should be used whenever possible. For early sepsis, penicillin or ampicillin and gentamicin can be obtained in most non-industrialized countries, and are appropriate whether Gram-negative organisms or group B streptococci predominate. Where drips can be used to give intravenous antibiotics, this is the preferable route, and the dosage regimens suggested in Appendix 2 are appropriate. If there are no butterfly needles available and intramuscular antibiotics have to be given, it is probably safe and a lot kinder to use once-daily gentamicin (4–6 mg/kg) for babies of any gestational age. There is insufficient evidence to recommend this for all newborns in industrialized countries, but good circumstantial evidence that it is safe.

Serum gentamicin levels are never measured in non-industrialized countries, yet worries about how to monitor levels are one of the main objections to once-daily daily dosing for term babies. It seems reasonable to recommend once-daily i.m. gentamicin in preference to thrice-daily i.m. gentamicin for babies in non-industrialized countries.

For late-onset sepsis, regimens will vary depending on availability and the nature and sensitivities of organisms causing sepsis. An antibiotic like chloramphenicol, which is now virtually never used in industrialized countries, may be all that is available. Chloramphenicol is cheap, better absorbed orally than other antibiotics (although the oral route is rarely indicated), and has activity against staphylococci and many other Gram-positive, as well as Gram-negative, organisms. Care must be taken with dosing of chloramphenicol since most cases of 'grey baby syndrome' are caused by overdosing [7].

Resistant organisms can readily be selected by prolonged antibiotic use, and are a common problem in neonatal units in non-industrialized countries, even those that do not artificially ventilate babies. To avoid this problem, it is important that antibiotics are stopped early when sepsis has been excluded or seems unlikely. It is not always possible to rely on blood cultures, either because blood was not taken prior to antibiotics, was not taken at all, did not reach the laboratory, or the lab is unreliable. A single-surface culture, e.g. an ear swab, may help in suspected early sepsis: if negative, it makes sepsis far less likely. However, if cultures are unavailable or unreliable, then decisions will have to be clinical.

For proven or strongly suspected sepsis, antibiotics should be given for the duration suggested in Chapter 6, not longer. For uncomplicated septicaemia without meningitis, 7 days of antibiotics usually suffice. Longer courses increase the risk of toxicity and of selecting for resistant organisms.

In general, follow the 'Start early, stop early' rule on antibiotic use.

UMBILICAL CORD CARE

Staphylococcal skin sepsis, often leading on to bone, joint and other systemic infections, is a major problem in some countries. Umbilical cord care is an important way to prevent such infection. Gentian violet is cheap, and has the advantage that it is instantly apparent whether or not cord care has been applied.

EYE CARE

Routine eye prophylaxis is not usually used in non-industrialized countries, as Credé's silver nitrate is too expensive. Povidone–iodine is an inexpensive alternative which has been proven to be effective in preventing ophthalmia neonatorum in Kenya [8] and is more effective than silver nitrate or erythromycin ointment in preventing *Chlamydia trachomatis* infection.

MOTHER AND BABY UNITS

At the Aga Khan University, Karachi, very low birthweight (VLBW) infants represent 1.5% of all live births, and 65% of them survive. In order to reduce the disproportionate care and time required by these babies, and to reduce their high rate of nosocomial sepsis, a mother and baby unit was opened in 1993. The purpose of this unit was to involve mothers in the active care of their babies, including breastfeeding and spoonfeeding babies to reduce the need for parenteral feeding and to encourage early discharge from hospital [9]. The outcome, shown in Figure 22.3, included a substantial reduction in nosocomial sepsis without any increase in mortality or morbidity rates.

SICK STAFF

Neonatal units are traditionally short-staffed. When a member of staff becomes unwell, they often feel obligated to their colleagues to continue working. If they initiate an outbreak of

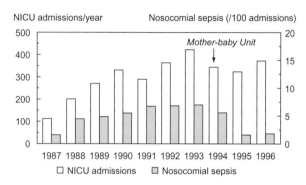

Figure 22.3 Reduction of nosocomial sepsis associated with the opening of a mother and baby unit at the Aga Khan University Hospital, Karachi [9]

infection, particularly gastroenteritis, their courage and loyalty will have been misguided. In general, staff should not work if they are sick, and should return only when they have recovered.

SPECIAL CONSIDERATIONS

Depending on local conditions, babies may be born with congenital tuberculosis or congenital malaria or may acquire malaria as a nosocomial infection (see Chapter 14). These organisms should be considered in the differential diagnosis of congenital infection and early-onset sepsis. Nosocomial malaria can be prevented by keeping mosquitoes out of the neonatal unit as much as possible, or by using bed-nets.

ANCILLARY CARE: TEMPERATURE REGULATION

Temperature regulation is an important consideration, particularly where babies are in danger of cold exposure, but to a lesser extent when high temperatures prevail. Cold damage has been shown to be closely associated with poor neonatal outcome, and, because enzymes function poorly at low temperatures, hypothermia can result in sepsis [10–12]. Babies in tropical countries are not immune to cold damage. Delivery is the main time of risk: wet babies rapidly become cold, particularly if they are growth-retarded, and should be dried quickly. The ambient temperature may fall enough at night in the tropics to pose a threat. In some parts of the world, the night temperature may fall to freezing point or below, and babies will die unless kept warm. Electrical incubators may not be available, or may break down from age and lack of engineers to maintain them. Alternative heat sources, such as lamps and even candles, are sometimes used to heat incubators. Whatever the methods used, it should be remembered that maintenance of the ambient temperature is an important and relatively simple way of preventing infections and poor outcome.

IMMUNIZATIONS

In non-industrialized countries, babies are given hepatitis B vaccine, BCG vaccine and oral polio vaccine at birth (see Chapter 21). Although OPV is not recommended for babies in neonatal units in industrialized countries, because of theoretical risks of spread to very preterm babies, in non-industrialized countries the wish to ensure immunity to poliovirus rightly over-rides such theoretical concerns.

SUMMARY

- At the first antenatal visit, the following should be performed, if possible:
  (a) blood for syphilis serology,
  (b) vaginal swab for bacterial vaginosis,
  (c) urine culture for bacteriuria, and
  (d) immunization against tetanus if not up-to-date.
- Intrapartum antibiotics, ampicillin, penicillin or erythromycin, are indicated for women in spontaneous preterm labour, or with fever >37.5°C, or with prolonged membrane rupture >18 hours, or with offensive liquor.

- Handwashing should be enforced, not just encouraged; soap and/or water bowls containing disinfectant must be available and be used before and after each baby contact.

- Breast milk, by breast or gavage (tube) feeds, reduces nosocomial infections and NEC.

- Antibiotics should be started early, but stopped early.

- Umbilical cord care reduces staphylococcal sepsis.

- Eye care with povidone–iodine reduces ophthalmia neonatorum.

- Staff who are unwell should not work.

- Mosquitoes should be kept out of the nursery or bed-nets should be used.

- Cold damage should be avoided by drying newborns rapidly after delivery and regulating ambient temperatures.

- Babies should be immunized at birth with hepatitis B vaccine, BCG and OPV.

References

1 Boyer KM & Gotoff SP. Prevention of early-onset neonatal group B streptococcal disease with selective intrapartum chemoprophylaxis. *N Engl J Med* 1986; **314**: 1665–9.

2 Larson E. A causal link between handwashing and risk of infection? Examination of the evidence. *Infect Control Hosp Epidemiol* 1988; **9**: 28–36.

3 Isaacs D, Catterson J, Hope PL *et al.* Factors influencing colonisation with gentamicin resistant Gram negative organisms in the neonatal unit. *Arch Dis Child* 1988; **63**: 533–5.

4 Tibballs J. Teaching hospital medical staff to handwash. *Med J Aust* 1996; **164**: 395–8.

5 Tan JCH & Jeffery HE. Factors that influence the choice of infant feeding. *J Paediatr Child Health* 1995; **31**: 375–8.

6 Relucio-Clavano N. The results of a change in hospital practices. A paediatrician's campaign for breast-feeding in the Philippines. *Assignment Children* 1981; **55/56**: 139–61.

7 Mulhall A, de Louvois J & Hurley R. Efficacy of chloramphenicol in the treatment of neonatal and infantile meningitis: a study of 70 cases. *Lancet* 1983; **i**: 284–7.

8 Isenberg SJ, Apt L & Wood MA. A controlled trial of povidone–iodine as prophylaxis against ophthalmia neonatorum. *N Engl J Med* 1995; **332**: 562–6.

9 Bhutto ZA, Yusuf K & Islam S. Survival and outcome of very low birth weight infants in a developing country: how feasible is early discharge? *Proceedings of the Royal College of Paediatrics and Child Health 1st Annual Meeting* 1997; **1**: 72, G 109.

10 Dagan R & Gorodischer R. Infections in hypothermic infants younger than 3 months old. *Am J Dis Child* 1984; **138**: 483.

11 Johnason RB, Spencer SA, Rolfe P *et al.* Effect of post-delivery care on neonatal body temperature. *Acta Paediatr* 1992; **81**: 859.

12 El-Radhy AS, Jawad M, Mansor N *et al.* Sepsis and hypothermia in the newborn infant: value of gastric aspirate examination. *J Pediatr* 1983; **104**: 300.

23 | Clinical pharmacology

INTRODUCTION

Neonates have been called 'therapeutic orphans' by Shirkey [1] because of the paucity of data on which their treatment is usually based. In the 1950s they were poisoned with chloramphenicol, which resulted in cardiovascular collapse – the 'grey baby syndrome' [2] – and with sulphonamides, which displaced albumin-bound bilirubin and resulted in kernicterus [3]. Although neonates are no longer treated therapeutically as miniaturized adults, nevertheless new drugs, including antibiotics, are introduced too often without adequate clinical trials. Pharmacokinetic data in preterm babies under 28 weeks' gestation are virtually absent. The few available studies show that absorption, distribution, protein binding, biotransformation and excretion of drugs by preterm babies differ significantly from that in older children. The metabolism and renal excretion of several drugs is initially poor, although it improves rapidly in the first month [4]. We believe that new antibiotics should be subjected to large-scale comparative trials in neonates before widespread use. Until such data on safety and efficacy are available, it is generally wise to be conservative. We, therefore, prefer to use antibiotics for which there is considerable experience, even if these drugs have known dose-related toxicity, as is the case for aminoglycosides.

MATERNAL ANTIBIOTICS

If the pregnant mother is treated with antibiotics which cross the placenta, the fetus is given antibiotics antenatally. This can be used therapeutically: passage of the drug across the placenta can treat the fetus, as in the treatment of maternal syphilis to prevent congenital syphilis. Treatment of the mother may prevent neonatal infection, as in intrapartum administration of ampicillin to prevent early-onset group B steptococcal (GBS) sepsis [5]. However, drugs administered to the pregnant woman can also cause untoward effects on the fetus. Tetracyclines readily cross the placenta and are deposited in fetal bone [6], resulting in impaired bone growth [7]. They are also deposited in the deciduous teeth of the fetus, resulting in later discoloration, enamel hypoplasia and malformation [8].

Nitrofurantoin, nalidixic acid and sulphonamides can cause haemolysis if the fetus has glucose-6-phosphate dehydrogenase (G6PD) deficiency and sulphonamides may displace bilirubin, causing hyperbilirubinaemia and possibly kernicterus [3]. Chloramphenicol given to the mother near parturition may cause neonatal circulatory collapse [2]. Aminoglycosides can be ototoxic to the developing fetus: streptomycin can definitely damage the eighth nerve [9,10], while kanamycin [11,12] and gentamicin [13] are potentially ototoxic.

Most antibiotics do not attain sufficient concentrations in breast milk to be toxic to the breastfed baby. However, tetracyclines should be avoided for lactating mothers because they may stain the baby's teeth, and sulphonamides [14] and nalidixic acid [15] have caused haemolysis in breastfed babies with G6PD deficiency. The AAP Committee on Drugs recommends stopping breastfeeding 12–24 hours before a woman is started on metronidazole [16].

ABSORPTION

Enteral administration of antibiotics is not generally recommended in the newborn period because of poor absorption. For example, serum levels of ampicillin 1 hour after oral administration of a 25 mg/kg dose to full-term infants were 2.6–7.2 µg/mL [17] compared with about 60 µg/ml 1 hour after thesame dose given i.v. [18,19], while oral nafcillin achieves blood levels about one-third of those with i.m. injection [20]. However, if the oral antibiotic achieves levels greatly in excess of the minimum inhibitory concentration (MIC) of the organism, and the response to treatment can be closely monitored, then enteral administration is a reasonable option. Infants of very low birthweight have erratic absorption of enteral drugs and poor muscle bulk for i.m. injection, so i.v. administration of antibiotics is almost always indicated [21].

ADMINISTRATION

Although relatively small doses of antibiotics are appropriate for neonates, antibiotics are often available only in vials for adult use, which require diluting. This can result in critical errors: in the study by Mulhall and colleagues, severe toxicity from chloramphenicol occurred due to errors in calculating the dilution factor [22].

Even when the manufacturers produce a neonatal formulation, this is calculated as an appropriate dose for a full-term infant, but the dose for an infant of very low birthweight may be considerably lower; either a very small volume has to be given or the antibiotic must be diluted.

Antibiotics are usually administered to neonates i.v. in small volumes and cannot be diluted too much, or flushed through too vigorously, because of the low total feed volume, the need for calories and the danger of over-hydration; delivery systems must therefore minimize dead space in syringes and tubing [23].

In non-industrialized countries, i.v. administration of antibiotics can be a problem: one colleague described i.v. lines as flowing either at maximum or not at all. This colleague is a strong advocate of the use of once-daily i.m. gentamicin, which is cheap, relatively safe, and avoids problems with i.v. infusions.

DISTRIBUTION

Antibiotics will become distributed in body tissues; the body can be considered as compartments comprising water, fat and protein. Hydrophilic drugs will distribute preferentially to the water compartment, hydrophobic drugs to fat, and heavily protein-bound drugs to protein. In the full-term newborn, water comprises about 75% of body weight, with extracellular water about 40% of body weight. At 28 weeks' gestation, however, total water is about 85% and extracellular water about 65% of body weight. After birth, total body water falls by up to 15% within 5 days [21].

Body fat is about 13% by weight of a full-term infant, but only 4% of a 1500-g baby and 1% of a 500-g baby. However, feeding leads to a rapid accretion of fat which comprises up to 30% of the baby's weight gain.

These variations in body composition indicate the difficulty in predicting drug disposition and the need for repeated assessments of serum levels of toxic drugs such as aminoglycosides.

PROTEIN BINDING

Many drugs are bound to serum proteins such as albumin, but the biological significance of this is uncertain. For example, although it is often stated that protein-bound antibiotics have little or no antibacterial activity, dicloxacillin is 98% protein bound, yet is no less effective than methicillin, which is 37% bound [24]. Sulphonamides [3] and some of the third-generation cephalosporins [25] bind avidly to albumin, will displace bilirubin from binding sites and potentially can cause hyperbilirubinaemia.

The serum albumin level is lower in full-term infants than later in childhood, and lower still in preterm infants. The resulting increase in unbound drug may result in greater therapeutic efficacy and toxicity. Serum protein levels rise with nutrition and with transfusions of blood or plasma.

METABOLISM

The liver is the main organ involved in metabolism of antibiotics, by way of microsomal enzyme systems. Non-synthetic hepatic biotransformation reactions, hydrolysis, hydroxylation, oxidation and reduction are all diminished in newborn compared with older children [21]. Of the synthetic biotransformation reactions, conjugation to glucuronide, which is the commonest conjugation pathway, is poor in neonates, whereas conjugation to sulphate and glycine is 'normal'. Oxidation and glucuronidation are the two metabolic pathways in which neonatal function is lowest compared with older children and adults. After 2–12 weeks, hepatic metabolism becomes more efficient. Lower doses of chloramphenicol are needed in neonates because of slow maturation in glucuronidation: the glucuronide form is inactive.

EXCRETION

Drugs are excreted mainly by the kidneys or in the bile; the former is the most important route of excretion and the better studied. Renal excretion of drugs is mediated by filtration by the glomeruli and by reabsorption and secretion by the renal tubules. The glomerular filtration rate (GFR) at term is about 25% of the adult value, and at 28 weeks' gestation is about 15% [26,27]. The GFR increases rapidly within 3 days of birth, but remains relatively low in preterm infants; it increases over several weeks and is directly related to postconceptional age [28].

Drugs such as the aminoglycosides and vancomycin, which are excreted by glomerular filtration, should therefore be given less frequently the more immature the baby. The GFR doubles by 2 weeks of age in term infants and dose intervals can be reduced, but this may not be appropriate for babies of very low birthweight [21].

Tubular reabsorption and secretion have been less well studied than GFR. Penicillins may be cleared slowly because their excretion depends on tubular secretion, which matures slower than GFR [29]. However, tubular reabsorption is also low in neonates and some antibiotics may be excreted more rapidly. Weak bases are likely to be excreted quicker, particularly by preterm infants, because acidification of the urine is relatively poor. Biliary excretion has not been intensively studied in neonates. Bile stasis is a recognized complication of total parenteral nutrition and also occurs in babies of very low birthweight. Drugs or metabolites excreted through bile might be expected to accumulate in babies with bile stasis.

SPECIFIC DRUGS

For dosage schedules, refer to the end of this chapter.

PENICILLINS

Penicillins interfere with bacterial cell wall mucopeptide synthesis, and block the cross-linking reaction which gives the bacterial peptidoglycan its rigidity. They bind to bacteria through penicillin-binding proteins in the cell wall. Gram-positive organisms exposed to β-lactam antibiotics (penicillins and cephalosporins) release lipoteichoic acid from the cell wall and this apparently contributes to cell lysis. If the concentration of antibiotic is increased above a critical level, there is a reduced bactericidal effect *in vitro* on Gram-positive organisms (the Eagle phenomenon); the relevance of this *in vivo* is unknown.

Penicillins are actively excreted by the renal tubules. The serum half-life is 5–6 hours in healthy newborn preterm babies and 2 hours in full-term babies over 1 week old.

Organisms are inherently resistant to penicillins if the structure of their cell wall differs from the classical structure, as in the case of mycobacteria.

Staphylococci, many Gram-negative bacilli and gonococci can produce β-lactamases which degrade the β-lactam ring common to all penicillins, which Greenwood has called their Achilles' heel [30]. Coliforms may also produce acylases, which have variable action against penicillins and cephalosporins. Resistance of pneumococci to penicillin is mediated by altered penicillin-binding proteins, not by β-lactamase production. Both Gram-positive and Gram-negative bacteria may be inhibited, but not killed, by β-lactam antibiotics: these 'persisters' will multiply when the antibiotic is stopped. Tolerance to penicillins, the phenomenon of inhibition greatly exceeding killing, is exhibited by some strains of staphylococci and streptococci. However, these phenomena which occur *in vitro* are of uncertain clinical significance.

Penicillin is the antibiotic of choice for infections attributable to group B streptococci, sensitive pneumococci, and most other streptococci. It is the only effective treatment for congenital syphilis. Penicillin G is also active against *Listeria*, although there is more experience with ampicillin. It is active against most anaerobes except *Bacteroides fragilis*.

Penicillin G is poorly absorbed when given orally. After parenteral administration, the half-life is inversely correlated with birthweight and postnatal age: in the first week after birth the half-life of aqueous (crystalline) penicillin G is 1.5 hours at term, but 10 hours in babies weighing <1500 g [24]. Procaine penicillin G produces serum levels >25 times the MIC of group B streptococci, 24 hours after a dose of 50 000 units/kg has been given to a full-term infant less than 1 week old [31]. The clearance of penicillin increases with increasing postnatal age. Benzathine penicillin G gives peak concentrations 12–24 hours after a single dose and serum levels are still equal to the MIC of group B streptococcus after 12 days [24]. There is evidence *in vitro*, but none *in vivo*, of synergy between penicillin and aminoglycosides.

Penicillin G does not penetrate well into the CSF, even if the baby has bacterial meningitis. Peak CSF levels are 2–5% of serum levels, but still exceed 50 times the MIC of group B streptococci. The recommended daily dose for group B streptococcal meningitis is 150 000–250 000 units/kg (see Appendix 2).

Ampicillin

Ampicillin is more active *in vitro* than penicillin G against enterococci (faecal streptococci), *Listeria monocytogenes* and some Gram-negative organisms, e.g. *Escherichia coli*, *Proteus*, *Salmonella*. On the other hand, penicillin G is more active *in vitro* than ampicillin against group B streptococcus and other streptococci (pneumococcus, group A streptococcus), although ampicillin is clinically effective.

Oral absorption of ampicillin is fairly good in well, full-term babies, achieving serum levels 2–24 times lower than after parenteral administration [17,20]. Amoxycillin achieves higher levels. There is little information on oral absorption of ampicillin by sick and preterm babies, to whom oral medications should not be given. CSF penetration of ampicillin is slightly better than that of penicillin G, particularly if the meninges are inflamed.

Ampicillin is actively excreted in the urine, and the half-life falls from 6 hours to 2 hours over the first 10 days after birth.

The advantage of ampicillin over penicillin G for empirical therapy of suspected early-onset sepsis is its somewhat broader spectrum. This is also a disadvantage, as ampicillin is more likely to select for colonization with *Candida* and Gram-negative enteric organisms [32]. Oral ampicillin can cause diarrhoea, which is less commonly seen following parenteral administration. Ampicillin very occasionally causes rashes in neonates. Mild blood eosinophilia may develop.

Anti-staphylococcal penicillins

The anti-staphylococcal penicillins are semi-synthetic penicillins with a side-chain that protects against binding of β-lactamases. Flucloxacillin and cloxacillin have been widely used in the UK, but there are no pharmacokinetic data for their use in neonates. Flucloxacillin is better absorbed enterally than cloxacillin by older children and adults. Oral nafcillin gives serum levels about one-third of those after intramuscular use [20]. Oxacillin and methicillin are very poorly absorbed enterally and are only given parenterally.

The pharmacokinetics of methicillin, oxacillin and nafcillin are similar to those of penicillin G in terms of half-life, increased clearance after the first postnatal week and with increasing postnatal age, and decreased clearance with lower birthweight [33]. The anti-staphylococcal agents all achieve CSF levels about 1.4–2% of serum levels when administered parenterally to rabbits with experimental meningitis [34]. There are no data on CSF penetration in neonates.

The anti-staphylococcal penicillins are active against sensitive *Staphylococcus aureus* and coagulase-negative staphylococci. They also have good activity against most penicillin-sensitive organisms such as streptococci, so it is not usually necessary to prescribe penicillin and flucloxacillin simultaneously. They have poor activity against *Treponema pallidum* and against anaerobes. Some strains of staphylococci are found to be 'tolerant' *in vitro,* in that the minimum bactericidal concentration (MBC) greatly exceeds the MIC. Although this suggests that organisms might be inhibited but not killed by flucloxacillin, there is little evidence to suggest that resistance attributable to tolerance is a significant clinical problem, except perhaps in endocarditis. On the other hand, multiply resistant strains of *S. aureus* and *S. epidermidis* that are resistant to anti-staphylococcal penicillins are an increasing problem (Chapter 14). Studies *in vitro* suggest synergy between anti-staphylococcal penicillins and aminoglycosides, but the only clinical evidence is that *S. aureus* bacteraemia due to endocarditis in adult drug addicts resolves more quickly with nafcillin and gentamicin than with nafcillin alone [35].

There is little toxicity with these drugs. Very occasionally they may cause neutropenia and drug eruptions. Oral use can cause diarrhoea. The severe hepatotoxicity of flucloxacillin described in elderly adults is not seen in neonates.

Other penicillins

Ticarcillin, the thienyl variant of carbenicillin, and the ureido-penicillins, azlocillin, mezlocillin and piperacillin, are the only penicillins with significant anti-pseudomonal activity.

CEPHALOSPORINS

The cephalosporins are antibiotics derived from cephalosporin C, which itself is a natural product of the *Cephalosporium* mould. Although they contain a β-lactam ring, they are relatively resistant to the action of β-lactamases. Their main mode of action is by interfering with bacterial cell wall synthesis.

Cephalosporin C was never marketed. The 'first generation' of cephalosporins, cephalothin and cephaloridine, were susceptible to Gram-negative β-lactamases, had variable nephrotoxicity and have been superseded for the treatment of systemic infections. The 'second-generation' cephalosporins include cefuroxime and cefoxitin, which are scarcely used in neonatal infections. They are more stable to β-lactamases and have a broad spectrum of activity against staphylococci, streptococci and some Gram-negative organisms. The 'third-generation' cephalosporins, however, are almost completely stable to β-lactamases. They have a broad spectrum of activity, although they are not the antibiotics of choice for staphylococcal or streptococcal infections. Cefotaxime is widely used in neonatal infections, but is inactive against *Pseudomonas*. Ceftazidime has by far the best anti-pseudomonal activity of the cephalosporins, but is less active against many coliforms. Ceftriaxone has the longest half-life, but can displace bilirubin from albumin *in vitro* [25] and is not recommended in neonates.

Moxalactam is strictly an oxacephem, having an oxygen instead of a sulphur in its ring. It has more activity against anaerobes. It, too, can displace albumin-bound bilirubin, but also interferes with vitamin K metabolism and can cause bleeding, which is a major drawback for preterm babies who are at risk of intraventricular haemorrhage, so is no longer used. Cef-tizoxime and cefmenoxime are similar to cefotaxime, but rarely used. Cefoperazone has anti-pseudomonal activity, but its activity against other organisms is otherwise less than that of cefotaxime. The cephalosporins have no activity against *Listeria* or enterococci (faecal streptococci) and should, therefore, not be used as sole agents (monotherapy) for empirical treatment of early or late neonatal sepsis.

The third-generation cephalosporins have excellent CSF penetration, even in the absence of meningeal inflammation [36]; when meningitis is present, the CSF level is 10–30% of serum levels for moxalactam [37] and 27–63% for cefotaxime [38]. However, they have not had the anticipated dramatic effect on morbidity and mortality of bacterial meningitis [39].

The second- and third-generation cephalosporins are safe and generally well tolerated by neonates, with the exceptions already outlined regarding bilirubin displacement and interference with vitamin K metabolism leading to hypoprothrombinaemia. Renal toxicity has not been a significant problem for neonates. Drug levels do not need to be monitored, which is a significant advantage. Some workers have found that rapid selection of cephalosporin-resistant organisms occurs after the introduction of third-generation cephalosporins [40], whereas others have used them for years without selection of resistant strains [41]: the difference may be in the duration of antibiotic 'courses' used in the institutions.

Excessive use of third-generation cephalosporins may encourage the selection of extended-spectrum β-lactamase-producing coliforms.

VANCOMYCIN

Vancomycin is a complex heterocyclic molecule classified as a glycopeptide antibiotic, and unrelated to the aminoglycosides. The molecule is too large to penetrate Gram-negative bacteria and vancomycin is active only against Gram-positive bacteria. Vancomycin was originally used in the 1950s to treat penicillin-resistant staphylococci and gained a reputation for toxicity. This was largely attributable to impurities, which have now been removed. It was reintroduced in 1978 because of the rise in methicillin-resistant *Staphylococcus aureus* (MRSA). It acts by interfering with cell wall synthesis and inhibiting RNA synthesis. It is excreted renally and is not metabolized.

Vancomycin is active against *S. aureus* and coagulase-negative staphylococci, streptococci and Gram-positive anaerobes, including *Clostridium difficile*, but not Gram-negative organisms. It is currently the treatment of choice for infections with methicillin-resistant strains of *S. aureus* and *S. epidermidis*. It is not absorbed orally, and can be given enterally to treat staphylococcal enterocolitis and *C. difficile* diarrhoea. When given parenterally, it must be infused slowly over at least 30 min, because faster infusions can cause a diffuse erythema over the head and upper trunk, the 'red man syndrome'. This is due to histamine release, not allergy, and is an erythroderma rather than a true rash. If a diffuse erythema does develop, it can be abolished by slowing the infusion rate. Vancomycin is potentially nephrotoxic and ototoxic, and drug levels must be monitored.

CSF levels are 10–15% of serum levels in shunt infections with mild inflammation [42]. Vancomycin can be given into a ventricular reservoir (such as a Rickham reservoir) in severe or persistent shunt infections, but may itself cause a chemical ventriculitis. Its use should be limited to proven infections because of the risk of selecting vancomycin-resistant enterococci.

TEICOPLANIN

Teicoplanin is a glycopeptide antibiotic developed in Europe. It has similar antibacterial activity to vancomycin. It is active against Gram-positive anaerobes, particularly *Clostridium* species, most *Listeria*, most enterococci and staphylococci, including methicillin-resistant strains, but is more bacteriostatic than bactericidal.

There is no cross-resistance with vancomycin, but resistance to teicoplanin is emerging. In one study, only 70% of coagulase-negative staphylococci were sensitive to teicoplanin [43].

Teicoplanin needs to be given only once daily, unlike vancomycin, and also unlike vancomycin can be given intramuscularly. It cannot be given by mouth. Relatively few side-effects have been described. Leucopenia, thrombocytopenia and abnormal liver functions have been described [44], but nephrotoxicity and ototoxicity may be less common than with vancomycin.

AMINOGLYCOSIDES

The first aminoglycoside, streptomycin, was discovered in 1943. Since then, various related antibiotics have been described: the main glycosides with 'mycin' (e.g. kanamycin) come from the mould *Streptomyces*, while those with 'micin' (e.g. gentamicin) come from the mould *Micromonospora* species. The exact mode of action is uncertain: streptomycin acts by binding to a ribosomal protein, whereas the other aminoglycosides appear to alter the bacterial messenger RNA, causing production of defective proteins [30].

The main activity of aminoglycosides is against Gram-negative organisms. However, their weak activity against staphylococci and streptococci may be clinically important because they act synergistically, at least *in vitro*, with penicillins.

Resistance to aminoglycosides is mainly attributable to plasmid-mediated enzymes which interfere with drug transport into the bacteria. Bacteria with resistance to one aminoglycoside due to a plasmid may be resistant also to one or more of the other aminoglycosides.

If an organism resistant to only one aminoglycoside is selected by antibiotic pressure and is causing sepsis, the resistant organism can often be eradicated by changing the antibiotic policy to use a different aminoglycoside [45,46].

There is relatively little evidence of significant nephrotoxicity and ototoxicity in neonates [47], even in babies accidentally overdosed with gentamicin [48], and neonates may be relatively resistant to toxic effects of aminoglycosides. Combinations of aminoglycosides, e.g. tobramycin and gentamicin, or amikacin and gentamicin, are more toxic to the vestibular nerve than is single-drug therapy [49]. Gentamicin accumulates in the body of neonates (mainly in the kidneys) even if serum levels are kept within the recommended ranges, as it does in adults, particularly when treatment is for more than 7 days [50]. Thus, it is advisable to stop aminoglycosides as early as possible. For example, if an aminoglycoside is being used for its synergistic activity with penicillin to treat babies with GBS sepsis, the aminoglycoside should be stopped when the baby shows sustained improvement, and certainly by 7 days. Frusemide can potentiate aminoglycoside toxicity and other drugs should be used in preference to aminoglycosides if frusemide is prescribed.

Monitoring of serum aminoglycoside levels has been strongly recommended for all babies receiving these antibiotics. Buchanan has advocated a more selective approach because of their low toxicity to neonates [47]. He suggests measuring levels only in certain high-risk situations: these include babies with renal dysfunction, babies responding poorly to therapy for a sensitive organism, babies on prolonged therapy, babies receiving two aminoglycosides simultaneously, and babies also receiving frusemide. Babies weighing <1500 g should also be included because their renal immaturity and variable fluid balance result in unpredictable aminoglycoside pharmacokinetics [33]. Indeed, most paediatricians would routinely monitor aminoglycoside levels in all babies requiring therapy for longer than 48 hours. Such monitoring would involve a trough level just before and a peak level 1 hour after the third or fourth dose of the aminoglycoside.

There is increasing use of once-daily aminoglycosides in adults and children, which is effective because of their significant 'post-antibiotic effect' and the fact that toxicity appears to relate not to high peak levels, but to the area under the curve [51]. Monitoring of aminoglycoside levels given once daily involves a level 1 hour and some 4–8 hours later to calculate the area under the curve.

Gentamicin, netilmicin, amikacin and tobramycin are widely used in neonates. There is relatively little to choose between them: tobramycin has more activity against *Pseudomonas*, whereas amikacin is preferred for *Serratia* infections. They are poorly absorbed enterally and are administered i.m., by slow i.v. injection or by i.v. infusion. Intravenous boluses are not recommended because of the possibility of very high levels being toxic. CSF penetration is poor, even in meningitis, yet the combination of ampicillin and an aminoglycoside has proved as effective as any other drug regimen so far tested in treating Gram-negative enteric meningitis. Aminoglycosides given by lumbar or intraventricular injection do not improve the outcome in bacterial meningitis, but aminoglycosides are often given into intraventricular reservoirs in persistent shunt infections, a practice that has not been critically evaluated. Aminoglycosides have been given orally as prophylaxis against necrotizing enterocolitis (see Chapter 13) but there is heavy selection for resistant organisms, so their use is discouraged.

CHLORAMPHENICOL

Chloramphenicol is a naturally occurring antibiotic produced by a *Streptomyces* strain, but can also readily be synthesized. Pro-drugs, inactive in themselves, but metabolized to chloramphenicol, are used to overcome problems with pure chloramphenicol: the succinate is soluble, unlike the pure drug, and can be used for injection, while the palmitate and stearate are less bitter for oral use.

Chloramphenicol inhibits bacterial protein synthesis competitive inhibition with messenger RNA for binding sites on the ribosome. Its spectrum includes most Gram-positive and Gram-negative bacteria. Although it is bacteriostatic for most enterobacteria, it is bactericidal for many other organisms. It has excellent CSF penetration and has been used extensively to treat bacterial meningitis. There are three main drawbacks to its use in the neonatal period. The first is its propensity to cause the 'grey baby syndrome' [2]. This condition, which can affect full-term as well as preterm babies, presents as vomiting, respiratory distress, poor feeding, abdominal distension and loose green stools. If chloramphenicol is continued, the babies develop circulatory collapse, becoming grey, poorly perfused and hypothermic, followed by death [36].

The second problem is that chloramphenicol levels are very unpredictable at standard doses and are greatly affected by concomitant use of phenytoin, which increases serum levels of chloramphenicol, and phenobarbitone, which reduces them. This is because chloramphenicol is metabolized by glucuronidation, and glucuronyl transferase is affected by these drugs. The third problem is that most coliforms are inhibited, but not killed, by chloramphenicol.

Additional problems are dose-related marrow suppression, mainly causing anaemia. Drug levels should be closely monitored if chloramphenicol is used in the neonatal period.

The reality of chloramphenicol use is that significant toxicity still occurs, despite wide recognition of the possible adverse effects [22]. There are far safer and probably more effective antibiotics than chloramphenicol for treating neonatal meningitis, and chloramphenicol should now only ever be used in exceptional circumstances.

ERYTHROMYCIN

Erythromycin is one of the macrolide antibiotics (named for their macrocyclic lactone ring) produced by a strain of *Streptomyces*. Erythromycin base is degraded by stomach acid and oral preparations are either enteric-coated (stearate) or are esters (erythromycin ethylsuccinate and estolate) which act as pro-drugs metabolized to active erythromycin. Erythromycin lactobionate and gluceptate are the intravenous preparations.

Erythromycin interferes with bacterial protein synthesis. It is active against Gram-positive organisms, including many penicillinase-producing staphylococci, and against mycoplasmas and ureaplasmas. It is also the drug of choice for chlamydial infections and for prophylaxis and treatment of *Bordetella pertussis* infections. Most Gram-negative organisms are not susceptible to erythromycin.

Erythromycin esters, particularly the estolate, can cause cholestatic jaundice. The pharmacokinetics of the oral preparations have been studied in neonates, but there are few or no data on intravenous use. However, i.v. erythromycin can rarely cause cardiac arrhymias or deafness.

CLINDAMYCIN

Clindamycin is a lincosamide, related to lincomycin, and both are produced by *Streptomyces lincolnensis*. They interfere with bacterial protein synthesis.

Clindamycin has somewhat better antibacterial activity and causes less marrow toxicity than lincomycin. It is active against staphylococci, streptococci and *Bacteroides fragilis*, as well as some other anaerobes. It has been used in the treatment of neonatal infections caused by anaerobes and by staphylococci, and in necrotizing enterocolitis [52]. There are no good pharmacokinetic data, and, although there have been few reports of toxicity, this may be because there are so few trials of its use.

TRIMETHOPRIM–SULPHAMETHOXAZOLE (COTRIMOXAZOLE)

Trimethoprim is a selective bacterial dihydrofolate reductase inhibitor. It acts synergistically with sulphonamides, which block an earlier stage in folate synthesis, so that lower concentrations of the two drugs can be used. As sulphonamides can displace bilirubin bound to albumin, it should always be considered, when prescribing for a neonate, whether trimethoprim alone might not be just as effective as cotrimoxazole (trimethoprim–sulphamethoxazole).

Trimethoprim is active against staphylococci, enterococci, *Escherichia coli*, *Proteus*, many coliforms, but not *Pseudomonas*. It diffuses well into the CSF and brain. Sulphamethoxazole has a spectrum of antibacterial activity similar to that of trimethoprim. Cotrimoxazole, but not trimethoprim alone, has occasionally been used in treating neonatal Gram-negative enteric bacillary meningitis [53,54], but there have been treatment failures. High-dose i.v. cotrimoxazole (20 mg/kg per day of trimethoprim) is the treatment of choice for *Pneumocystis carinii* pneumonia. Cotrimoxazole has been given p. o. and i.v. and, although few adverse reactions have been reported, even with high-dose i.v. use, the use of the drug has not been studied systematically. Trimethoprim given to the mother will cross the placenta and diffuse into breast milk at high concentrations [33].

METRONIDAZOLE

Metronidazole is a nitroamidazole antibiotic with excellent activity against anaerobes, including *Bacteroides fragilis*. It is active against *Entamoeba histolytica*, but has no important action against aerobes. The half-life is 23–25 hours in full-term infants, but is prolonged to 59–109 hours in preterm infants [55,56].

Peak levels decrease with duration of treatment and there is controversy as to whether or not the half-life becomes shorter with treatment. CSF penetration is excellent and metronidazole has been used successfully to treat *B. fragilis* meningitis [57]. It is commonly used in the UK in combination with antibacterial agents to treat necrotizing enterocolitis. Toxicity has not been described, although high doses can cause reversible neuropathy in adults.

AZTREONAM

As multiply resistant Gram-negative organisms become an increasing problem, newer antibiotics are being developed. Aztreonam is a monocyclic β-lactam antibiotic with activity against Gram-negative enteric bacilli, including *Pseudomonas aeruginosa*. The pharmacokinetics of aztreonam have been studied in neonates [58,59] and it appears to be of low toxicity. It will penetrate inflamed meninges. It has been used synergistically with gentamicin to treat *Pseudomonas* infections and infections with other Gram-negative organisms. Hypersensitivity reactions including rash and urticaria can occur.

CIPROFLOXACIN

Ciprofloxacin, a nalidixic acid derivative with a spectrum similar to that of aztreonam, has been used with limited success to treat infections with resistant *Enterobacter cloacae* [60] and has been used successfully to treat a baby with a CSF shunt infection caused by a multiresistant *Pseudomonas aeruginosa* [61], although CSF penetration is only moderate [60,61]. Ciprofloxacin can damage cartilage in laboratory animals and is not generally recommended in childhood, so should be used only when there is no suitable alternative.

IMIPENEM–CILASTATIN

Imipenem is a carbapenem produced by a strain of *Streptomyces*, and is always used in combination with cilastatin, a renal dipeptidase inhibitor with no intrinsic antibacterial activity. It is active *in vitro* against *Staphylococcus aureus*, *S. epidermidis*, streptococci excluding *S. faecium*, and a wide range of Gram-negative organisms. It will penetrate inflamed, but not uninflamed, meninges. Because of CNS toxicity, is it not recommended for the treatment of meningitis. Imipenem–cilastatin has been evaluated in children [62] and in newborns [63,64]. The drug is a very powerful inducer of β-lactamases and, although these do not act on imipenem, they can result in the selection of organisms resistant to penicillins and cephalosporins.

Side-effects include thrombophlebitis, diarrhoea and, in children with CNS abnormality, convulsions. The new carbapenem, meropenem, may have fewer side-effects [65], but there are no data yet on its use in neonates.

References

1 Shirkey HC. Therapeutic orphans: who speaks for children? *South Med J* 1970; **63**: 1361–3.
2 Burns LE, Hodgman JE & Cass AB. Fatal circulatory collapse in premature infants receiving chloramphenicol. *N Engl J Med* 1959; **261**: 1318–21.
3 Silverman WA, Andersen DM, Blanc WA *et al.* A difference in mortality rate and incidence of kernicterus among premature

infants allotted to two prophylactic antibacterial regimens. *Pediatrics* 1956; **18**: 614–24.

4 van den Anker JN. Pharmacokinetics and renal function in preterm infants. *Acta Paediatr* 1966; **85**: 1393–9.

5 Boyer KM & Gotoff SP. Prevention of early-onset neonatal group B streptococcal disease with selective intrapartum chemoprophylaxis. *N Engl J Med* 1986; **314**: 1665–9.

6 Totterman LE & Saxen L. Incorporation of tetracycline into human foetal bones after maternal drug administration. *Acta Obstet Gynaecol Scand* 1969; **48**: 542–9.

7 Cohlan SQ, Bevelander G & Tiamsic T. Growth inhibition of prematures receiving tetracycline. *Am J Dis Child* 1963; **105**: 453–61.

8 Kline AH, Blattner RJ & Lunin M. Transplacental effect of tetracyclines on teeth. *JAMA* 1964; **188**: 178–80.

9 Robinson GC & Cambon KG. Hearing loss in infants of tuberculous mothers treated with streptomycin in pregnancy. *N Engl J Med* 1964; **271**: 949–51.

10 Conway N & Birt DN. Streptomycin in pregnancy: effect on the foetal ear. *BMJ* 1965; **2**: 260–3.

11 Yow MD, Tengg NE, Bangs J *et al.* The ototoxic effects of kanamycin sulfate in infants and in children. *J Pediatr* 1962; **60**: 230–42.

12 Jones HC. Intrauterine ototoxicity: a case report and review of literature. *J Natl Med Assoc* 1973; **65**: 201–4.

13 McCracken GH, Mize SG & Threlkeld N. Intraventricular gentamicin therapy in Gram-negative bacillary meningitis of infancy. *Lancet* 1980; **i**: 787–91.

14 Harley JD & Robin H. 'Late ' neonatal jaundice in infants with glucose-6-phosphate dehydrogenase deficient erythrocytes. *Aust Ann Med* 1962; **11**: 148–55.

15 Belton EM & Jones RV. Haemolytic anaemia due to nalidixic acid. *Lancet* 1965; **ii**: 691.

16 AAP Committee on Drugs. *Pediatrics* 1994; **93**: 137.

17 McCracken GH, Ginsberg CM, Clahsen JC & Thomas ML. Pharmacologic evaluation of orally administered antibiotics in the newborn infant. *Antimicrob Agents Chemother* 1978; **5**: 214–19.

18 Axline SG, Yaffee SJ & Simon HJ. Clinical pharmacology of antimicrobials in premature infants. II. Ampicillin, oxacillin, neomycin and colistin. *Pediatrics* **39**: 97–107.

19 Boe RW, Williams CPS, Bennet JV & Oliver TK. Serum levels of methicillin and ampicillin in newborn and premature infants in relation to postnatal age. *Pediatrics* 1967; **39**: 194–201.

20 Grossman M & Ticknor W. Serum levels of ampicillin,

cephalothin, cloxacillin and nafcillin in the newborn infant. *Antimicrob Agents Chemother* 1965; **5**: 214–19.

21 Prober CG, Stevenson DK & Benitz WE. The use of antibiotics in neonates weighing less than 1200 grams. *Pediatr Infect Dis J* 1990; **9**: 111–21.

22 Mulhall A, de Louvois J & Hurley R. Chloramphenicol toxicity in neonates: its incidence and prevention. *BMJ* 1983; **287**: 1424–7.

23 Rajchgot P, Prober CG, Soldin SJ *et al.* Toward optimization of therapy in the neonate. *Clin Pharmacol Ther* 1983; **33**: 551–5.

24 McCracken GH & Freij BJ. Clinical pharmacology of antimicrobial agents. In: Remington JS & Klein JO (eds) *Infectious Diseases of the Fetus and Newborn Infant*, 3rd edn. Philadelphia: WB Saunders, 1990: 1020–78.

25 Robertson A, Fink S & Karp W. Effect of cephalosporins on bilirubin–albumin binding. *J Pediatr* 1988; **112**: 291–4.

26 Aperia A & Zetterstrom R. Renal control of fluid homeostasis in the newborn infant. *Clin Perinatol* 1982; **9**: 523–33.

27 Guignard JP & John EG. Renal function in the tiny, premature infant. *Clin Perinatol* 1986; **13**: 377–401.

28 Oh W. Renal functions and clinical disorders in the neonate. *Clin Perinatol* 1981; **8**: 215–23.

29 Besunder JB, Reed MD & Blumer JL. Principles of drug biodisposition in the neonate. *Clin Pharmacokinet* 1988; **14**: 189–216.

30 Greenwood D. *Antimicrobial Chemotherapy*, 2nd edn. Oxford: Oxford University Press, 1989.

31 McCracken GH, Ginsberg C, Chrane DF *et al.* Clinical pharmacology of penicillin in newborn infants. *Pediatrics* 1973; **82**: 692–8.

32 Tullus K & Burman LG. Ecological impact of ampicillin and cefuroxime in neonatal units. *Lancet* 1989; **i**: 1405–7.

33 Saez-Lorens X & McCracken GH Jr. Clinical pharmacology of antibacterial agents. In: Remington JS & Klein JO. *Infectious Diseases of the Fetus and Newborn Infant*, 4th edn. Philadelphia: WB Saunders, 1995: 1287–336.

34 Strausbaugh LJ, Murray TW & Sande MA. Comparative penetration of six antibiotics into the cerebrospinal fluid of rabbits with experimental staphylococcal meningitis. *J Antimicrob Chemother* 1980; **6**: 363–71.

35 Korzeniowski O & Sande MA. Combination antimicrobial therapy for *Staphylococcus aureus* endocarditis in patients addicted to parenteral drugs and in non-addicts. A prospective study. *Ann Intern Med* 1982; **97**: 496–503.

36 McCracken GH & Nelson JD. *Antimicrobial Therapy for Newborns*, 2nd edn. New York: Grune & Stratton, 1983.

37 Schaad UB, McCracken GH, Threlkeld N *et al*. Clinical evaluation of a new broad-spectrum oxa-beta-lactam, moxalactam, in neonates and infants. *J Pediatr* 1981; **98**: 129–36.

38 Kafetzis DA, Brater DC, Kapiki AN *et al*. Treatment of severe neonatal infections with cefotaxime: efficacy and pharmacokinetics. *J Pediatr* 1982; **100**: 438–9.

39 McCracken GH, Threlkeld N, Mize S *et al*. Moxalactam therapy for neonatal meningitis due to Gram-negative enteric bacilli. A prospective controlled evaluation. *JAMA* 1984; **252**: 1427–32.

40 Modi N, Damjanovic V & Cooke RW. Outbreak of cephalosporin resistant *Enterobacter cloacae* infection in a neonatal intensive care unit. *Arch Dis Child* 1987; **62**: 148–51.

41 Spritzer R, Kamp HJVD, Dzolvic G & Sauer PJJ. Five years of cefotaxime use in a neonatal intensive care unit. *Pediatr Infect Dis J* 1990; **9**: 92–6.

42 Schaad UB, McCracken GH & Nelson JD. Clinical pharmacology and efficacy of vancomycin in pediatrics. *J Pediatr* 1980; **96**: 119–26.

43 Neumeister B, Kastner S, Conrad S, Klotz G & Bartmann P. Characterization of coagulase-negative staphylococci causing nosocomial infections in preterm infants. *Eur J Clin Microbiol Infect Dis* 1995; **14**: 856–63.

44 Padovani EM, Khoory BJ, Beghini R, Chiaffoni GP & Fanos V. Teicoplanin: clinical efficacy, antibacterial activity and tolerance in the treatment of staphylococcal infections in the newborn. *Ann Exp Clin Med* 1994; **i**: 111–15.

45 Raz R, Sharir R, Shmilowitz L *et al*. The elimination of gentamicin-resistant Gram-negative bacteria in a newborn intensive care unit. *Infection* 1987; **15**: 32–4.

46 Isaacs D, Catterson J, Hope PL *et al*. Factors influencing colonisation with gentamicin resistant Gram negative organisms in the neonatal unit. *Arch Dis Child* 1988; **63**: 533–5.

47 Buchanan N. Aminoglycoside monitoring in neonates – a reappraisal. *Aust NZ J Med* 1985; **15**: 457–9.

48 Fuquay D, Koup J & Smith AL. Management of neonatal gentamicin over-dosage. *J Pediatr* 1981; **99**: 473–6.

49 Eviatar L & Eviatar E. Development of head control and vestibular responses in infants treated with aminoglycosides. *Dev Med Child Neurol* 1982; **24**: 372–9.

50 Assael BM, Cavanna G, Jusko WJ *et al*. Multiexponential elimination of gentamicin. A kinetic study during development. *Dev Pharmacol Ther* 1980; **1**: 171–81.

51 Skopnik H, Wallraf R, Nies B *et al*. Pharmacokinetics and antibacterial activity of daily gentamicin. *Arch Dis Child* 1992; **67**: 57–61.

52 Faix RG, Polley TZ & Grasela TH. A randomized, controlled trial of parenteral clindamycin in neonatal necrotizing enterocolitis. *J Pediatr* 1988; **112**: 271–7.

53 Sabel KG & Brandberg A. Treatment of meningitis and septicemia in infancy with a sulfamethoxazole–trimethoprim combination. *Acta Paediatr Scand* 1975; **64**: 25–32.

54 Ardati KO, Thirumoorthi MC & Dajani AS. Intravenous trimethoprim–sulfamethoxazole in the treatment of serious infections in children. *J Pediatr* 1979; **95**: 801–6.

55 Jager-Roman E, Doyle PE, Baird-Lambert J *et al.* Pharmacokinetics and tissue distribution of metronidazole in the newborn infant. *J Pediatr* 1982; **100**: 651–4.

56 Hall P, Kaye CM, McIntosh N & Steele J Intravenous metronidazole in the newborn. *Arch Dis Child* 1983; **58**: 529–31.

57 Feldman WE. *Bacteroides fragilis* ventriculitis and meningitis. *Am J Dis Child* 1976; **13**: 880–3.

58 Likitnukul S, McCracken GH, Threlkeld N *et al.* Pharmacokinetics and plasma bactericidal activity of aztreonam in low birth weight infants. *Antimicrob Agents Chemother* 1987; **31**: 81–3.

59 Umana MA, Odio CM, Castro E *et al.* Evaluation of aztreonam and ampicillin vs. amikacin and ampicillin for treatment of neonatal bacterial infections. *Pediatr Infect Dis J* 1990; **9**: 175–80.

60 Bannon MJ, Stutchfield PR, Weindling AM & Damjanovic V. Ciprofloxacin in neonatal *Enterobacter cloacae* septicaemia. *Arch Dis Child* 1989; **64**: 1388–91.

61 Isaacs D, Slack, MPE, Wilkinson AR & Westwood AW. Successful treatment of pseudomonas ventriculitis with ciprofloxacin. *J Antimicrob Chemother* 1986; **17**: 535–8.

62 Ahonkhai VI, Cyhan GM, Wilson SE & Brown KR. Imipene–cilastatin in pediatric patients: an overview of safety and efficacy studies conducted in the United States. *Pediatr Infect Dis J* 1989; **8**: 740–4.

63 Reed MD, Kleigman RM, Yamashita TS, Myers CM & Blumer JL. Clinical pharmacology of imipenem and cilastatin in premature infants during the first week of life. *Antimicrob Agents Chemother* 1990; **34**: 1172–7.

64 Stuart RL, Turnidge J & Grayson ML. Safety of imipenem in neonates. *Pediatr Infect Dis J* 1995; **14**: 804–5.

65 Bradley JS. Meropenem: a new, extremely broad spectrum beta-lactam antibiotic for serious infections in paediatrics. *Pediatr Infect Dis J* 1997; **16**: 263–8.

Appendix 1: Definitions of neonatal infections

Dubious	Probable	Definite
Pneumonia		
Transient pulmonary shadowing resolving within 48 hours	Clinical picture of respiratory distress consistent with pneumonia and radiographical appearance of streaky densities or confluent lobar opacification persisting for >48 hours. Possible causative organisms: grown from endotracheal aspirate.	As for probable pneumonia but with positive blood cultures for a respiratory pathogen or post-mortem confirmation of the diagnosis.
Necrotizing enterocolitis (NEC)		
I. Blood in stools; normal clotting screen. II. Abdominal distension, suspicious abdominal radiograph but no blood and no intramural gas. I and II tolerate early reintroduction of enteral feeds.	III. Bloody stools, abdominal distension and suspicious abdominal radiograph without intramural gas.	IV. As for III but with pneumatosis intestinalis. V. Per-operative or post-mortem diagnosis.
Bacteraemia/ septicaemia		
Contaminant: growth of *Staphylococcus epidermidis*, fastidious streptococcus or other aerobic or anaerobic organism(s) from blood cultures taken from a neonate with possible sepsis, but in whom the clinical picture subsequently suggests the organism was a contaminant.	Group B streptococcus: Early RDS or persistent fetal circulation and colonization with group B streptococcus but no positive systemic cultures. Pneumococcus, *Haemophilus*, *Listeria*, etc. Clinical sepsis with colonization at birth but no positive systemic cultures.	Pure growth of pathogen from one or more blood culture bottles or antigen detection associated with clinical picture of sepsis. Includes *S. epidermidis*, etc., when risk of infection high (e.g. when a long line is *in situ*) or strong clinical evidence of sepsis *and* abnormal white count or low platelets.
Meningitis		
Contaminant: growth of possible CSF pathogen from CSF, only on		Pure growth of pathogen from CSF; or CSF pleocytosis and positive

Dubious	Probable	Definite
Meningitis (*cont.*)		
enrichment culture, and without CSF pleocytosis, with subsequent clinical picture not truly suggestive of meningitis.		blood cultures; or virus isolated from CSF or other site with aseptic meningitis.
Conjunctivitis		Purulent discharge from one or both eyes with presence of pus cells and pure growth of bacterial pathogen, virus or *C. trachomatis* (or antigen detection of the latter).
Skin: septic spots (micro-abscess)		Discrete pustules containing pus cells and a pure growth of *S. aureus* or other pathogens.
Cellulitis	Spreading area of skin inflammation.	Spreading area of skin inflammation *and* positive bacteriology on needle aspiration or blood cultures.
Skin abscess		Raised, often fluctuant, swelling yielding pure growth of a bacterial or fungal pathogen.
Omphalitis	Inflammation around umbilicus.	Inflammation around umbilicus *and* pure growth of an organism from the umbilicus.
Wound infection		Inflammation of skin incision with discharge of pus from wound.
Urinary tract infection	Pure growth $\geq 10^5$ organisms/mL of urine from bag specimen (needs SPA).	Pure growth of pathogen from SPA or clean catch of urine. (Pyelonephritis may be diagnosed at autopsy.)
Osteomyelitis		Clinical evidence and/or radiographical changes (lytic lesions, bone scan, etc.) with or without microbiological confirmation.

Dubious	Probable	Definite
Gastroenteritis		Loose or watery stools persisting for >24 hours associated with presence of an intestinal pathogen.
Peritonitis		Growth of organism(s) from peritoneal fluid.
Bacterial endocarditis		Characteristic clinical picture, usually in assocation with persistently positive blood cultures and vegetations on echocardiogram.
Systemic fungal infection		CSF, SPA urine and/or positive blood cultures. Culture from SPA urine alone may merely be renal candidiasis.
Congenital infections		Laboratory evidence (specific IgM or culture of organism), often supported by clinical picture.
Upper respiratory tract infection		Rhinorrhoea, cough, increased ventilatory requirements, apnoea, fever associated with respiratory virus identification.
Asymptomatic virus shedding		Positive virus identification but no attributable symptoms.
Systemic viral infections		Hepatitis, myocarditis, meningitis, encephalitis *and* virus identification.
Localized viral infections		Skin (HSV, enterovirus), eye or other site not previously covered.
Deep abscess		Abscess in lung, liver, spleen, etc.
Pleural empyema		Purulent pleural exudate.
Fungal dermatitis		Skin rash with isolation of fungus.

Appendix 2: Dosage schedules for antimicrobial agents

These regimens are based largely on those in the *Neonatal Formulary* (Northern Neonatal Pharmacopoeia. *Neonatal Formulary*, 9th edn. London: BMJ Publishing Group, 1996). Please check doses carefully before prescribing antibiotics, as these are up-to-date at time of writing, but recommendations may have changed. The dosages are given as the amount in a single dose unless otherwise specified.

We are particularly grateful to Dr Edmund Hey and the Northern Neonatal Network for permission to use data from the *Neonatal Formulary*. This excellent publication is continuously updated and the latest version can be obtained from the Pharmacy Information Service, Royal Victoria Infirmary, Newcastle-upon-Tyne, UK (Tel: (0191) 232 5131 × 24469, Fax: (0191) 221 0081).

Penicillins

Drug	Dosage (dose/kg)	Timing	Duration
Penicillin G	30 mg (50 000 U) i.v. or i.m. 60 mg (100 000 U) for meningitis	12-hourly ($\leq$ 7 days old) 8-hourly (1–3 weeks old) 6-hourly ($\geq$ 4 weeks old)	7–10 days for septicaemia 10–14 days for congenital syphilis 3 weeks for meningitis
Ampicillin	50 mg i.v. or i.m. 100 mg for meningitis	(As for penicillin G)	7–10 days for septicaemia 3 weeks for meningitis
Flucloxacillin	50–100 mg i.v. or i.m.	(As for penicillin G)	7–10 days for septicaemia 3 weeks for staphylococcal meningitis or osteomyelitis
Methicillin	25–50 mg i.v. or i.m.	(As for penicillin G)	(As for flucloxacillin)
Oxacillin	25–50 mg i.v. or i.m.	(As for penicillin G)	(As for flucloxacillin)

Aminoglycosides

Drug	Dosage (dose/kg)	Timing	Therapeutic range (mg/L)	
			Trough	Peak
Gentamicin	2.5–3.5 mg i.v. or i.m. Once daily: 4 mg (<35 weeks gestation) 5 mg ($\geq$ 35 weeks)	12-hourly 24-hourly 24-hourly	<2 <1 <1	6–8 6–8 6–8
Amikacin	12 mg (<35 weeks gestation) i.v. or i.m. 15 mg ($\geq$ 35 weeks)	24-hourly 24-hourly	<8 <8	20–30 20–30
Netilmicin	4 mg i.v. or i.m. 5 mg (<35 weeks gestation) 6 mg ($\geq$ 35 weeks)	12-hourly 24-hourly 24-hourly	<2 <2 <2	9–12 9–12 9–12
Tobramycin	3.5 mg i.v. or i.m. 4 mg (<35 weeks gestation) 5 mg ($\geq$ 35 weeks)	12-hourly 24-hourly 24-hourly	1–2 1–2 1–2	5–8 5–8 5–8

Cephalosporins

Drug	Dosage (dose/kg)	Timing	Notes
Cefuroxime	25 mg i.v. or i.m.	12-hourly ($\leq$ 7 days old) 8-hourly (1–3 weeks old) 6-hourly ($\geq$ 4 weeks old)	Increase dose interval for renal failure (serum creatinine >200 mmol/L)
Cefotaxime	50 mg	(As for cefuroxime)	
Ceftazidime	25–50 mg	12-hourly (< 1 month old) 8-hourly (> 1 month)	
Ceftriaxone	50 mg	24-hourly	

Other parenteral antibacterials

Drug	Dosage (dose/kg)	Timing	Notes
Azlocillin	50 mg i.v. or i.m. ($\leq$ 2 weeks old) 100 mg (>2 weeks old)	Preterm 12-hourly Term 8-hourly	Reduce dose frequency in renal failure
Aztreonam	30 mg i.v. or i.m.	12-hourly ($\leq$ 7 days old) 8-hourly (1–3 weeks old) 6-hourly ($\geq$ 4 weeks old)	Reduce dose frequency in renal failure
Chloramphenicol	12 mg i.v. or i.m.	12-hourly ($\leq$ 10 days old) 8-hourly (> 10 days old)	Loading dose 20 mg/kg i.v. Monitor drug levels
Ciprofloxacin	5 mg i.v. or i.m.	12-hourly	Beware of toxicity
Clindamycin	5–15 mg/kg i.v.	8-hourly	
Cotrimoxazole	24 mg/kg slow i.v. (4 mg trim + 20 mg sulpha) 120 mg/kg i.v.	12-hourly 12-hourly	For meningitis For PCP
Erythromycin	15 mg/kg i.v.	8-hourly	
Metronidazole	7.5 mg/kg i.v.	12-hourly 8-hourly (>4 weeks old)	Can give 15 mg/kg i.v. loading dose
Piperacillin	100 mg/kg i.v. or i.m.	12-hourly	
Rifampicin	6 mg/kg i.v.	12-hourly	
Teicoplanin	8 mg/kg i.v. or i.m.	24-hourly	15 mg/kg i.v. loading dose
Ticarcillin	75 mg/kg i.v. or i.m.	6–12-hourly	

Other parenteral antibacterials (cont.)

Drug	Dosage (dose/kg)	Timing	Notes
Trimethoprim	1 mg/kg i.v. or oral	12-hourly	Loading dose 3 mg/kg i.v. or oral
Vancomycin	15 mg/kg i.v.	24-hourly (<28 weeks) postconceptional age	Trough <10 mg/L, Peak 25–40
		12-hourly (29–35 weeks) 8-hourly (>35 weeks)	Intrathecal, 5 mg daily

Oral antibiotics

Drug	Dosage (dose/kg)	Timing	Notes
Amoxycillin	20–35 mg/kg	8-hourly	
Chloramphenicol	25 mg/kg	8-hourly	Not recommended under 6 weeks old
Ciprofloxacin	7.5 mg/kg	12-hourly	
Cotrimoxazole (trimethoprim-sulphamethoxazole)	24 mg/kg (4 mg trim + 20 mg sulpha)	12-hourly	
	24 mg/kg	24-hourly	For PCP prophylaxis
Erythromycin	10 mg/kg	6-hourly	
Pyrimethamine	1 mg/kg	24-hourly	For congenital toxoplasmosis. Loading dose 1 mg/kg 12-hourly for 2 days orally
Spiramycin	50 mg/kg	12-hourly	For congenital toxoplasmosis
Sulphadiazine	100 mg/kg	24-hourly	For congenital toxoplasmosis
Trimethoprim	1–2 mg/kg	12-hourly	Loading dose 3 mg/kg. Double dose over 6 weeks old

Antituberculous drugs

Drug	Dosage (dose/kg)	Timing	Notes
Isoniazid	10–15 mg/kg oral	24-hourly	
Rifampicin	10–15 mg/kg oral	24-hourly	
Pyrazinamide	15–30 mg/kg oral	24-hourly	
Ethambutol	15–25 mg/kg oral	24-hourly	Not recommended < 6 years or if renal function impaired, but may have to be used for resistant tuberculosis
Streptomycin	15 mg/kg i.m.	12-hourly	

Antifungals

Drug	Dosage (dose/kg)	Timing	Notes
Amphotericin B	1 mg/kg i.v. infusion	24-hourly	Total dose 20–30 mg/kg for systemic candidiasis
Fluconazole	5–6 mg/kg i.v. or oral	24-hourly	10 mg/kg i.v. or oral loading dose
Flucytosine (5-fluorocytosine)	25–50 mg/kg i.v. or oral	6-hourly	Monitor levels (aim for 50–80 mg/L 2 hours post-dose). Should not be used without another antifungal
Miconazole	25 mg/kg oral gel	12-hourly	
Nystatin	100 000 U (1 mL) orally	4-hourly	

Antivirals

Drug	Dosage (dose/kg)	Timing	Notes
Aciclovir	10 mg/kg i.v.	8-hourly	Up to 20 mg/kg/dose VZV
Ganciclovir	5 mg/kg i.v.	8-hourly	

Index

Note – Page numbers in *italic* type refer to illustrations and tables.